T0226548

NEUROFEEDBACK AND NEUROMODULATION TECHNIQUES AND APPLICATIONS

NEUROFEEDBACK AND NEUROMODULATION TECHNIQUES AND APPLICATIONS

Edited by

ROBERT COBEN

JAMES R. EVANS

Amsterdam • Boston • Heidelberg • London • New York • Oxford
Paris • San Diego • San Francisco • Singapore • Sydney • Tokyo

Academic press is an imprint of Elsevier

Academic Press is an imprint of Elsevier
32 Jamestown Road, London NW1 7BY, UK
30 Corporate Drive, Suite 400, Burlington, MA 01803, USA
525 B Street, Suite 1900, San Diego, CA 92101-4495, USA

First edition 2011

Notice

No responsibility is assumed by the publisher for any injury and/or damage to persons or
property as a matter of products liability, negligence or otherwise, or from any use or
operation of any methods, products, instructions or ideas contained in the material herein.
Because of rapid advances in the medical sciences, in particular, independent verification
of diagnoses and drug dosages should be made.

British Library Cataloguing-in-Publication Data
A catalogue record for this book is available from the British Library

Library of Congress Cataloging-in-Publication Data
A catalog record for this book is available from the Library of Congress

ISBN: 978-0-12-382235-2

For information on all Academic Press publications
visit our website at www.elsevierdirect.com

Typeset by MPS Limited, a Macmillan Company, Chennai, India
www.macmillansolutions.com

Printed and bound by CPI Group (UK) Ltd, Croydon, CR0 4YY

**Working together to grow
libraries in developing countries**

www.elsevier.com | www.bookaid.org | www.sabre.org

ELSEVIER   BOOK AID
            International   Sabre Foundation

CONTENTS

**4. EEG Vigilance and Phenotypes in Neuropsychiatry:
   Implications for Intervention**   79
Martijn Arns, Jay Gunkelman, Sebastian Olbrich, Christian Sander,
and Ulrich Hegerl

Part Two: Endogenous Neuromodulation Strategies   125

**5. Neurofeedback with Children with Attention Deficit
   Hyperactivity Disorder: A Randomized Double-Blind
   Placebo-Controlled Study**   127
Roger J. deBeus and David A. Kaiser

CONTRIBUTORS

Martijn Arns
Research Institute Brainclinics, Nijmegen, and Utrecht University, Department of Experimental Psychology, Utrecht, The Netherlands

Mario Beauregard
Centre de Recherche en Neuropsychologie et Cognition (CERNEC), Département de Psychologie, Université de Montréal; Département de Radiologie, Université de Montréal; Centre de Recherche en Sciences Neurologiques (CRSN), Université de Montréal, and Centre de Recherche du Centre Hospitalier de l'Université de Montréal (CRCHUM), Canada

Niels Birbaumer
Institute of Medical Psychology and Behavioral Neurobiology, University of Tübingen, Tübingen, Germany; and Ospedale San Camillo, Istituto di Ricovero e Cura a Carattere Scientifico, Venezia – Lido, Italy

Ellen Broelz
Institute of Medical Psychology and Behavioral Neurobiology, University of Tübingen, Tübingen, Germany

Robert Coben
Neurorehabilitation and Neuropsychological Services, Massapequa Park, New York, USA

Marco Congedo
ViBS Team (Vision and Brain Signal Processing), GIPSA-Lab, National Center for Scientific Research (CNRS), Grenoble University, Grenoble, France

Dirk de Ridder
TRI Tinnitus Clinic, BRAI^{2}N and Department of Neurosurgery, University of Antwerp, Antwerp, Belgium

Roger J. deBeus
Department of Psychiatry and Behavioral Sciences, Quillen College of Medicine, East Tennessee State University, Johnson City, Tennessee, USA

Paul B. Fitzgerald
Monash Alfred Psychiatry Research Center (MAPrc), The Alfred and Monash University, School of Psychology and Psychiatry, Melbourne, Victoria, Australia

Felipe Fregni
Laboratory of Neuromodulation, Spaulding Rehabilitation Hospital, Harvard Medical School, Boston, Massachusetts, and Berenson-Allen Center for Noninvasive Brain Stimulation, Beth Israel Deaconess Medical Center, Harvard Medical School, Boston, Massachusetts, USA

John H. Gruzelier
Department of Psychology, Goldsmiths, University of London, London, UK

Jay Gunkelman
Q-Pro Worldwide, Crockett, California, USA

D. Corydon Hammond
University of Utah School of Medicine, Salt Lake City, Utah, USA

Ulrich Hegerl
University of Leipzig, Leipzig, Germany

Jack Johnstone
Q-Metrx, Inc., Burbank, California, and Department of Psychology, University of California Los Angeles, Los Angeles, California, USA

David A. Kaiser
Wavestate Inc., Marina Del Ray, California, USA

Mirjam E.J. Kouijzer
Behavioral Science Institute, Radboud University Nijmegen, Nijmegen, The Netherlands

Juri D. Kropotov
Institute of the Human Brain of the Russian Academy of Sciences, St Petersburg, Russia; and Institute of Psychology, Norwegian University of Science and Technology, Trondheim, Norway

Berthold Langguth
Department of Psychiatry and Psychotherapy and Tinnitus Clinic, University of Regensburg, Regensburg, Germany

Sangkyun Lee
Institute of Medical Psychology and Behavioral Neurobiology, University of Tübingen, Tübingen, and Graduate School of Neural and Behavioural Sciences, International Max Planck Research School, Tübingen, Germany

Johanne Lévesque
Institut PsychoNeuro, Laval, Canada

Joy Lunt
Brain Potential, Inc., Burbank, California, USA

Andreas Mueller
Brain and Trauma Foundation, Grison, and Praxis für Kind, Organisation und Entwicklung, Chur, Switzerland

Sebastian Olbrich
University of Leipzig, Leipzig, Germany

Valery A. Ponomarev
Institute of the Human Brain of the Russian Academy of Sciences, St Petersburg, Russia

Jay S. Reidler
Laboratory of Neuromodulation, Spaulding Rehabilitation Hospital, Harvard Medical School, Boston, Massachusetts, USA

Tomas Ros
Department of Psychology, Goldsmiths, University of London, London, UK

Sergio Ruiz
Institute of Medical Psychology and Behavioral Neurobiology, University of Tübingen, Tübingen, and Graduate School of Neural and Behavioral Sciences, International Max Planck Research School, Tübingen, Germany, and Department of Psychiatry, Faculty of Medicine, Pontificia Universidad Católica de Chile, Santiago, Chile

Christian Sander
University of Leipzig, Leipzig, Germany

Leslie Sherlin
Neurotopia, Inc., Los Angeles, California; Nova Tech EEG, Inc., Mesa, Arizona, and Southwest College of Naturopathic Medicine, Tempe, Arizona, USA

Ranganatha Sitaram
Institute of Medical Psychology and Behavioral Neurobiology, University of Tübingen, Tübingen, Germany

Desirée Spronk
Research Institute Brainclinics, Nijmegen, The Netherlands

Ute Strehl
Institute of Medical Psychology and Behavioral Neurobiology, University of Tübingen, Tübingen, Germany

Gabriel Tan
Michael E. DeBakey Veterans Affairs Medical Center, Houston, Texas, and Baylor College of Medicine, Houston, Texas, USA

Lori A. Wagner
Neurorehabilitation and Neuropsychological Services, Massapequa Park, New York, USA

Jonathan Walker
Neurotherapy Center of Dallas, Dallas, Texas, USA

Sarah Wyckoff
Institute of Medical Psychology and Behavioral Neurobiology, University of Tübingen, Tübingen, Germany

Soroush Zaghi
Laboratory of Neuromodulation, Spaulding Rehabilitation Hospital, Harvard Medical School, Boston, Massachusetts, and Berenson-Allen Center for Noninvasive Brain Stimulation, Beth Israel Deaconess Medical Center, Harvard Medical School, Boston, Massachusetts, USA

It was not many years ago that the term "neuromodulation" would have been considered a contradictory term by many — at least in regard to modification of a damaged or dysfunctional central nervous system. Although it generally had been assumed that learning and memory somehow resulted in relatively permanent modifications of brain structure and/or function, the notion persisted that neural function and structure basically were set by genetics and were relatively immune to change. However, within the past couple of decades developments in neuroimaging have enabled scientific research providing evidence of neural plasticity far greater than previously had been imagined. Research on neural plasticity is burgeoning, along with a plethora of scientifically unsubstantiated claims by practitioners from many different professions for "brain-based" methods for remediation of various medical, psychological, and educational problems.

Despite the fact that, until recently, brain plasticity was not a generally accepted concept, for many years there have been remedial approaches where advocates make either explicit or implied claims that their use results in modulation of brain function. Some involve intensive, graduated practice of functions that had been impaired by brain damage, e.g., cognitive rehabilitation. Some involve exposure of clients to various types of stimuli, which usually are rhythmic or of specified frequency (e.g., auditory/visual stimulation with light/sound machines, music therapy). Often this is done with the assumption that rhythms of the brain are entrained or otherwise modified by such exogenous stimuli. Some consider electroshock therapy and transcranial magnetic stimulation to fall into this category. Still others emphasize self-directed activity, such as making precise movements in synchrony with a metronome, or learning self-control of one's brain rhythms (EEG) with the aid of electronic equipment that provides feedback concerning specific aspects of those endogenous rhythms, i.e., EEG biofeedback or neurofeedback. Practitioners of such remedial approaches generally have been marginalized by mainstream medicine, psychology, and education, partially due to the aforementioned belief in immutability of brain structure/function, but also due to perceived, or real, lack of scientific support for efficacy of the methods involved.

It is the editors' opinion that two procedures for neuromodulation hold special promise due to emerging scientific evidence of their enduring effectiveness with a variety of conditions that are known, or believed, to be due to brain damage and/or dysfunction. These are neurofeedback (NF) and transcranial magnetic stimulation (TMS) in their various forms. Research and clinical practice in NF began in earnest in the 1960s and 1970s, decreased considerably for a while thereafter, but, since the early 1990s, have grown rapidly. There are NF practitioners in many countries around the world, professional NF associations have been formed on three continents, at least ten books have been published dealing primarily with NF, and a professional journal devoted almost exclusively to NF (*Journal of Neurotherapy*) has been published regularly since 1995. Unlike many other groups with claims of facilitation of neuromodulation, the field of NF actively promotes scientific research; and in Australia, Belgium, Canada, England, Germany, the Netherlands, Russia and the United States (as well as some other countries) rigorous scientific research on the mechanisms and efficacy of NF is being actively pursued. The field has evolved far from its beginnings when research participants or patients could be provided feedback concerning only degree of power or percentage of power in a specific EEG frequency band at a single scalp electrode site. Today, feedback can be adjusted to reflect not only EEG power at all frequency/site combinations (now including even ultra low frequencies such as 0.001 Hertz), but also degree of connectivity (e.g., coherence) between all site combinations. Using low resolution electromagnetic tomography (LORETA) procedures, feedback concerning EEG activity in various subcortical areas and cortical networks or "hubs" presently is possible. And, feedback of information concerning activity in cortical and subcortical regions using functional MRI (fMRI) is receiving considerable research attention as an alternative or supplement to EEG biofeedback.

TMS, as usually defined today, is a relative newcomer to the field of neuromodulation. In this approach weak electrical currents are produced in brain tissues by applying rapidly changing magnetic fields to specific scalp locations. In some contrast to NF, which historically has been associated mainly with the field of psychology, TMS primarily is associated with medical research and practice. Also in some contrast to NF, where laboratory discoveries quickly were applied to clinical practice, the field of TMS appears to be moving more cautiously, building upon solid research findings prior to making claims for clinical efficacy. As with NF, scientific research on TMS and its potential clinical uses is occurring in many parts of the world.

Despite growing clinical use of TMS, and especially of NF, and despite emerging research results supporting their efficacy, both remain on the fringes of medical, psychological, and education practice. Charges of "show me the data" often are made by critics who claim there is no solid scientific support for these approaches. Such evidence exists, but heretofore has been scattered among many different professional journals and other sources. The editors perceived a need for the latest and best theorizing and research findings concerning these neuromodulation techniques to be brought together in a single source to which professionals and other interested persons would have ready access. We believe that this book accomplishes that goal. Although there certainly are others, it could be argued that the chapter authors of this text constitute the majority of the leading NF and TMS theoreticians and scientists of today's world. Several books have been published on the general topic of neuromodulation or specifically on neurofeedback. While a few have chapters detailing supportive research, most were oriented primarily toward theories of efficacy, descriptions of various approaches to NF, and/or details of clinical practice. This book is unique in its emphasis on solid scientific support as it brings together for the first time the neuromodulation fields of NF and TMS.

Rob Coben
Jim Evans

PART One

Neuromodulation: Analysis Techniques

CHAPTER 1

Use of Quantitative EEG to Predict Therapeutic Outcome in Neuropsychiatric Disorders

Jack Johnstone[1] and Joy Lunt[2]
[1]Q-Metrx, Inc., Burbank, California, and Department of Psychology, University of California Los Angeles, Los Angeles, California, USA
[2]Brain Potential, Inc., Burbank, California, USA

Contents

INTRODUCTION

The thesis of this chapter is that recording and analysis of EEG signals can be used in more productive ways than to identify and categorize behavioral disorders. More recent applications of EEG have been directed toward prediction of outcome of therapeutic intervention. Here we review use of EEG to guide interventions using medication, neurofeedback, and transcranial magnetic stimulation.

Clinical electroencephalography (EEG) typically involves visual examination of multichannel waveform displays by an experienced clinician, usually a neurologist, to detect and characterize seizure disorders and encephalopathies. EEG is the technique of choice for this purpose because it is noninvasive and cost-effective. Further, EEG provides sub-millisecond time resolution so that changes in neurophysiological activity can be studied in detail over time, far exceeding the time resolution available with

Neurofeedback and Neuromodulation Techniques and Applications
DOI: 10.1016/B978-0-12-382235-2.00001-9

3

other functional neuroimaging measures such as functional magnetic resonance imaging (fMRI), single positron emission tomography (SPECT), and positron emission tomography (PET). A large body of work documents the general acceptance of EEG in the medical literature (for a comprehensive review see Niedermeyer & Lopes da Silva, 2004).

FOUNDATIONS OF CLINICAL EEG: RELIABILITY

When EEG is read visually by experienced experts there is often considerable lack of agreement on the presence and significance of EEG "abnormalities" and many patterns are considered "normal variants" or "maturational". There have been numerous studies of the inter- and intra-rater reliability in evaluation of EEG signals. An early study by Williams et al. (1985) investigated inter-observer reliability in a random sample of 100 electroencephalographers. Ten-second samples of EEG records were evaluated from 12 EEGs. They concluded that there is considerable variability in EEG interpretation and that characteristics of the individual performing the interpretation were an important factor. Spencer et al. (1985) included review of 144 scalp ictal EEGs from 54 patients by three electroencephalographers. They found approximately 60% agreement in determination of the lobe of the brain involved in seizure onset and approximately 70% agreement for side of onset. They concluded that reliable determination of localization in scalp ictal records requires additional formal criteria.

A more recent study by Williams et al. (1990) showed that prior clinical diagnosis was an influential factor in EEG interpretation. Piccinelli et al. (2005) studied inter-rater reliability in patients with childhood idiopathic epilepsy. They report that experienced electroencephalographers have an "at least moderate agreement" on the majority of features of a wake and sleep EEG. Importantly, they also conclude that agreement was "unsatisfactory" when assessing background EEG activity. Gerber et al. (2008) studied inter-observer agreement in EEG interpretation in critically ill adults. They found moderate agreement "beyond chance" for the presence of rhythmic and periodic patterns. Agreement for other features was "slight to fair".

Boutros et al. (2005) reviewed the basis for determining EEG as "normal", and, specifically, how normal adults are selected for studies using EEG in neuropsychiatric research. They noted that EEG abnormalities have been reported in as many as 57.5% of normal adults (Struve, 1985). The authors defined seven criteria for normalcy, including (1) absence of systemic disorders with CNS involvement (metabolic, endocrine), (2) absence of traumatic brain injury, childhood neurologic disorders, and dementia, (3) absence of Axis I psychiatric disorders, excluding alcohol and drug abuse, (4) absence of alcohol abuse or dependence, (5) absence of psychotropic medications, (6) absence of first-degree relatives with psychiatric disorders, and (7) Axis II personality disorder or mental subnormality. These criteria were reviewed in 38 studies reported in the literature using visual EEG interpretation. They showed that the majority of studies met no criteria, or only one or two criteria. The overall conclusion is that boundaries for normal, unquantified EEG are poorly defined.

It is clear that because of the ambiguity about the definition of "normal", and lack of agreement among clinicians regarding the presence or absence of significant EEG abnormalities, either epileptic or abnormal rhythmicity, use of qualitative EEG alone does not have sufficient predictive power to effectively guide intervention in patients with neuropsychiatric disorders. The addition of quantitative EEG analysis increases both reliability and predictive power.

QUANTITATIVE EEG

The term "quantitative EEG" (qEEG) refers to quantitative signal analysis of the digitized electroencephalogram. The use of Fourier or Wavelet analysis is most often used to estimate the frequency spectrum. Many studies using qEEG compare an individual pattern of features such as absolute and relative EEG power, coherence, peak alpha frequency, asymmetry, and related measures to a reference database. Statistical deviations from the database can then be examined for clinical significance. A number of such databases are commercially available (see reviews by Johnstone & Gunkelman, 2003; Thatcher & Lubar, 2009). These databases each have strengths and weaknesses but overall were developed taking into account the criteria for normalcy suggested by Boutros et al. (2005), described above.

A number of studies indicate robust test–retest reliability for quantified EEG, and are reviewed below. The excellent reproducibility of findings in qEEG studies argues that the poor reliability seen for qualitative EEG is due to differences in interpretation rather than error of measurement or other technical factors.

An early qEEG reliability study by Fein et al. (1983) investigated the test–retest reliability of EEG spectral analysis in groups of dyslexic and control children. They measured the coefficient of variation within subjects over two repetitions of 3-minute recordings with eyes closed and with eyes open. This technique showed significant second-to-second variability of EEG without a consistent pattern of effects of group, reference used, task or repetition. EEG spectra were averaged over the 3-minute segment and compared to a similar segment recorded following a battery of behavioral tasks, approximately 4 hours later. Intra-class correlations (ICC) were computed to assess stability comparing the two 3-minute segments. The ICCs were typically above 0.9 for control subjects. Similar analyses with dyslexics showed somewhat lower reliability in specific leads and reference configurations, but EEG spectral profiles also were stable over a 4—5 hour period. These results were consistent for measures of absolute power as well as relative power. The authors conclude that, overall, these data demonstrate a high degree of reliability in EEG spectra in children under well-controlled recording conditions.

A follow-up study (Fein, Galin, Yingling, Johnstone, & Nelson, 1984) with the same subjects indicated that despite differences in recording equipment and procedures, the EEG spectra were found to be highly stable over a period of 1—3 years. Subsequent studies confirm the generally robust test—retest reliability of qEEG analyses (Burgess & Gruzelier, 1993; Fernandez et al., 1993; Gasser, Bacher, & Steinberg, 1985; Harmony et al., 1993; Lund, Sponheim, Iacono, & Clementz, 1995; Salinsky et al., 1991; see also Thatcher, Biver, & North, 2003). It is clear that qEEG evaluation when based on standardized and well-controlled recording and analysis procedures can produce replicable and, therefore, potentially useful clinical results.

The utility of a method for producing valid and useful clinical findings is based on a foundation of accurate and reliable measurement. It is also relevant to address the clinical applications and "intended use" of the method, for example, EEG considered as a valid diagnostic procedure, aiding in placing individuals into distinct diagnostic categories with well-defined behavioral boundaries. Indeed, quantitative EEG has been criticized for not being diagnostic of complex neurobehavioral syndromes and was considered by the American Academy of Neurology to be "investigational for clinical use in post-concussion syndrome, mild or moderate head injury, learning disability, attention disorders, schizophrenia, depression, alcoholism, and drug abuse" (Nuwer, 1997). Many other authors disagree, however, providing evidence that application of qEEG to diagnose psychiatric disorders does have clinical utility (for reviews see Coburn et al., 2006; Hughes & John, 1999).

Clinical applications of qEEG now are also being explored in medication management, development of neurofeedback protocols, and guiding transcranial magnetic stimulation therapy. Visual interpretation of EEG waveforms alone has not been found to be useful in these important applications, likely because of the poor reliability of interpretation, as discussed above. In a recent comprehensive review of the topic, Thatcher (2010) reaches similar conclusions and also suggests that increased reliability allows for better predictive validity. Combining visual examination of the EEG waveforms by an experienced expert with quantitative EEG analyses, however, will likely improve overall predictive accuracy compared to each of these procedures used separately.

An alternate approach to using brain electrical activity to diagnose psychiatric disorders is consideration of individual EEG patterns as "intermediate phenotypes." Johnstone, Gunkelman, & Lunt (2005) suggested that since qEEG patterns are highly reliable and stable and often show a genetic basis, yet are not isomorphic with behavioral categories, these patterns may be useful as predictors of clinical response. Candidate phenotypes have been offered, and will be described in this chapter along with possible intervention strategies for medication and EEG biofeedback (neurofeedback) based on these phenotypes. Such use of qEEG to predict and guide therapeutic outcome is recent, and appears to the authors to be more promising than the often-used clinical diagnostic approach.

Different diagnostic categories are differentially represented in phenotype categories. Further, it should be recognized that individuals may manifest features of several phenotypes, and that features distinguishing phenotypes are on a continuum without distinct boundaries. For example, many children with attention deficit disorder show an excess of frontocentral activity in the theta frequency range, 4–7 Hz. However, not all individuals show this pattern and certain individuals show a pattern of excessive fast activity anteriorly. Therefore, although it is possible to accurately measure the amount of anterior theta or beta activity, these measures are not specifically "diagnostic" of the disorder. It is believed to be more effective to use the neurophysiological markers to guide neurophysiological intervention than to diagnose a behavioral category and use it as a guide.

QUANTITATIVE EEG/ERP AND MEDICATION MANAGEMENT

A large body of literature often referred to as "Pharmaco-EEG" has shown effects of most of the commonly used psychopharmacologic agents

Table 1.1 Effects of common psychiatric medications on EEG

Class	Medications (examples)	Effects on EEG
Psychostimulants	Ritalin, Dexedrine, Adderall	Decreases slow activity (delta and theta frequencies); increases fast activity (beta frequencies)
Benzodiazepines	Xanax, Valium, Ativan	Increased 14—25 Hz Anticonvulsant properties
Barbiturates	Phenobarbitol	Increases delta activity and increases 18—35 Hz beta spindles. High dosage produces "burst-suppression"
Tricyclic antidepressants	Elavil, Tofanil, Norpramin, Sinequan, Pamelor	Increases both slow and fast activity and decreases alpha frequency activity (sedating)
SSRIs	Prozac, Effexor, Zoloft, Luvox, Paxil, Lexipro, Celexa	Produces less delta, decreases alpha, and increases beta (less sedating)
Other antidepressants	Wellbutrin (Zyban)	Reduces seizure threshold, non-sedating
Mood stabilizers (anticyclics)	Lithium, Tegretol	Increases theta frequency activity. Overdose produces marked slowing and triphasic discharges

on most measures of brain electrical activity. The most commonly used psychopharmacologic agents have been shown to have specific effects on EEG. Table 1.1 shows a summary of known medication effects on EEG (for review see Saletu, Anderer, & Saletu-Zyhlarz, 2006).

More recently, quantitative EEG features have been used to predict therapeutic response to medication, and more effectively manage psychiatric medication clinically ("predictive model"). Suffin and Emory (1995) recorded baseline EEG after patients were washed out of all psychoactive medication. Two groups of patients were selected: One group of patients was diagnosed with attentional disorders without affective symptoms and another group with affective disorders without attentional symptoms. These patients were medicated according to standard clinical practice and the Clinical Global Improvement scale (CGI) was used to assess outcome.

There were clear associations between specific EEG features at baseline and effects of medications: Individuals with slow EEG patterns tended to respond better to stimulant medication. Individuals with excessive frontal alpha activity responded better to antidepressant medications and those with deviations in EEG coherence responded better to anticonvulsants or anticyclics, *independent of clinical diagnosis.* The authors concluded that the pattern of deviations from the reference database was a better predictor of clinical response than was clinical diagnosis. A prospective follow-up study compared clinical outcome with medication selection based on patterns of deviations from a reference database compared to standard clinical practice (Suffin et al., 2007). Clinical outcome was significantly improved using qEEG guidance in medication selection. Based on these findings physicians were encouraged to select psychopharmacologic agents based on similarity with qEEG profiles of known responders to specific agents. The phenotype model, described above, was used by Arns, Gunkelman, Breteler, and Spronk (2008) in a study demonstrating the utility of the intermediate EEG phenotype model in selecting stimulant medications for treatment of children with ADHD.

Use of qEEG methods to guide selection and management of psychiatric medication has been studied extensively, and recently was reviewed by Leuchter, Cook, Hunter, and Korb (2009). These authors consider several EEG features as potential biomarkers of medication response in major depression, including some results from low resolution electromagnetic tomography, LORETA (see also Mulert et al., 2007). LORETA results are consistent with other imaging modalities such as PET, in suggesting that elevated theta activity in anterior cingulate cortex is measurable from prefrontal scalp recording electrodes and can be used as a biomarker for response to antidepressant medication.

Evoked and event-related potentials are related measures based on averaging EEG in response to sensory stimuli or other specific internal or external events. An evoked potential method that shows promise as a biomarker for antidepressant response is the loudness-dependent auditory evoked response (LDAEP). This evoked response originates in primary auditory cortex and appears to be sensitive to central serotonergic activity (Juckel, Molnar, Hegert, Csepe, & Karmos, 1997). When stimuli are presented with increasing intensity, individuals with diminished serotonergic activity show an increased or more sensitive response to increasing auditory stimulus intensity than individuals formerly diagnosed with depression and taking SSRI (selective serotonin reuptake inhibitor) medication. The presence of a strong LDAEP has been shown to predict treatment outcome with antidepressant medication in major depression (Juckel et al., 2007). Juckel et al. (2010) also provide evidence that the mechanism of the LDAEP has a genetic basis.

Auditory evoked potentials have also been used extensively in pharmaco-logic treatment in schizophrenia. The method most often used in evoked potential studies of schizophrenia is the auditory paired click paradigm, pioneered in the work of Freedman and Adler (see Adler et al., 1982; Freedman et al., 1983). This technique is the subject of a recent review (Patterson et al., 2008). Many studies have found a difference in the amplitude of the response to the first compared to the second click in closely timed paired stimuli, and that this decrement is smaller in schizophrenics. This has been widely interpreted as reflecting defective sensory gating in schizophrenics. There is considerable variability across studies, and the technique is sensitive to a number of technical factors, including electrode location, band pass filtering, number of trials averaged, age, and rules regarding inclusion of the P30 component (the preceding positive peak in the auditory evoked potential waveform).

Olincy et al. (2006) administered a low and a high dose of an α-7 nicotinic agonist to a group of 12 non-smoking schizophrenics and studied changes in the P50 component and neurocognitive performance. The drug produced inhibition of the response to the second click in paired stimuli. Improvements in neurocognitive measures of attention were documented for the low drug dose. This study showed not only the utility of the P50 biomarker in assessing change in the central nervous system associated with a specific agent, but also that the magnitude of changes in response could assist in determining the most effective dose.

Large clinical trials have now been carried out and published on the use of frontal EEG measures to manage antidepressant medications (Leuchter et al., 2009a; Leuchter et al., 2009b). The Biomarkers for Rapid Identification of Treatment Response in Major Depression ("BRITE-MD") was a large multi-site trial (N = 220 participants completing the study) that used a neurophysiological biomarker to predict treatment response. Changes in the Hamilton-D scale were used to measure clinical outcome. An antidepressant treatment response index ("ATR") was derived from the power spectrum at baseline compared to the end of one week of the antidepressant escitalopram. The index is "a weighted combination of the relative theta and alpha power at week 1, and the difference between alpha 1 power (8.5–12 Hz) at baseline and alpha 2 power (9–11.5 Hz) at week 1".

Patients received quantitative EEG assessments at baseline and following one week of treatment with escitalopram. Patients were then randomized into treatment groups with (1) continued administration of escitalopram, (2) addition of bupropion to escitalopram, or (3) switch to bupropion. The

ATR predicted both response and remission at 8 weeks with 74% accuracy. Prediction of outcome based on genotyping, physician assessment, and serum drug levels were not significant (see Leuchter et al., 2009a). These authors reported that the ATR was also able to predict differential response to antidepressant medication. Patients with ATR values below a specific threshold were likely to respond to escitalopram and above the threshold were more likely to respond to bupropion.

Another large-scale study (N = 89) compared selection of medication for major depression based on algorithms developed in the "Sequenced Treatment Alternatives to Relieve Depression" (STARD) study that did not use EEG as a predictor (Rush et al., 2006), with medication guided by use of quantitative EEG features (DeBattista et al., 2009). There was a clear improvement on a number of measures of clinical outcome, including the Quick Inventory of Depressive Symptomatology and the Montgomery−Asberg Depression Rating Scale, with qEEG-guided intervention compared to STARD algorithms.

Overall, a number of qEEG and evoked potential procedures have been described that have significant potential for guiding therapeutic intervention with medication. The main use for quantitative EEG and evoked potential technology in this regard has been in studies of major depression and schizophrenia. In addition, however, quantitative EEG methods are being actively used in other neurophysiological interventions. A particularly productive line of inquiry involves consideration of changes in evoked potentials due to phase reset mechanisms (as opposed to the averaged activity of fixed generators of evoked potential components). Since it is our opinion that this could have major implications for guiding intervention strategies, we describe here some details of the procedure.

Evoked potentials are usually recorded by means of averaging segments or trials of EEG following the presentation of sensory stimuli. These potentials are generally considered to be fixed latency, fixed polarity, responses that appear superimposed on the background EEG. This is the basis of the "evoked" model. Recent literature has emphasized the need to consider that ERPs are generated at least in part by a reset of on-going oscillations, i.e., phase reset (Klimesch, Sauseng, Hanslmayr, Gruber, & Freunberger, 2007), the so-called "phase reset" model. Reduction in amplitude from the first to the second stimulus in a pair may be due to alterations in phase-locking. The role of phase-locking has been studied using intracranial recording in epilepsy patients (Rosburg et al., 2009). Poor gators showed less phase-locked beta frequency oscillation (20−30 Hz) in the 200−315 msec region following the first stimulus. This was found to be related to poorer memory encoding.

The relation between brain oscillations and auditory evoked potentials has been studied directly in schizophrenia (Brockhaus-Dumke, Mueller, Faigle, & Klosterkoetter, 2008). This work included 32 schizophrenic patients and 32 controls with EEG continuously recorded during an auditory paired click paradigm. The authors concluded that analyzing phase and amplitude in single trials provides more information on auditory information processing and reflects differences between schizophrenic patients and controls better than analyzing averaged ERP responses. Unfortunately this study found group differences in the N100 component which was predicted by phase-locking in the theta and alpha frequency ranges, but not the commonly reported findings with the P50 component which was predicted by phase-locking in the beta and gamma frequencies.

PREDICTION OF NEUROFEEDBACK PROTOCOL EFFICACY

Neurofeedback involves recording, analyzing, and presenting results of quantitative EEG analyses in near real-time to individuals in order to promote changes in brain electrical activity. There is no requirement for conscious awareness in neurofeedback training. In fact, a need for conscious awareness would limit the applicability of training in real-world situations. Following neurofeedback training, individuals do not need to willfully and consciously modify specific EEG patterns in order to effect behavioral change.

In the past, most training criteria have been set for individuals based on evaluation of behavior using a concept of arousal or symptom presentation. Now, increasingly, training incorporates characterization of neurophysiologic status using EEG and quantitative EEG, and evoked potentials to help predict outcome.

There are different ways to examine "arousal". Physiologically, our arousal level is usually considered in terms of the sleep/wake cycle. It is not unusual to see individuals who have problems regulating this activity. People who fall asleep as soon as they sit still, or people who cannot fall asleep as they lay in bed are examples of what happens when there are difficulties managing arousal. Prominent EEG changes seen with decreased arousal are easy to detect with recordings from the sensorimotor strip. These changes are used to assess depth of sleep: For example, differential appearances of discharges at the vertex (Cz) signal progression to Stage II sleep. Historically, neurofeedback practitioners began using protocols that remained on or near the sensorimotor strip (Lubar, 1985; Sterman & Friar, 1972; Tansey, 1984) with the goal of regulating arousal. Protocols often included Cz, C3 or C4, each with an ear reference.

The mechanism of arousal of the cortex by subcortical activity can be measured by sensors placed on the sensorimotor strip. When this mechanism is dysfunctional, we may observe particular aberrant behaviors. However, this remains a very subjective process and clinicians are not always able to make an accurate prediction of treatment efficacy based on this information alone. As clinicians employ more complicated protocols to help individuals modulate their arousal level, it is important to include objective information that can provide more guidance about the physiology of an individual's brain and how this might impact their level of arousal, and, hence, their response to treatment.

Early neurofeedback work with autism is a good example of the importance of modulation of general arousal. It was often thought that autistic children were highly over-aroused. This was based on their behaviors (e.g., "stimming"), and protocols were used to "calm" these children (Jarusiewicz, 2002). However, as more of these children had qEEG analyses done, it was noted that the pattern of brain electrical activity included far more slow content as compared to normative databases. It seemed that there was a mismatch between the observed "over-aroused" behaviors and the slower EEG patterns.

It is useful to think of the dimensions of arousal on an x, y graph. If we track the physiological arousal level on the y axis and the behavioral arousal on the x axis, we will find that there are times that these two match and times when they clearly do not. When neurofeedback practitioners have both pieces of information, they often better predict successful protocols that address issues of arousal.

At this point in the development of neurofeedback methods, neurofeedback clinicians need not limit themselves to the work on the sensorimotor strip, and, therefore, more comprehensive models have been considered. Johnstone (2008) suggested a role for qEEG in assisting in neurofeedback protocol development. Three main concerns were addressed: (1) general regulatory or arousal-based symptoms, (2) identifying focal regions of interest for training, and (3) evaluating connectivity among brain regions, both between and within hemispheres.

Assessment of general arousal is not as relevant and offers little guidance when looking at problems in localized areas of the brain. It is under these circumstances that evaluation of regional brain function is needed. Identification of focal or regional abnormality using qEEG, when considered in the context of behavioral symptoms and neurocognitive function, can more specifically guide protocol development. Examples of behaviors that are often correlated with regional abnormality in qEEG include language disability, difficulty with perception of emotional expression, avoidance behaviors in sensory integration disorders, specific memory difficulties, poor impulse control, lack of judgment, and numerous others. While changes in behavior can be helpful in tracking progress, more information can be very useful prior to neurofeedback training in finding neurophysiological causes or correlates of symptoms. qEEG analysis can be especially helpful in these circumstances. Specific information about frequency ranges, locations and connectivity issues can then be matched with behavioral symptoms in developing neurofeedback protocols to address regionally based issues.

qEEG analysis can be used not only to ascertain the need to modulate arousal and regional activation, but also neural connectivity. Certain clinical presentations are best characterized as "disconnection syndromes", and in such cases detection and remediation of abnormalities in EEG coherence are often clinically effective. The importance of disconnection syndromes in clinical neuropsychology is well known and coherence abnormalities have been documented in many studies of pathological conditions (Leocani & Comi, 1999). Neurofeedback training to increase and decrease connectivity has been recently shown to be useful in studies of autistic individuals (Coben, 2007; Coben & Padolsky, 2007).

The most direct method for using qEEG information to guide neurofeedback training involves feedback of information based on the extent of the z-score deviation for a specific feature, often called "live z-score training". One of the most intriguing aspects of this method is the apparent capacity of the brain to respond to multiple z-score training demands simultaneously. If this aspect of the method can be further validated, it suggests a more efficient way to carry out complex protocols within a brief period of time. It is important that the selection of z-scores to be trained are based on clinical criteria and take into account artifact, drowsiness, and transients, which are best identified in the raw EEG signal. In addition, selection of z-scores to be modified should not be based exclusively on the magnitude of z-score deviations because this can lead to ineffective or negative outcomes. The case history presented below is an example of when *not* to train certain patterns of z-score deviations. We emphasize the importance of clinical correlation with symptoms, complaints, and results of other diagnostic testing, including psychometric evaluation, in protocol development.

Also important is the dynamic information that can be gathered from the raw EEG signal. Identification of transient events and paroxysmal bursts are examples of information that can be helpful in protocol development. Neurofeedback training, both on the sensorimotor strip and in regions identified by visual inspection of EEG have been shown to be efficacious in treatment of epileptic disorders (Sterman, 2000), using such techniques as threshold adjustment. The threshold adjustment routine allows the clinician to provide feedback about transient paroxysmal events that are best identified in the raw EEG and can be characterized within a specific frequency range for feedback. These transient events may be of considerable clinical significance but are generally poorly resolved in time-averaged qEEG analyses.

EEG patterns, or phenotypes, have been identified that often can be linked to behavioral patterns (Johnstone et al., 2005). For example, excess frontal theta frequency activity is one of the phenotypes seen in individuals who suffer from attentional difficulties. However, it is important for clinicians to understand that this pattern does not exist exclusively as a biomarker for attention, and cannot be considered diagnostic. It is seen in other presentations as well. It can be seen in cases of brain injury, depression, and other difficulties. So, it remains important to know the specific behaviors and symptom presentation of each client to best make use of the objective data that can be collected from the raw EEG signal and the qEEG analysis.

Other measurement and analysis tools are emerging that are likely to enhance successful prediction of favorable outcome by helping in selection of specific neurofeedback protocols. For example, magnetoencephalography (MEG) provides additional information about sources of brain activity. EEG databases can be developed to specifically address predicting outcome in neurofeedback. Integration of neurocognitive assessment will provide a better understanding of the psychological correlates of phenotype patterns, and should allow more accurate prediction of therapeutic outcome using neurofeedback methods.

A case study demonstrating the utility of using the information in the raw EEG signal, results of a qEEG report, and the information gathered in a clinical interview follows.

Case Study

A 14-year-old male presents with multiple complaints that have not been resolved in treatment by two separate psychiatrists and a clinical psychologist. Parents began to seek treatment for him when his generalized anxiety escalated in the 6th grade. He would often be so anxious that he would crawl under either his, or the teacher's desk. He also experienced severe separation anxiety if his mother left the room for more than 5 minutes, and would repeatedly ask where she was and insist that he had to go find her. He was unable to go to sleep unless his mother sat at his bedside, and, even so, it would often take more than 2 hours for him to fall asleep. He was difficult to wake in the morning regardless of how long he had been allowed to sleep. Several times a week, he would sleepwalk to other areas of the house and often get into a bed, not his own, to sleep for the rest of the night. He was very hyperactive and was unable to sit at a table for a meal or sit still in a classroom. He constantly "drummed" on anything, including his own arms and legs. Recording his first EEG was a challenge. He displayed an extremely low frustration tolerance and poor impulse control. He often lashed out physically at his sister and also had physically aggressive episodes at school. Due to the unpredictably of his behaviors, his family rarely knew what to expect from him and he was unable to establish friendships.

Responses to medications were poor and/or adverse. Administration of Ativan for anxiety was followed by the patient putting his fist through a plate of glass and needing physical restraint to transport him to the hospital for care. Use of Ambien and Lunesta for sleep was followed by significant agitation. Following a small dose of Remeron, parents noted a slight improvement as it "took the edge off" and "subdued him slightly". But, there was no improvement in initiation of sleep or parasomnias. The patient used a low dose of Remeron for about 6 months. Because of negative or minimal response to medication the parents decided to begin neurofeedback training. Prior to training, a full clinical evaluation and an EEG/qEEG study was performed.

Visual inspection of his clinical EEG showed that there were bursts of spindling beta activity in the left frontal and right frontal regions, that were seen both bisynchronously and with shifting laterality. Results of qEEG analyses showed excessive beta activity in frontal regions bilaterally and an associated marked lack of interhemispheric beta coherence, particularly in prefrontal leads. These findings suggested the need to suppress beta activity in both hemispheres, and specifically *not* increase the significantly decreased z-scores for interhemispheric beta coherence. This approach has been described previously (Johnstone & Lunt, 2007). Neurofeedback protocols were developed emphasizing two-channel sum training to suppress frequently occurring beta bursts over frontal regions of both hemispheres.

Following approximately 60 sessions of training using frontal beta suppression and additional protocols to modulate centroparietal activity, a repeat qEEG was performed. The EEG was now read as within normal limits and difference topographs comparing the two recordings show a marked decrease in anterior beta. Database comparisons indicated that there was no longer significantly elevated anterior beta or significantly decreased anterior beta coherence. This was accompanied by marked clinical improvement documented by parents and teachers.

The outcome following qEEG guided neurofeedback is summarized below:

Before	After
Chronic generalized anxiety	Occasional moments of anxiety that are appropriate to the situation
Separation anxiety	Gone — now able to be away from home for several days with friends or family
Chronic insomnia	Able to fall asleep easily without anyone staying with him
Sleep disturbances (sleep walking)	No longer does this
Hyperactivity "drumming"	Physical activity is now purposeful and within normal limits, no more drumming
Frustration tolerance	Now able to tolerate more frustrating circumstances without over reacting
Lack of impulse control	Now able to stop and consider consequences
Unable to establish friendships	Now has several good friends

It cannot be concluded that neurofeedback was the sole reason for clinical improvement but given prior repeated trials with medication and behavioral counseling, it is clear that neurofeedback had an important influence on favorable clinical outcome.

USING EEG TO GUIDE TRANSCRANIAL MAGNETIC STIMULATION

Puri and Lewis (1996) suggested that transcranial magnetic stimulation (TMS) is a viable and important tool for diagnosis and therapy in psychiatric disorders. Subsequently, transcranial magnetic stimulation has been the subject of many hundreds of research studies over the past decade. Two main types of stimulation typically are used: low frequency stimulation (<1 Hz, "TMS") and high frequency stimulation (>5 Hz, "repetitive TMS", or "rTMS"). Low frequency high field stimulation generally produces inhibitory effects and higher frequency stimulation produces excitatory effects. TMS is currently being studied as a potential treatment for many disorders including epilepsy, depression, bipolar disorder, schizophrenia, posttraumatic stress disorder, obsessive—compulsive disorder, anxiety, stroke, and chronic pain. Numerous reviews of the technology and applications are now available (see George & Belmaker, 2006; Wassermann, Epstein, & Ziemann, 2008).

Most clinical work has been directed toward the treatment of depression, using rTMS over the left dorsolateral prefrontal cortex. In a recent review Brunelin et al. (2007) stated "the antidepressive properties of rTMS now appear obvious". Rosenberg et al. (2002) studied rTMS to left frontal cortex in patients with major depression. Stimulation was focused 5 cm anterior to the site of optimal motor stimulation. Seventy-five percent of the patients had a significant antidepressant response to rTMS, and 50% had sustained response at 2-month follow-up.

Overall, research shows the technique to be safe (Janicak et al., 2008). Lisanby et al. (2009) demonstrated efficacy using daily rTMS in a population of 164 individuals with major depression, showing a 22% reduction in symptoms compared to 9% with a sham control. It is clear that although rTMS may be clinically useful, it is not yet an optimal treatment, and techniques are needed to improve efficacy, particularly with treatment-resistant depression. One method used to improve efficacy was individualized placement of the stimulating coil by means of structural MRI (Fitzgerald et al., 2009). These researchers report significantly improved depression scales following 4 weeks of rTMS by using coil placement based on individual MRI compared to standard placement based on the motor response.

Jin et al. (2006) used measurement of individual alpha frequency to set stimulation rates in an rTMS study of schizophrenics. A series of 27 subjects with predominantly negative symptoms of schizophrenia received daily rTMS to midfrontal cortex for a period of 2 weeks. The authors documented that rTMS based on individualized alpha frequency ("αTMS"), significantly improved the therapeutic effect compared to lower frequency, higher frequency, and sham stimulation. In addition, therapeutic improvement was highly correlated with increased frontal alpha activity.

Magno-EEG resonant therapy (MERT) is an innovative form of TMS developed by Jin (personal communication, 2010). The MERT technique uses EEG to identify stimulus intensity, frequency, location, and duration needed to normalize EEG activity, particularly the dominant alpha frequency. Most rTMS protocols use the same frequency, location, and duration of stimulation on all patients, and do not consider intrinsic EEG frequency. With MERT, a customized treatment is developed for each individual based on analysis of the resting EEG.

MERT has been used primarily to target the dominant background EEG activity. The amount and frequency of EEG alpha activity, typically in the 8–13 Hz range, has been shown to be associated with overall brain metabolism, as well as cognitive functions generally, and a variety of types of mental disorders. Research is now being directed towards study of depression, anxiety, schizophrenia, and addiction. Further work obviously will be needed to specify optimal frequencies and stimulation techniques for different disorders.

CONCLUSION

A growing body of literature suggests there is significant value in using EEG information for guiding clinical intervention with medication, neurofeedback, and TMS. Studies of medication have largely focused on applications in depression and schizophrenia. Further work should extend this approach to additional clinical populations. Further development of predictive algorithms should emphasize newer pharmaceutical and neutraceuticals, used separately and in combination with other agents of the same or different classes. In addition, more detailed outcome measures beyond clinical global improvement scales should be employed in studies that use a combination of agents.

Research on neurofeedback would also benefit from development of predictive algorithms that combine behavioral analysis, neurocognitive assessment, and neurophysiological methods. It is expected that specific constellations of these features could be identified to more objectively guide development of successful neurofeedback protocols.

Much research is under way to apply transcranial magnetic stimulation to problems in neurology and psychiatry. Basic research to facilitate our understanding of intracranial current flow is likely to be helpful in optimizing rTMS procedures. Further individualization of stimulation rates and stimulation site(s) based on EEG and ERP features will also likely increase clinical efficacy of these techniques.

REFERENCES

Adler, L. E., Pachtman, E., Franks, R. D., Pecevich, M. C., Waldo, M., & Freedman, R. (1982). Neurophysiological evidence for a defect in neuronal mechanisms involved in sensory gating in schizophrenia. *Biological Psychiatry, 17,* 639–655.

Arns, M., Gunkelman, J., Breteler, M., & Spronk, D. (2008). EEG phenotypes predict treatment outcome to stimulants in children with ADHD. *Journal of Integrative Neuroscience, 7,* 421–438.

Boutros, N., Mirolo, H. A., & Struve, F. (2005). Normative data for the unquantified EEG: Examination of adequacy for neuropsychiatric research. *Journal of Neuropsychiatry and Clinical Neuroscience, 17,* 84–90.

Brockhaus-Dumke, A., Mueller, R., Faigle, U., & Klosterkoetter, J. (2008). Sensory gating revisited: Relation between brain oscillations and auditory evoked potentials in schizophrenia. *Schizophrenia Research, 99,* 238–249.

Brunelin, J., Poulet, E., Boeuve, C., Zeroug-vial, H., d'Amato, T., & Saoud, M. (2007). Efficacy of repetitive transcranial magnetic stimulation (rTMS) in major depression: A review. *L'Encéphale* (abstract in English), *33,* 126–134.

Burgess, A., & Gruzelier, J. (1993). Individual reliability of amplitude distribution in topographic mapping of EEG. *Electroencephalography and Clinical Neurophysiology, 86,* 219–223.

Coben, R. (2007). Connectivity guided neurofeedback for autistic spectrum disorder. *Biofeedback, 35,* 131–135.

Coben, R., & Padolsky, I. (2007). Assessment guided neurofeedback for autistic spectrum disorder. *Journal of Neurotherapy, 11,* 5–23.

Coburn, K. L., Lauterbach, E. C., Boutros, N. N, Black, K. J., Arciniegas, D. B., & Coffet, C. E. (2006). The value of quantitative electroencephalography in clinical psychiatry: Committee on research of the American Neuropsychiatric Association. *Journal of Neuropsychiatry and Clinical Neuroscience, 18,* 460–500.

DeBattista, C., Kinrys, G., & Hoffman, D. (2009). Referenced-EEG® (rEEG®) efficacy compared to STARD for patients with depression treatment failure. Presented at US Psychiatric and Mental Health Congress, 2009.

Fein, G., Galin, D., Johnstone, J., Yingling, C. D., Marcus, M., & Kiersch, M. (1983). EEG power spectra in normal and dyslexic children: I. Reliability during passive conditions. *Electroencephalography and Clinical Neurophysiology, 55,* 399–405.

Fein, G., Galin, D., Yingling, C. D., Johnstone, J., & Nelson, M. A. (1984). EEG spectra in 9-13 year old boys are stable over 1-3 years. *Electroencephalography and Clinical Neurophysiology, 58,* 517–518.

Fernandez, T., Harmony, T., Rodriguez, M., Reyes, A., Marosi, E., & Bernal, J. (1993). Test–retest reliability of EEG spectral parameters during cognitive tasks: I. Absolute and relative power. *International Journal of Neuroscience, 68,* 255–261.

Fitzgerald, P. B., Hoy, K., McQueen, S., Maller, J. J., Herring, S., Segrave, R., et al. (2009). A randomized trial of rTMS targeted with MRI based neuro-navigation in treatment-resistant depression. *Neuropsychopharmacology, 34,* 1255–1262.

Freedman, R., Adler, L., Waldo, M., Pachtman, E., & Franks, R. (1983). Neurophysiological evidence for a defect in inhibitory pathways in schizophrenia: A comparison of medicated and drug-free patients. *Biological Psychiatry, 18,* 989–1005.

Gasser, T., Bacher, P., & Steinberg, H. (1985). Test—retest reliability of spectral parameters of the EEG. *Electroencephalography and Clinical Neurophysiology, 60,* 312—319.

George, M. S., & Belmaker, R. H. (Eds.), (2006). *Transcranial magnetic stimulation in clinical psychiatry.* Arlington, VA: American Psychiatric Publishing.

Gerber, P. A., Chapman, K. E., Chung, S. S., Drees, C., Maganti, R. K., Ng, Y., et al. (2008). Interobserver agreement in the interpretation of EEG patterns in critically ill adults. *Journal of Clinical Neurophysiology, 25,* 241—249.

Harmony, T., Fernandez, T., Rodriguez, M., Reyes, A., Marosi, E., & Bernal, J. (1993). Test—retest reliability of spectral parameters during cognitive tasks: II. Coherence. *International Journal of Neuroscience, 68,* 263—271.

Hughes, J. R., & John, E. R. (1999). Conventional and quantitative electroencephalography in psychiatry. *Journal of Neuropsychiatry and Clinical Neurosciences, 11,* 190—208.

Janicak, P. G., O'Reardon, J. P., Sampson, S. M., Husain, M. M., Lisanby, S. H., Rado, J. T., et al. (2008). Transcranial magnetic stimulation (TMS) in the treatment of major depression: A comprehensive summary of safety experience from acute exposure, extended exposure and during reintroduction treatment. *Journal of Clinical Psychiatry, 69,* 222—232.

Jarusiewicz, B. (2002). Efficacy of neurofeedback for children in the autistic spectrum: A pilot study. *Journal of Neurotherapy, 6,* 39—49.

Jin, Y., Potkin, S. G., Kemp, A. S., Huerta, S. T., Alva, G., Thai, T. M., et al. (2006). Therapeutic effects of individualized alpha frequency transcranial magnetic stimulation (αTMS) on the negative symptoms of schizophrenia. *Schizophrenia Bulletin, 32,* 556—561.

Johnstone, J. (2008). A three-stage neuropsychological model of neurofeedback: Historical perspectives. *Biofeedback, 36,* 142—147.

Johnstone, J., & Gunkelman, J. (2003). Use of databases in qEEG evaluation. *Journal of Neurotherapy, 7,* 31—52.

Johnstone, J., Gunkelman, J., & Lunt, J. (2005). Clinical database development: Characterization of EEG phenotypes. *Clinical Electroencephalography and Neuroscience, 36,* 99—107.

Johnstone, J., & Lunt, J. (2007). NF sum training for patterns with shifting laterality. Oral presentation, International Society for Research and Neurofeedback Annual Meeting, San Diego, CA, September 7, 2007.

Juckel, G., Molnar, M., Hegert, U., Csepe, V., & Karmos, G. (1997). Auditory evoked potentials as indicator of brain serotonergic activity: First evidence in behaving cats. *Biological Psychiatry, 41,* 1181—1195.

Juckel, G., Pogarell, O., Augustin, H., Mulert, C., & Muller-Siecheneder, F. (2007). Differential prediction of first clinical response to serotongergic and norandrenergic antidepressants using the loudness dependence of auditory evoked potentials in patients with major depressive disorder. *Journal of Clinical Psychiatry, 68,* 1206—1212.

Juckel, G., Schumacher, C., Giegling, I., Assion, H-J., Mavrogiorgou, P., Pogarell, O., et al. (2010). Serotonergic functioning as measured by the loudness dependence of auditory evoked potentials is related to a haplotype in the brain-derived neurotrophic factor (BDNF) gene. *Journal of Psychiatric Research, 44,* 541—546.

Klimesch, W., Sauseng, P., Hanslmayr, S., Gruber, W., & Freunberger, R. (2007). Event-related phase reorganization may explain evoked neural dynamics. *Neuroscience and Behavioral Reviews, 31,* 1003—1016.

Leocani, L., & Comi, G. (1999). EEG coherence in pathological conditions. *Journal of Clinical Neurophysiology, 16,* 548—555.

Leuchter, A. F., Cook, I., Hunter, A., & Korb, A. (2009). Use of clinical electrophysiology for the selection of medication in the treatment of major depressive disorder: The state of the evidence. *Clinical Electroencephalography and Neuroscience, 49,* 78—83.

Leuchter, A. F., Cook, I., Marangell, L. B., Gilmer, W. S., Burgoyne, K. S., Howland, R. H., et al. (2009a). Comparative effectiveness of biomarkers and clinical indicators for predicting outcomes of SSRI treatment in Major Depressive Disorder: Results of the BRITE-MD study. *Psychiatry Research, 169*, 124–131.

Leuchter, A. F., Cook, I., Gilmer, W. S., Marangell, L. B., Burgoyne, K. S., Howland, R. H., et al. (2009b). Effectiveness of a quantitative electroencephalographic biomarker for predicting differential response or remission with escitalopram and bupropion in major depressive disorder. *Psychiatry Research, 169*, 132–138.

Lisanby, S. H., Husain, M. M., Rosenquist, P. B., Maixner, D., Gutierrez, R., Krystal, A., et al. (2009). Daily left prefrontal repetitive transcranial magnetic stimulation (rTMS) in the acute treatment of major depression: Clinical predictors of outcome in a multisite, randomized controlled clinical trial. *Neuropsychopharmacology, 34*, 522–534.

Lubar, J. (1985). EEG biofeedback and learning disabilities. *Theory into Practice, 26*, 106–111.

Lund, T. R., Sponheim, S. R., Iacono, W. G., & Clementz, B. A. (1995). Internal consistency reliability of resting EEG power spectra in schizophrenic and normal subjects. *Psychophysiology, 32*, 66–71.

Niedermeyer, E., & Lopes da Silva, F. (Eds.), (2004). *Electroencephalography: Basic principles, clinical applications, and related fields* (5th ed.). Philadelphia: Lippincott Williams & Wilkins.

Nuwer, M. (1997). Assessment of digital EEG, quantitative EEG, and EEG brain mapping: Report of the American Academy of Neurology and the American Clinical Neurophysiology Society. *Neurology, 49*, 277–292.

Mulert, C., Juckel, G., Brunnmeier, M., Karch, S., Leicht, G., Mergi, R., et al. (2007). Rostral anterior cingulate cortex activity in the theta band predicts response to antidepressant medication. *Clinical Electroencephalography and Neuroscience, 38*, 78–81.

Olincy, A., Harris, J. G., Johnson, L. L., Pender, V., Kongs, S., Allensworth, D., et al. (2006). Proof-of-concept trial of an α7 nicotinic agonist in schizophrenia. *Archives of General Psychiatry, 63*, 630–638.

Patterson, J. V., Hetrick, W. P., Boutros, N. N., Jin, Y., Sandman, C., Stern, H., et al. (2008). P50 Sensory gating ratios in schizophrenics and controls: A review and data analysis. *Psychiatry Research, 158*, 226–247.

Piccinelli, P., Viri, M., Zucca, C., Borgatti, R., Romeo, A., Giordano, L., et al. (2005). Inter-rater reliability of the EEG reading in patients with childhood idiopathic epilepsy. *Epilepsy Research, 66*, 195–198.

Puri, B. K., & Lewis, S. W. (1996). Transcranial magnetic stimulation in psychiatric research. *British Journal of Psychiatry, 169*, 675–677.

Rosenberg, P. B., Mehndiratta, R. B., Mehndiratta, Y. P., Wamer, A., Rosse, R. B., & Balish, M. (2002). Repetitive transcranial magnetic stimulation treatment of comorbid posttraumatic stress disorder and major depression. *Journal of Neuropsychiatry and Clinical Neurosciences, 14*, 270–276.

Rosburg, T., Trautner, P., Fell, J., Moxon, K. A., Elger, C. E., & Boutros, N. N. (2009). Sensory gating in intracranial recording: The role of phase locking. *NeuroImage, 44*, 1041–1049.

Rush, A. J., Trivedi, M. H., Wisniewski, S. R., Nierenberg, A. A., Stewart, J. W., Warden, D., et al. (2006). Acute and longer-term outcomes in depressed outpatients requiring one or several treatment steps: A STARD report. *American Journal of Psychiatry, 163*, 1905–1917.

Saletu, B., Anderer, P., & Saletu-Zyhlarz, G. M. (2006). EEG topography and tomography (LORETA) in the classification and evaluation of the pharmacodynamics of psychotropic drugs. *Clinical Electroencephalography and Neuroscience, 37*, 66–80.

Salinsky, M. C., Oken, B. S., & Morehead, L. (1991). Test−retest reliability in EEG frequency analysis. *Electroencephalography and Clinical Neurophysiology, 79*, 382−392.

Spencer, S. S., Williamson, P. D., Bridgers, S. L., Mattson, R. H., Cicchetti, D. V., & Spencer, D. D. (1985). Reliability and accuracy of localization by scalp ictal EEG. *Neurology, 35*, 1567−1575.

Sterman, M. B. (2000). Basic concepts and clinical findings in the treatment of seizure disorders with EEG operant conditioning. *Clinical Electroencephalography, 31*, 45−55.

Sterman, M. B., & Friar, L. (1972). Suppression of seizures in epileptics following sensorimotor EEG feedback training. *Electroencephalography and Clinical Neurophysiology, 33*, 89−95.

Struve, F. A. (1985). Clinical electroencephalography as an assessment method in psychiatric patients. In R. C. Hall, & T. P. Beresford (Eds.), *Handbook of psychiatric diagnostic procedures* (Vol. 2, pp. 1−48). New York: Spectrum Publications.

Suffin, S. C., & Emory, W. H. (1995). Neurometric subgroups in attentional and affective disorders and their association with pharmacotherapeutic outcome. *Clinical Electroencephalography, 26*, 76−83.

Suffin, S. C., Gutierrez, N. M., Karan, S., Aurora, G., Emory, W. H., & Kling, A. (2007). A QEEG database method for predicting pharmacotherapeutic outcome in refractory major depressive disorders. *Journal of American Physicians and Surgeons, 12*, 104−108.

Tansey, M. A. (1984). EEG sensorimotor rhythm biofeedback training: Some effects on the neurological precursors of learning disabilities. *International Journal of Psychophysiology, 3*, 85−99.

Thatcher, R. W. (2010). Validity and reliability of quantitative electroencephalography. *Journal of Neurotherapy, 14*, 122−152.

Thatcher, R. W., Biver, C., & North, D. (2003). Quantitative EEG and the Frye and Daubert standards of admissibility. *Clinical Electroencephalography, 34*, 39−53.

Thatcher, R. W., & Lubar, J. F. (2009). History of the scientific standards of qEEG normative databases. In T. H. Budzynski, H. K. Budzynski, J. R. Evans, & A. Abarbanel (Eds.), *Introduction to quantitative EEG and neurofeedback* (2nd ed., pp. 29−62). New York: Academic Press.

Wassermann, E., Epstein, C., & Ziemann, U. (Eds.), (2008). *Oxford handbook of transcranial stimulation*. New York: Oxford University Press.

Williams, G. W., Luders, H. O., Brickner, A., Goormastic, M., & Klass, D. W. (1985). Interobserver variability in EEG interpretation. *Neurology, 35*, 1714−1719.

Williams, G. W., Lesser, R. P., Silvers, J. B., Brickner, A., Goormastic, M., Fatica, K. J., et al. (1990). Clinical diagnoses and EEG interpretation. *Cleveland Clinic Journal of Medicine, 57*, 437−440.

CHAPTER 2

EEG Source Analysis: Methods and Clinical Implications

Marco Congedo[1] and Leslie Sherlin[2]

[1]ViBS Team (Vision and Brain Signal Processing), GIPSA-Lab, National Center for Scientific Research (CNRS), Grenoble University, Grenoble, France

[2]Neurotopia, Inc., Los Angeles, California; Nova Tech EEG, Inc., Mesa, Arizona, and Southwest College of Naturopathic Medicine, Tempe, Arizona, USA

Contents

INTRODUCTION

Over the past two decades analysis of electroencephalographic (EEG) recordings has received a strong growth thanks to the discovery of "source analysis". By this we mean moving from the sensor space, the data as recorded from the extracranial electrodes, into the source space, representing some form of intracranial current source that generates the observed measurement. This movement has somewhat compensated for the poor spatial resolution of EEG, and therefore this neuroimaging modality has been rediscovered and is now among the much more sophisticated and newer modalities such as MEG (magnetoencephalography), fMRI (functional magnetic resonance imaging), PET (positron emission tomography), and nIRS (near infra-red spectroscopy).

Neurofeedback and Neuromodulation Techniques and Applications
DOI: 10.1016/B978-0-12-382235-2.00002-0

EEG source analysis has been applied purposefully in cognitive and clinical studies. More recently it has also become prominent in *real-time EEG applications* such as *neurofeedback* and *brain—computer interface*. Those applications best exploit the high-temporal resolution of EEG, due to the high sampling rate of EEG (in the order of milliseconds) and the fact that EEG signals instantaneously grasp electrical current variations in the brain. But what do we mean in practice by "source analysis"? Two major families of EEG source analysis methods can be found currently in the literature: (1) the methods based on a head model and an inverse solution (e.g., Pascual-Marqui, Michel, & Lehmann, 1994), which attempt to localize the current source in the brain; and (2) the so-called "blind" or "semi-blind" methods (e.g., Congedo, Gouy-Pailler & Jutten, 2008), which attempt to recover the source time course without explicitly modeling the subject's head. We have been using both the first (Lubar, Congedo, & Askew, 2003; Sherlin & Congedo, 2005; Sherlin et al., 2007) and second kind of methods (Gouy-Pailler, Congedo, Brunner, Jutten, & Pfurtscheller, 2010; Van der Loo et al., 2009). The two families can be fruitfully combined by applying a blind method before the source localization (Congedo, Lotte, & Lécuyer, 2006). In this chapter we will concentrate on the second family of methods mentioned, the blind source separation (BSS), and, more particularly, on a unified flexible technique that has proven to be useful in many different experimental and clinical situations.

The goal of this chapter is to explain and illustrate the appeal of BSS for EEG data, focusing on neurofeedback applications. We explicitly address readers without a strong mathematical background, mainly medical doctors and clinicians, preferring an intuitive understanding of the material rather than a formal one. This chapter can be conceived as a journey starting from the physical basis of EEG recordings, the concept of correlation, passing through the understanding of the blind source separation concept, to finally see why and how the technique turns out to be very useful in neurofeedback. We hope that at the end of this chapter the reader will be left with a conceptual understanding of the BSS concepts, which usually are treated formally by and for engineers. We intentionally refrain from using linear algebra notation, the natural language for the multivariate EEG source analysis. For a more formal treatment of the material presented here we refer to the review paper by Congedo et al. (2008). The main ideas expressed in this chapter have been foreseen in Congedo and Joffe (2007).

METHOD

Principles of EEG Physics

EEG source analysis methods can be understood considering the theory of brain volume conduction, that is, how the current in the brain reaches the electrode sensors. It is well established that the generators of brain electric fields recordable from the scalp are macroscopic post-synaptic potentials created by assemblies of pyramidal cells of the neocortex (Speckmann & Elger, 2005). Pyramidal cells are aligned and oriented perpendicularly to the cortical surface. Synchronous firing of these cells is possible thanks to a dense net of local horizontal connections (mostly <1 mm). At recording distances larger than about three/four times the diameter of the synchronized assemblies the resulting post-synaptic potential behaves as if it were produced by electric dipoles, that is, as if in a propagating medium we were recording from a distance the potential variations created by batteries of alternating current. More formally stated, in the multipole expansion higher terms vanish and we may be satisfied by such dipole approximation (Lopes da Silva & Van Rotterdam, 2005; Nunez & Srinivasan, 2006, Ch. 3). As is well known, electromagnetic phenomena are governed by the four Maxwell equations. Three physical phenomena justify a tremendous simplification of such electromagnetic equations in the case of scalp EEG:

1. Unless dipoles are moving there is no appreciable delay in the scalp sensor measurement (Lopes da Silva & Van Rotterdam, 2005), i.e., all sensors record the current of all dipoles simultaneously and instantaneously.

2. In brain electric fields there is no appreciable electromagnetic coupling (magnetic induction) in frequencies up to about 1 MHz, thus the quasi-static approximation of Maxwell equations holds throughout the spectrum of interest (Nunez & Srinivasan, 2006, pp. 535-540).

3. For source oscillations below 40 Hz it has been verified experimentally that capacitive effects are also negligible, implying that potential difference is in phase with the corresponding generator (Nunez & Srinivasan, 2006, p. 61).

These three phenomena strongly support the *linear superposition principle*, according to which the relation between neocortical dipolar fields and scalp potentials may be approximated by a system of linear equations (see Sarvas, 1987 for the equations for MEG), which we will explain next. Despite this being a great simplification, we need to keep in mind that scalp EEG may reflect only macroscopic cerebral phenomena, that is, a current field extending over a several centimeter-sized cube. We say that these phenomena have a low spatial frequency, meaning that they change slowly along cortical regions. Such spatial frequency should not be confounded with the frequency of the EEG oscillations, although a relationship between the two is established by the physiology of the brain. For example, massive assemblies in the human brain synchronize at low frequencies (up to about 35 Hz), whereas local synchronizations in higher frequencies are confined to small neocortical areas. Thus, it turns out that with continuous recording (the basis for neurofeedback) we can monitor only low frequency oscillations with a sufficient signal-to-noise ratio. Gamma activity in the brain is best studied averaging time-locked recordings or by intracranial recordings.

Volume Conduction and EEG

The generative model of scalp EEG is called *linear instantaneous time-invariant mixing* and it is illustrated in Figure 2.1 (refer to caption for details).

The main point we need to stress is this: every active dipole is diffused to most, if not all, electrodes, that is, the observed measurement (scalp voltage) is a *mixing* of the underlying sources. The current diffusion from source to sensor is *instantaneous*. The generative model is therefore *linear*,

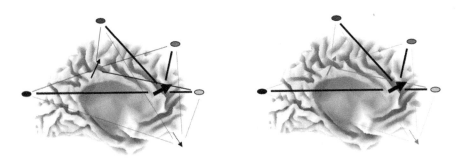

Figure 2.1 Left: schematic representation of the linear instantaneous mixing of three equivalent dipoles on four sensors. The thick arrows represent dipoles (cerebral sources) while the dotted dipole represents an extracerebral source corresponding, for example, to current produced by eye movements. Grey ovals represent EEG electrodes. Lines connecting dipoles to electrodes represent their current diffusion. Right: schematic representation of a spatial filter by the blind source separation method, the effect of which in this example is to suppress two of the three dipoles (grey connecting lines for these sources represent suppession); the data would now contain only the contribution of one dipole (bold thick arrow).

meaning that we can write the voltage of the *i*th electrode as a linear combination (weighted sum) of source activity, such as

$$x_i(t) = a_{i1} \cdot s_1(t) + a_{i2} \cdot s_2(t) + \ldots + a_{iM} \cdot s_M(t) \tag{2.1}$$

where $x_i(t)$ is the *i*th electrode measurement at time instant t, $s_1(t)\ldots s_M(t)$ are the contributions of M visible sources at the same time instant and the $a_{i1}\ldots a_{iM}$ are the mixing coefficients uniquely expressing the relation between source $s_1(t)\ldots s_M(t)$ and the *i*th electrode. Note that some mixing coefficients may be null, thus the above generative model is quite general, having the ability to relate the sensor measurement to any number and configuration of underlying sources. Also, note that in this particular model the mixing coefficients do not depend on time, that is, they are fixed. That is why we call the model *time-invariant*. Above all, keep in mind that the mixing coefficients will depend on source position, intensity, pole separation, and orientation. The smaller the distance between the source and the electrode, the higher the coefficients will be. The coefficients will also be higher for dipoles pointing in the direction of the electrode and vanishing as the dipole is perpendicular to such direction (Nunez & Srinivasan, 2006). This phenomenon, explains why "source localization" cannot be attained using scalp topographical maps, and is illustrated in Figure 2.2 (refer to caption for details).

In summary, in addition to the simplification of the superposition principle aforementioned, our generative model implicitly assumes that the dipoles have fixed location and orientation during the observation period. However, their activity may be intermittent during the observation period. These are reasonable assumptions as the dipole location and orientation are fixed by cortical anatomy. With these assumptions in mind, let us now explore the concept of correlation, which will open the way to understanding the blind source separation (BSS) process.

The Concept of Statistical Correlation

The *Pearson product-moment correlation* is a well-known concept. Two variables are said to be positively correlated if when one increases the other tends to increase as well. They are said to be negatively correlated when one increases and the other tends to decrease. They are said to be non-correlated if there is neither of these tendencies. An important characteristic of correlation is that it is a *dimensionless* measure (standardized), meaning that correlations obtained on different pairs of variables are comparable, regardless of the unit

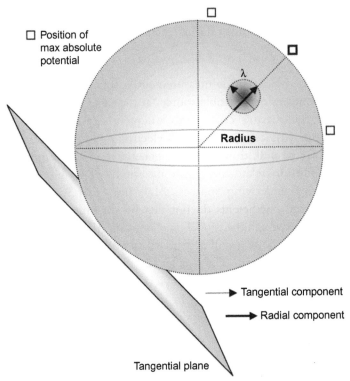

Figure 2.2 Schematic representation of the current diffusion for radial and tangential dipoles in an infinite homogeneous isotropic conductive spherical medium, which only roughly approximates the human head. The dipoles extend within the small sphere labeled as "λ". If the direction of the dipole is radial (indicated by the bold arrow) the maximum observed voltage on the surface of the sphere will be in the position indicated by the bold square. If the direction of the dipole is tangential (indicated by a light arrow), the maximum absolute observed voltage on the surface of the sphere will be approximately in the position indicated by the two light squares. Thus, whereas the radial dipole will result in a monopolar scalp map, the tangential dipole will result in a bipolar scalp map, although the position of the dipole is exactly the same.

in which the variables are expressed. For example, suppose we suspect that there is a relationship between age and weight of individuals. Figure 2.3 shows the scatter plot of 456 random cases taken from the NHANES database (see caption for details). As can be seen from the plot, there is a significant positive correlation between age and weight up until about age 20, then the correlation disappears. If instead of the weight in kilograms we take the weight in pounds, we obtain exactly the same correlation values. Furthermore if we

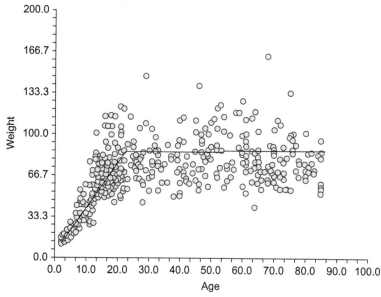

Figure 2.3 Scatter plot age/weight of 456 random cases taken from the NHANES (National Health and Nutrition Examination Survey) database. (*Source: http://www. denofinquiry.com/nhanes/source/choose.php.*)

consider next the correlation between age and height and the two values of correlations differ, we can compare the two correlations and say that one is stronger then the other. The perfect negative correlation is equal to -1 and the perfect positive correlation is equal to $+1$, while two variables are said to be perfectly uncorrelated if the correlation equals zero. Perfect correlation is obtained if the points of the scatter plot align perfectly; the more the data points are dispersed the smaller the correlation. If the data are normally distributed, a spherical cloud of data points always indicates the absence of correlation. Correlation exists only if the cloud assumes an ellipsoidal shape with inclined axes. The concept of correlation is entangled with the concepts of *linear regression* and *prediction*. In fact, if two variables are correlated we may obtain a prediction of the value of either variable knowing the value of the other; i.e., if the correlation is significant, the linear regression is necessarily significant (the slope of the line best fitting the scatter plot is significantly different from zero). For instance, in Figure 2.3 it appears obvious that knowing the age of an individual after age 20 does not give us an indication about what his/her weight would be, but a reasonable weight range can be predicted for age 0–20. Indeed, such ranges

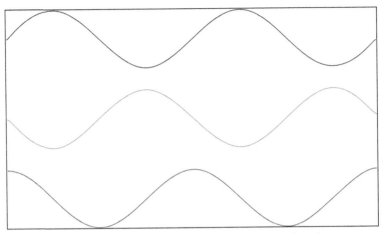

Figure 2.4 Two cycles of three sinusoidal waves. As compared to the top wave, the middle wave has a 180° phase shift and the bottom wave a 90° phase shift. See text for further properties.

are given to pediatric doctors in the form of percentiles (confidence intervals) to check the normal growth of our children.

When it comes to time-series, particularly sinusoidal time-series (which is the case with EEG oscillations), the correlation depends on the *phase* of the sinusoids. Figure 2.4 depicts two periods of three sinusoids with identical frequency, but different phase. The phase difference or shift between any one of the three sinusoids and itself is zero, thus the *autocorrelation* is obviously exactly +1. The phase shift between the sinusoids shown top and middle is 180° (half of a cycle). That is, the middle wave is the top wave with the sign switched; thus their correlation is exactly equal to −1. You can check from the plot that as one wave rises the other falls, and vice versa, with no exception. Needless to say, you can *predict exactly* the value of the middle wave knowing the value of the top wave, that is, there is *no additional information at all* in the middle wave. The phase shift between the top and bottom sinusoids is 90° (one-quarter of a cycle), and it happens that at this particular phase shift the correlation is exactly zero. This relationship is so important that the names *sine* and *cosine*, respectively, have been assigned to these two sinusoids. From what we have said it follows that a wave with the same frequency and any other phase shift will be correlated somehow to the sine and to the cosine. Actually, we can go further and say that any other such wave can be written as a linear combination of the sine and cosine. For this reason we say that the sine and the cosine form an *orthogonal basis*. This idea informed the great intuition of Joseph Fourier (1768–1830), who demonstrated that under rather general conditions *any* periodic time-series, regardless of its complexity, and even if it is not at all sinusoidal, can be written as an infinite sum of sines and cosines at different frequencies. When you compute the power spectrum of the EEG by Fast Fourier Transform (FFT), you actually compute a non-standardized version of the correlation between your data and the sine and cosine wave at each discrete frequency for which you want to compute the power. You do not need to check the amount of sinusoidal components in your time-series at any phase shift; you just need to do that for the sine and cosine. Then you add up the two to obtain the power. It turns out that those two particular waves, being orthogonal, and thus spanning the whole phase cycle, account by themselves for *any possible phase shift in your data*.

The Concept of Blind Source Separation (BSS)

One way to perform BSS of human EEG is to require a linear transformation of the data canceling the correlation between sensor measurements. What does that mean? In Figure 2.1 we have shown that each electrode records a mixing of source activity. This would imply that electrode time-series are correlated, *even if the dipole time-series are not correlated*. This happens because the sensor measurements at different electrodes share a portion of the same sources. Indeed, this is what we observe in continuous EEG recordings. A typical example is given in Figure 2.5 (refer to caption for details). Arranging all pair-wise correlations between the 19 time-series of Figure 2.5 in a matrix we obtain the correlation matrix, also shown in graphical form in Figure 2.5. The correlation matrix is far from being diagonal, that is to say, there is a lot of correlation between electrodes. An expert eye would see this already in the raw EEG data. Note also the similarity of the power spectra, autocorrelation functions, and Hurst exponents of the channels, pointing out, again, the similarity of the EEG time courses at different electrodes. Turning back to what we have said about correlation and prediction, let us state that since the correlation among electrodes is high, there is a great deal of *redundant* information in scalp EEG. Redundancy is presented at the scalp electrodes due to the volume conduction and the fact that the scalp sensors are recording the summation of all sources, previously described as mixing of signals, under the electrode site. Such redundancy is a waste, in the sense that we

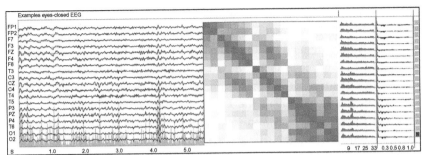

Figure 2.5 (*See Color Plate Section*) From left to right: about 5.5 s of eyes-closed EEG recorded at the standard 19 leads described by the 10–20 electrode placement system, the 19 × 19 correlation matrix of EEG time-series, the power spectra (red plot: 1 Hz–32 Hz), autocorrelation function (blue plot: lag = 0–1 s) and Hurst exponent (green bars) of the 19 EEG signals. The entries of the correlation matrix are color coded, with white coding correlation equal to zero and red (blue) coding correlation equal to 1 (−1). The entries in diagonal are the autocorrelations, hence they all equal 1. Note that electrode T3 is much less correlated to other electrodes as compared to the others. This is because it contains a considerable amount of muscle artifacts (as seen also from the high-frequency content of the power spectrum and the flat autocorrelation function), which does not distribute through the head to other electrodes.

can explain the data with less than 19 time-series, by identifying the *unique information* carried by each, just as the sine and cosine alone explain sinusoids with any phase shift. It is additionally a distraction, because the signal at two correlated electrodes is less *clear*, much like listening to two speeches mixed together as compared to listening to them separately. Now, assume the dipolar activity itself is *uncorrelated*, and let us ask, for instance, whether we can in some way "filter" the input of the 19 time-series and receive as output a smaller number of uncorrelated time-series. And even further, would this filter be able to recover the source activity itself? The answer to these questions is exactly what BSS attempts to achieve. Next, we will see how it works and what conditions are necessary for its success.

Performing BSS by Decorrelation

Consider the equation $8 = 4/2$. We can invert the 4 and multiply it at both sides to get $1/4 \times 8 = 2$. Similarly, referring to our mixing model in Eq 2.1, we want to invert the equations and solve for a given source $s_j(t)$ starting from N scalp electrodes to recover M sources such as

$$s_j(t) = b_{j1} \cdot x_1(t) + b_{j2} \cdot x_2(t) + \ldots + b_{jN} \cdot x_N(t) \tag{2.2}$$

In Eq 2.2 the coefficients $b_{j1}\ldots b_{jN}$ are called *demixing coefficients*. They are found "inverting" the mixing coefficients in Eq 2.1 and provide "weights" to be applied to scalp electrode samples to recover the source, that is, to suppress all the others. The basic idea of BSS neurofeedback is to use one or more chosen sources $s_j(t)$ as the basis for the feedback signal and not the raw sensor data. In doing so we obtain two advantages: first, if the source is successfully extracted the feedback signal truly reflects neocortical oscillations. This is not necessarily true for scalp sensor measurement. Second, by selecting a number of sources we implicitly filter out all the remaining ones, that is, the feedback signal will not be affected by irrelevant brain activity and separated artifacts. These two advantages are often referred to as increased *sensitivity* and *specificity*, respectively.

In order to solve Eq 2.2 the mixing coefficients or the demixing coefficients must be estimated. If we estimate them using only the observed data the method is named "blind" because those coefficients are not modeled using head geometry. As a matter of fact, we want to estimate both the mixing (or demixing) coefficients and the sources from the data only. At first, this sounds a little too ambitious. Nonetheless, it can be shown that such estimation is possible under some mild assumptions on the sources, which we will list further on, preserving the *waveform* of the sources. However, there is a price to pay, which is known as the *three BSS indeterminacies: order, sign, and energy*. The order indeterminacy means that the sources are extracted in an arbitrary order. This implies that, for example, if we run the algorithm on different segments of the data we have to make sure to match the sources in order to compare them. The sign indeterminacy means that the actual sign of the sources cannot be known. Typically this is not a limitation because the relevant information is in the waveform, not in its sign and measures such as power are invariant under sign switching. The energy (power) indeterminacy means that the actual power (in absolute terms) of the sources is not known. Again, typically, this is not a limitation as, for example in neurofeedback, we are interested only in the relative power change of the source over time. The sign and energy indeterminacy have been separated for ease of exposition, however in reality they amount to the same indeterminacy, referred to together as the *scaling indeterminacy*. In fact, multiplying the source time-series for a scaling factor, which can be positive or negative, we account for both the sign and energy indeterminacy. Referring to Eq 2.1, let us take the example of multiplying each source by a number and its coefficient by its inverse. The final resulting scalp voltage would not change. If the number is negative the source will switch sign. Hence, all we can do in seeking a solution to Eq. 2.2 is to artificially fix the scaling of the source, for example, by requiring that the output source will have unitary energy, it does not matter what the sign is.

Assuming that the sources are decorrelated, one may require a linear transformation of the EEG data resulting in a diagonal correlation matrix (see Figure 2.5). However, it is well known that a decorrelation of the EEG time-series alone does *not* solve the problem. The method to decorrelate a multiple time-series is known as principal component analysis (PCA). PCA has been known since the time of Karl Pearson (1857−1936), and more recently has been formalized by Harold Hotelling (1895−1973). For many years researchers have tried to apply PCA to EEG data with inaccurate results in terms of source extraction. The reason is that there are infinite numbers of such decorrelating matrices with unitary output that can be found by PCA. That is, PCA does not estimate the actual sources, it finds only an economical representation of the data by decorrelating the input. It is said that PCA solves "half" of the ICA problem. In fact, once decorrelation is attained by PCA, another transformation is required in order to obtain the sought solution. This fact can be understood intuitively in geometrical terms: suppose we have two sensors and two sources and the data are normally distributed. Once we have decorrelated the sensor data and forced unitary energy, we see that the scatter plot will form a circle-shaped cloud of points. Now, you can rotate (a special kind of linear transformation) the cloud as you wish and the shape will not change, that is, the data will still be uncorrelated. Every possible rotation will provide a different linear transformation of the data. The crucial question is, what is the unique rotation that will recover the actual sources? The same argument applies for any number of sensors. With three sensors and three sources the cloud will form a sphere that can be rotated in three dimensions, but the argument is the same. With more than three dimensions the argument is the same, just; the visualization of the phenomenon becomes impossible (the cloud will form a hyper-sphere).

A method estimating the actual (de)mixing coefficients under an independence assumption, not just an arbitrary decorrelating transformation, was found in the 1980s by some colleagues of the first author in Grenoble (Hérault & Jutten, 1986; Jutten & Hérault, 1991). The method was called independent component analysis (ICA). This discovery has resulted in a great deal of research. ICA today is a special case of the broadest family of BSS algorithms, which are applied in several fields of engineering such as speech enhancement, image processing, geophysical data analysis, wireless communications, and biological signal analysis.

In this chapter we do not focus on ICA, but on BSS decorrelating methods. In Congedo, Gouy-Pailler and Jutten (2008) we have argued that these methods are well adapted to continuously recorded EEG.

Conditions for Successful BSS

The secret to achieving BSS by decorrelation methods is in a theorem (Afsari, 2008), a detailed explanation of which is beyond the scope of this chapter. For our purposes, let us accept that we need to find a set of demixing coefficients respecting data decorrelation plus at least one more decorrelating condition. According to the principles we have previously described, the data decorrelation will make the data hyperspherical and the additional decorrelation condition(s) will find the unique rotation requested to *identify* the sources. Data decorrelation implies that the transformed data correlation matrix is diagonal. A suitable transformation of the data as per Eq 2.2 must diagonalize also at least another matrix of statistics describing the dependence between the EEG time-series. The two most important ways these additional statistics can be defined are:

1. Considering two or more data segments and requiring that the transformation diagonalize the correlation matrix for all of them.
2. Filter the data in two or more band-pass regions and require that the transformation diagonalize the correlation matrix for all of them.

The first procedure will succeed if the source energy in the two or more segments is not constant, but will change in a way that is unique to each source. For instance, if the subject takes part in two experimental conditions, those sources activating in one of the two conditions can be found by this BSS procedure. Another example is the recovering of the generators of particular EEG rhythms. It will suffice to select two segments, one in which the rhythm is present and the other where it is absent or substantially reduced, and diagonalize the correlation matrix for both of them. The second procedure will recover sources as long as their power spectrum is not proportional. In this case the unique "variation" of the source necessary for its identification is not the energy over time or across conditions, but the power spectral profile itself. The two procedures can be combined to succeed if either of the two conditions are respected (see Congedo et al., 2008). In practice, the BSS is more efficient when more than two matrices are jointly diagonalized. The method to perform such a joint diagonalization has been named

Approximate Joint Diagonalization (AJD: Congedo & Pham, 2009; Pham & Congedo, 2009; Tichavsky & Yeredor, 2009) and will not be detailed here. In summary, BSS can be obtained by diagonalizing simultaneously a set of correlation matrices, which may be estimated at different time segments and/or experimental conditions and/or frequencies. The choice of the matrix set to be diagonalized is instrumental to the success of the BSS. A validation of BSS obtained with the second procedure (Van der Loo et al., 2007) is given in Figure 2.6 (see text for details).

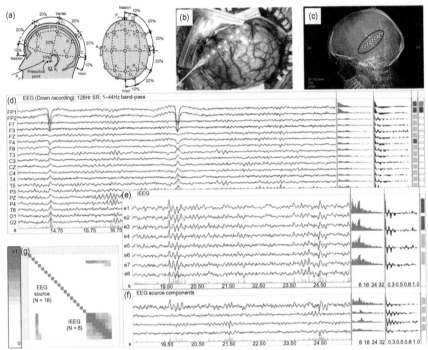

Figure 2.6 (*See Color Plate Section*) A tinnitus patient was implanted with two rows of eight extradural intracranial recording electrodes. Nineteen scalp electrodes (EEG) and the intracranial electrodes (iEEG) were recorded simultaneously with a common reference positioned on the vertex. (a) Position of the 19 electrodes on the scalp (10–20 system). (b) Demonstration of the surgical procedure to insert the extradural electrodes. (c) Computerized tomography of the patient's head showing the location of the electrodes (over the left secondary auditory cortex). (d) Example 9 seconds of the scalp EEG data. (e) Example 7 seconds of the intracranial data. (f) Four of the 18 sources estimated from scalp EEG data only with time-course corresponding exactly to the extradural recording in (e). (g) Correlation matrix between the 18 sources estimated from the scalp EEG and the eight extradural recordings (iEEG). The first source in (f) is strongly correlated with the iEEG, which can be seen also from the time-course. The source localization of the first source by sLORETA confirmed that the source is generated by the secondary auditory cortex (data not shown here; see Van der Loo et al., 2007).

CLINICAL EXAMPLES

In this section we demonstrate how and why BSS may prove to be useful in neurofeedback by giving real data examples.

This first example demonstrates how BSS may be used to isolate and extract frontal theta activity. Figure 2.7 (top) shows a 4-second epoch

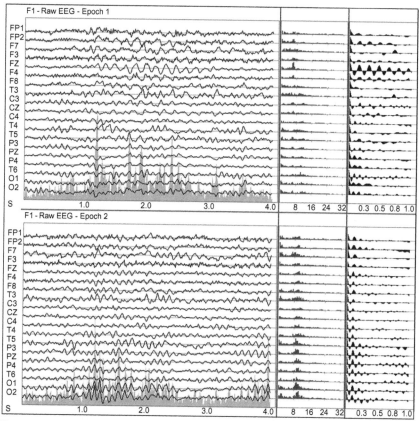

Figure 2.7 Top: A 4 s epoch (epoch 1) extracted from the raw eyes-open EEG recording of a 16-year-old female patient with a diagnosis of attention deficit hyperactivity disorder (inattentive type). From left to right: electrode labels according to the 10−20 international system, raw EEG tracing (upward deflection is negative potential; the space between two horizontal centering lines is 75 μV), average power spectrum (from zero to 32 Hz; arbitrary units) and autocorrelation function (the space between two horizontal centering lines is autocorrelation = 1 in the upward direction and −1 in the downward direction). The gray-shaded area in the background of EEG tracings is the global field power, the sum of the square of potentials across electrodes for each sample (arbitrary units). Bottom: As top but for another 4 s epoch (epoch 2).

(epoch 1) extracted from an eyes-open recording of a 16-year-old female patient with a diagnosis of attention deficit hyperactivity disorder (inattentive type). Notice the burst of theta sinusoidal activity (around 6−7 Hz), easily visible at electrode FZ from around second 1 to 3.2. Elsewhere in the epoch, the dipole layer is almost silent, with low-amplitude patternless tracing (noise). Figure 2.7 (bottom) shows another 4-second epoch extracted from the same recording a few seconds later (epoch 2). At this time the frontal activity of the patient is dominated by more persistent and weaker oscillations with dominant frequency around 9−10 Hz, which are visible to a somewhat lesser degree at electrode FZ. Frontal theta activity is virtually absent in epoch 2, which is instead characterized by strong occipital dominant rhythms at 10−11 Hz (occipital alpha) also spreading frontally (a possible indication of abnormal brain functioning). It appears obvious that the two brain states portrayed by these EEG tracings are quite different. Visual inspection of the entire recording from this patient (not shown) reveals that the theta burst of epoch 1 is infrequent, whereas generalized alpha, such as in epoch 2, is more frequent. Attention deficit disorder may manifest itself with several characteristic patterns of abnormal brain electrical activity, typically involving the frontal lobe in medial regions. Slowing in the theta and/or alpha range, depending on age, has been repeatedly reported as a marker of this disorder (Lubar, 1997). We now show how BSS can help with characterizing the dipole layer responsible for the theta burst visible in epoch 1.

Figure 2.8 shows the 17 source components estimated by the BSS algorithm using the second approach aforementioned, here named AJDC (approximate joint diagonalization of cospectra) and described in detail in Congedo, Gouy-Pailler and Jutten (2008). Notice that we are using these two epochs only to estimate the demixing matrix. In Figure 2.8 the components are sorted in descending order of explained variance for epoch 1 in the frequency range 1−20 Hz. The first component describes accurately the theta burst of epoch 1, as can be seen by comparing its time course, power spectrum, and autocorrelation function to the raw tracing at electrode FZ, its power spectrum and autocorrelation function (Figure 2.7, top). Notice that in this instance the component does not seem to have much better SNR (signal-to-noise ratio) as compared to the raw tracing at FZ. This is due to the fact that the raw tracing has already a very high SNR; in fact this was the reason to choose this epoch for estimating the source component of interest.

Next, we illustrate on an unknown epoch the gain in SNR and interference suppression that we can reach via BSS. Figure 2.9 (top) shows

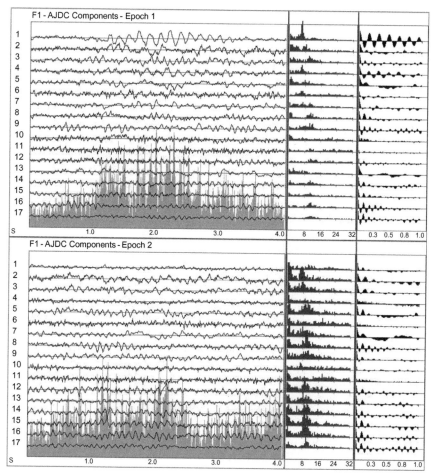

Figure 2.8 Top: Source components for epoch 1 in Figure 2.7 top (epoch 1). From left to right: component serial number labels, component tracing (black curves; arbitrary units), average power spectrum (from zero to 32 Hz; arbitrary units) and autocorrelation function (the space between two horizontal centering lines is auto-correlation = 1 in the upward direction and −1 in the downward direction). The gray shaded area in the background of source component tracings is the global field power, the sum of the square of source amplitude across components for each sample (arbitrary units). Bottom: Same as top, but for epoch 2 shown at bottom in Figure 2.7.

another 4 s epoch from the same recording (epoch 3). Figure 2.9 (bottom) shows the estimated components using the same demixing matrix used to estimate source components in Figure 2.8. In the raw EEG the tracing at FZ for this epoch is a mixture of theta and alpha activity, plus a slow

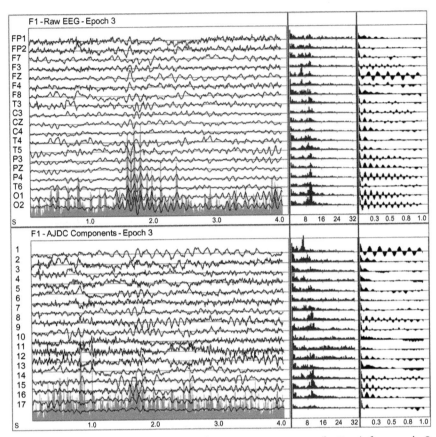

Figure 2.9 Raw EEG tracing (top) and source components (bottom) for epoch 3 extracted from the recording of the patient. See captions for Figures 2.7 and 2.8.

(<4 Hz) component, as can be seen with help of the power-spectrum. Compare this time course with the first component extracted by BSS. This is our component extraction pointing to the dipole layer responsible for the theta burst in Figure 2.7 (top), which the waveform clearly resembles. Evidently, for this epoch the extracted component as compared to the FZ tracing displays a much higher SNR, and the alpha oscillation has been almost completely suppressed.

This example illustrates an important point: each row vector of the demixing matrix can be conceived as a *spatial filter* extracting dipole layers from *specific brain regions*. BSS components may result in higher SNR and in the suppression of interference generated in other regions, which affects the scalp measurement because of volume conduction. The effect of volume conduction is appreciated comparing the diversity of source components as compared to raw EEG tracings. Notice also the diversity of power spectra in the bottom of Figure 2.9 as compared to the top, that is, of the sources as compared to the raw tracings. The application of this concept is straightforward. For instance, suppose the experimenter or the clinician wishes to monitor off-line or on-line the occurrence of frontal midline theta bursts. Then, instead of using EEG data band-pass filtered in the frequency region of interest at electrode FZ, he/she may use the extracted source $s(t)$. At the expense of using more electrodes, he/she would gain in SNR and/or interference suppression. In this sense, BSS may be used instead of inverse solutions for monitoring real-time brain electrical fields (Congedo, Lubar, & Joffe, 2004; Congedo, 2006). Notice that, in contrast to frequency band-pass filters, BSS spatial filters can suppress interference also if it has the same spectral content as the component of interest. In contrast to spatial filters based on EEG inverse solution, the weighting vector estimated by BSS does not depend on a head model or on electrode placement. Moreover, it estimates the orientation of the dipolar field, with considerable gain in its separation power.

Interestingly, we have performed BSS analysis estimating co-spectral matrices on as little as 3.5 s of EEG featuring the activity of interest (epoch 1). This is a demonstration of the efficiency of some BSS algorithms, particularly; those based on second order statistics (Congedo et al., 2008).

DISCUSSION

In this chapter we have made a journey through physics, electrophysiology and statistics to explain on an intuitive level the concept of blind source separation (BSS). We have argued that BSS can become very useful for neurofeedback, improving upon existing methods for extracting brain activity of interest in real-time. BSS-neurofeedback and inverse solution-neurofeedback are attracting increased interest in the neurofeedback community. Presently, however, very few neurofeedback software designs allow these advanced techniques. In order to promote real-time EEG applications such as those discussed here, a consortium of French Institutions has developed the Open-ViBE platform (Open Virtual Brain Environment; Renard et al., 2010). Several neurofeedback scenarios are already available for Open-ViBE. Open-ViBE is completely free and open-source and can be downloaded at http://openvibe.inria.fr/.

REFERENCES

Afsari, B. (2008). Sensitivity analysis for the problem of matrix joint diagonalization, SIAM. *Journal on Matrix Analysis and Applications, 30*(3), 1148–1171.

Congedo, M. (2006). Subspace projection filters for real-time electromagnetic brain imaging. *IEEE Transactions on Biomedical Engineering, 53*(8), 1624–1634.

Congedo, M., Gouy-Pailler, C., & Jutten, C. (2008). On the blind source separation of human electroencephalogram by approximate joint diagonalization of second order statistics. *Clinical Neurophysiology, 119*, 2677–2686.

Congedo, M., & Joffe, D. (2007). Multi-channel spatial filters for neurofeedback. In J. Evans (Ed.), *Neurofeedback: Dynamics and clinical applications*. New York: Haworth Press.

Congedo, M., Lotte, F., & Lécuyer, A. (2006). Classification of movement intention by spatially filtered electromagnetic inverse solutions. *Physics in Medicine and Biology, 51*, 1971–1989.

Congedo, M., Lubar, J. F., & Joffe, D. (2004). Low-resolution electromagnetic tomography neurofeedback. *IEEE Transactions on Neuronal Systems & Rehabilitation Engineering, 12*(4), 387–397.

Congedo, M., & Pham, D.-T. (2009). Least-squares joint diagonalization of a matrix set by a congruence transformation, SinFra'09 (Singaporean-French IPAL Symposium), Singapore, February 18–20.

Gouy-Pailler, C., Congedo, M, Brunner, C., Jutten, C., & Pfurtscheller, G. (2010). Nonstationary brain source separation for multiclass motor imagery. *IEEE Transactions on Biomedical Engineering, 57*(2), 469–478.

Hérault, J. & Jutten, C. (1986). Space or time adaptive signal processing by neural network models. In: *Proceedings of the International Conference on Neural Networks for Computing*, Snowbird (Utah), 151, 206–211.

Jutten, C., & Hérault, J. (1991). Blind separation of sources, Part 1: an adaptive algorithm based on neuromimetic architecture. *Signal Process, 24*(1), 1–10.

Lopes da Silva, F., & Van Rotterdam, A. (2005). Biophysical aspects of EEG and magneto-encephalogram generation. In E. Niedermeyer, & F. Lopes da Silva (Eds.), *Electroencephalography. Basic principles, clinical applications, and related fields* (5th ed., pp. 107–125). New York: Lippincott Williams & Wilkins.

Lubar, J. F. (1997). Neocortical dynamics: Implications for understanding the role of neurofeedback and related techniques for the enhancement of attention. *Applied Psychophysiology and Biofeedback, 22*(2), 111–126.

Lubar, J. F., Congedo, M., & Askew, J. H. (2003). Low-resolution electromagnetic tomography (LORETA) of cerebral activity in chronic depressive disorder. *International Journal of Psychophysiology, 49*, 175–185.

Nunez, P. L., & Srinivasan, R. (2006). *Electric field of the brain* (2nd ed.). New York: Oxford University Press.

Pascual-Marqui, R. D., Michel, C. M., & Lehmann, D. (1994). Low resolution electromagnetic tomography: A new method for localizing electrical activity in the brain. *International Journal of Psychophysiology, 18*(1), 49–65.

Pham, D.-T., & Congedo, M. (2009). Least square joint diagonalization of matrices under an intrinsic scale constraint, ICA 2009 (8th International Conference on Independent Component Analysis and Signal Separation), March 15–18, Paraty, Brasil, 298-305.

Renard, Y., Lotte, F., Gibert, G., Congedo, M., Maby, E., Delannoy, V., et al. (2010). OpenViBE: An open-source software platform to design, test and use brain–computer interfaces in real and virtual environments. *PRESENCE: Teleoperators and Virtual Environments, 19*(1), 35–53.

Sarvas, J. (1987). Basic mathematical and electromagnetic concepts of the biomagnetic inverse problem. *Physics in Medicine and Biology, 32*(1), 11–22.

Sherlin, L., Budzynski, T., Kogan-Budzynski, H., Congedo, M., Fischer, M. E., & Buchwald, D. (2007). Low-resolution electromagnetic brain tomography (LORETA) of monozygotic twins discordant for chronic fatigue syndrome. *Neuroimage, 34*(4), 1438–1442.

Sherlin, L., & Congedo, M. (2005). Obsessive compulsive dimension localized using low resolution electromagnetic tomography (LORETA). *Neuroscience Letters, 387*(2), 72–74.

Speckmann, E.-J., & Elger, C. E. (2005). Introduction to the neurophysiological basis of the EEG and DC potentials. In E. Niedermeyer, & F. Lopes da Silva (Eds.), *Electroencephalography. Basic principles, clinical applications, and related fields* (5th ed., pp. 17–29). New York: Lippincott Williams & Wilkins.

Tichavsky, P., & Yeredor, A. (2009). Fast approximate joint diagonalization incorporating weight matrices. *IEEE Transactions on Signal Process, 57*(3), 878–891.

Van der Loo, E., Congedo, M., Plazier, M., Van De Heyning, P., & De Ridder, D. (2007). Correlation between independent components of scalp EEG and intracranial EEG (iEEG) time series. *International Journal of Bioelectromagnetism, 9*(4), 270–275.

Van der Loo, E., Gais, S., Congedo, M., Vanneste, S., & Plazier, M. (2009). Tinnitus intensity dependent gamma oscillations of the contralateral auditory cortex. *PLoS ONE, 4*(10), e7396 doi:10.1371/journal.pone.0007396.

CHAPTER 3

ERP-Based Endophenotypes: Application in Diagnosis and Neurotherapy

Juri D. Kropotov[1,2], Andreas Mueller[3], and Valery A. Ponomarev[1]

[1]Institute of the Human Brain of the Russian Academy of Sciences, St Petersburg, Russia
[2]Institute of Psychology, Norwegian University of Science and Technology, Trondheim, Norway
[3]Brain and Trauma Foundation, Grison, and Praxis für Kind, Organisation und Entwicklung, Chur, Switzerland

Contents

INTRODUCTION

In a narrow sense brain neuromodulation includes methods of transcranial Direct Current Stimulation (tDCS) and neurofeedback. These two methods are based on knowledge regarding underlying neurophysiological processes. It is obvious that before doing any neuromodulatory approach on a client we need to know how his/her cortex is self-regulated and how

Neurofeedback and Neuromodulation Techniques and Applications
DOI: 10.1016/B978-0-12-382235-2.00003-2

information is processed in the cortex. A recently emerged branch of neuroscience, called *neurometrics*, helps in answering these two questions.

According to E. Roy John, the founder of this field, neurometrics is

a method of quantitative EEG that provides a precise, reproducible estimate of the deviation of an individual record from norm. This computer analysis makes it possible to detect and quantify abnormal brain organization, to give a quantitative definition of the severity of brain disease, and to identify subgroups of pathophysiological abnormalities within groups of patients with similar clinical symptoms.

(John, 1990)

Several normative EEG-based databases exist (NxLink, introduced in John, 1977; Neuroguide, described in Thatcher et al., 1999; Brain Resource Company presented in Gordon, Cooper, Rennie, Hermens, & Williams, 2005). These databases were very helpful in defining neuronal correlates of some brain dysfunctions such as ADHD (Arns, de Ridder, Strehl, Breteler, & Coenen, 2009), traumatic brain injury (Thatcher et al., 1999), and dementia (Prichep et al., 1994).

One of the parameters measured in these databases is EEG power in a certain frequency band. Spectral characteristics of spontaneous EEG used in all normative databases include absolute and relative EEG power in different frequency bands, at different electrode sites, as well as measures of coherence between EEG recorded from pairs of electrodes. Spontaneous EEG in a healthy brain represents a mixture of different rhythmicities which are conventionally separated into alpha, theta, and beta rhythms. Recent research shows that each of these rhythmicities is generated by a specific neuronal network: posterior and central alpha rhythms are generated by thalamo-cortical networks, beta rhythms appear to be generated by local cortical networks, while the frontal midline theta rhythm (the only healthy theta rhythm in the human brain) is hypothetically generated by the septo-hippocampal neuronal network (for a recent review see Kropotov, 2009). In general terms, spontaneous oscillations reflect mechanisms of cortical self-regulation implemented by distinct neuronal mechanisms.

EVENT-RELATED POTENTIALS (ERPs)

Another important aspect of brain functioning is the response of the brain to stimuli, and actions evoked by those stimuli. This electrical brain response is measured by event-related potentials (ERPs). Technically, ERPs are obtained by simple averaging of all EEG epochs in many sequentially presented trials in a single subject and for a single electrode. Consequently, ERPs can be considered as voltage deflections, generated by cortical neurons that are time-locked to specific events and associated with stages of information flow in specific cortical areas.

It should be stressed here that ERPs, even in a simple behavioral paradigm, are generated by multiple neuronal sources. The sources are associated with ERP components which, in practice, are defined by their positive or negative polarity, latency, scalp distribution, and relationship to experimental variables (Duncan et al., 2009). Research during the past 50 years has separated several ERP components such as mismatch negativity, N400, error-related negativities, different types of P300, etc.

The guidelines for the use of ERPs in clinical research are presented in a recent paper by a group of distinguished researchers in the field (Duncan et al., 2009). The methodological issues emphasized in the paper are as follows: (1) minimizing eye movements in order to get a signal-to-noise ratio as high as possible; (2) measuring components defined as "the contribution of the recorded waveform of a particular generator process, such as the activation of a localized area of cerebral cortex by a specific pattern of input." Components can be disentangled by means of experimental manipulation if they are differentially sensitive in amplitude and latency to different manipulations (Donchin et al., 1986).

THEORETICAL CONSIDERATIONS

As we know from research in neuroscience, behavior is determined by multiple brain systems playing different roles in planning, execution, and memorization of human sensorimotor actions. These brain systems in turn are determined by genes and their complex interactions with each other and the environment. So, in contrast to genotype, behavior can be considered as a phenotype of a subject. In the past, psychiatry mainly relied on behavior. Recently, however, a concept of endophenotype was introduced in psychiatry (Gottesman & Gould, 2003). Endophenotypes are heritable, quantifiable traits (such as EEG power in specific frequency bands, or components of event-related potentials) that index an individual's liability to develop or manifest a given disease or behavioral trait. Endophenotypes represent simpler clues to genetic mechanisms than the behavioral symptoms. The whole idea of introducing this concept is based on the assumption that a more accurate psychiatric diagnosis can be made using knowledge about brain systems (such as the executive system) and brain operations (such as action selection and action monitoring). The term comes from the Greek word *endos,* meaning "interior, within". In another words, endophenotype denotes a measurable component along the pathway between phenotype and genotype). An example of a physiological endophenotype could be given by a late positive fluctuation (the P3b waveform) of ERPs elicited in the oddball paradigm in response to target stimuli. This waveform appears to reflect the context updating (Donchin, 1981) and can be considered as an index of working memory.

In this chapter we present a theory according to which the brain is divided into several functional systems, playing different roles in organization of behavior: sensory system, affective system, executive system, memory systems, and attentional networks (Kropotov, 2009). Each of these brain functional systems can be considered as a set of overlapping neuronal networks, each performing a specific computation associated with a distinct psychological operation.

Neuronal elements in a neuronal network receive multiple inputs and transfer them into action potentials. The transfer operation performed by a neuron (output versus input) represents a non-linear relationship described by a sigmoid function. Similarly, the transfer function of a neuronal net as a whole also can be described by the sigmoid function presented in Figure 3.1(a). The shape of this function means that: (1) the neuronal network is poorly activated by a low input because the inputs in the majority of neurons do not exceed thresholds; (2) the neuronal network changes activity almost linearly to a moderate input; (3) the activation of the neuronal network reaches a plateau at higher levels of input — a so-called "ceiling" effect.

We can further suggest that the performance of the system is defined by the ability of the system to react to a small change in the input. Mathematically, the performance of the system is defined by the first derivative dO/dI (Figure 3.1b). The first derivative is represented by a so-called inverted-U shape. In psychophysiology it is known as the Yerkes—Dodson Law (Curtin, 1984).

So, the neural network is characterized by two parameters: level of activation (that is, the input signal which drives the system), and the responsiveness of the system (reaction of the system to a small change in the input). In neurophysiological studies these two parameters are usually named *tonic* and *phasic* activities respectively. We speculate that, for the brain, tonic and phasic activities have two different functional meanings, the first associated with the state and the second with the response. For

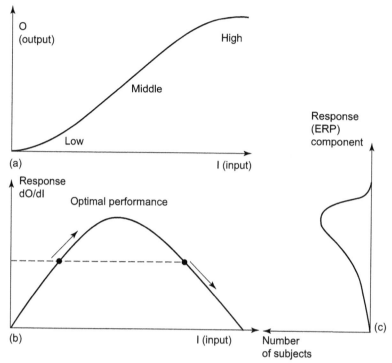

Figure 3.1 Reactivity of neuronal network. (a) Schematic representation of the dependence of the overall activity of a hypothetical neuronal network on the input driving the system. (b) Schematic representation of the dependence of the response of the system on its input. The response is defined as a reaction of the system to a small and elementary increase of the input. (c) Distribution of subjects over reactivity of the system. The distribution is closer to the Gausisan, in which smaller amplitudes correspond to poor performance.

example, for the attentional network the tonic activity can be associated with non-specific arousal, while the phasic activity can be associated with selective attention. We presume that the reactivity of a certain functional network is reflected in a distinct ERP component. So, when we measure an ERP component in a population of subjects the distribution of the subjects over the component would be expected to look like that depicted in Figure 3.1(c). Indeed, the majority of the population of healthy subjects would have the component with amplitude around an average level and only few would have the component deviant from normality thus forming a normal or log-normal distribution.

In reality, response of a neuronal network consists of reactions of excitatory and inhibitory neurons that produce potentials of different polarities.

Moreover, the neuronal reaction evolves in time in a hierarchically orga-
nized network. The process of shaping the component is determined by a
complex interaction between feed-forward and feed-back pathways inter-
connecting lower and higher level layers of the network.

NEW METHODS IN ERP ANALYSIS

Recently, the practical application of ERPs was accelerated by introducing
new mathematical techniques for ERP analysis. One of these techniques
is independent component analysis (ICA). ICA is a decomposition technique which is regarded as a solution of the "blind source separation
(BSS)" problem (James & Hesse, 2005). ICA decomposes data such that
the resulting component activities have minimal mutual information. The
mutual information is considered as a measure of statistical independence
of the components (Congedo et al., 2008).

It should be stressed here that the concept of statistical independence
goes far beyond statistical orthogonality. Independence implies that two or
more variables are not only orthogonal (uncorrelated), but also that all
higher order moments are zero. In this respect the ICA differs from principal component analysis (PCA), which assumes only statistical orthogonality (Bugli & Lambert, 2007). From a more practical point of view,
another advantage of ICA is that this approach can be applied to low density EEG data (Makeig et al., 2002). In research involving ERPs, ICA has
been applied for separating the observed signals into both physiologically
and behaviorally distinct components.

There are at least three different methods of applying ICA to ERP
analysis which deal with different input and output datasets, and which
allow different questions to be addressed: (1) the input data for the first
method represent single-trial ERP epochs from a single subject: the ICA
components are defined either separately for each subject, with subsequent
cluster analysis (Makeig et al., 2004; Zeman, Till, Livingston, Tanaka, &
Driessen, 2007), or for all trials in all subjects (Debener, Makeig, Delorme, &
Engel, 2005; Mehta, Jerger, Jerger, & Martin, 2009); (2) the input data
for the second method are averaged ERPs recorded in response to
many stimulus types and many task conditions (Makeig et al., 1999);
and (3) the input data for the third method are from averaged ERPs
recoded in a few task conditions, but for many subjects (Liu et al.,
2009; Olbrich, Maes, Valerius, Langosch, & Feige, 2005).

HBI REFERENCE DATABASE

In this chapter we introduce a methodology that was recently implemented in the HBI (Human Brain Index) reference database. The database includes 19-channel EEG recordings of more than 1000 healthy subjects in resting conditions with eyes open and eyes closed as well as in six task conditions. Subjects were recruited from students of St Petersburg State University (recordings were made by I. S. Nikishena), the staff of the Institute of the Human Brain of Russian Academy of Sciences (recordings were made by E. A. Yakovenko), students of the Norwegian University of Science and Technology, Trondheim (recordings were made by S. Hollup), and healthy subjects from Chur, Switzerland, recruited by Dr Andreas Mueller (recordings were made by E. P. Tereshchenko, I. Terent'ev, and G. Candrian). The investigation was carried out in accordance with the Declaration of Helsinki, and all subjects provided informed consent. The tasks were specifically developed for recording components associated with visual and auditory processing, facial emotion recognition, working memory, engagement (GO) and disengagement (NO-GO) operations, mathematical- and speech-related operations, and novelty reactions.

Exclusion criteria were: (1) an eventful perinatal period; (2) presence of head injury with cerebral symptoms; (3) history of neurological or psychiatric diseases; (4) history of convulsion; and (5) current medication or drugs. Inclusion also required normal mental and physical development, as well as average or better grades in school.

GO/NO-GO TASK

Here we provide details of the two-stimulus GO/NO-GO task that was developed to study sensory and executive functions in the human brain. Three categories of visual stimuli were selected: (1) 20 different images of animals, referred to later as "A"; (2) 20 different images of plants, referred to as "P"; (3) 20 different images of people of different professions, presented together with an artificial "novel" sound, referred to as "H + Sound". All visual stimuli were selected to have similar size and luminosity. The randomly varying novel sounds consisted of five 20 ms fragments filled with tones of different frequencies (500, 1000, 1500, 2000, and 2500 Hz). Each time a new combination of tones was used and the novel sounds appeared unexpectedly (probability of appearance: 12.5%). Stimulus intensity was about 75 dB SPL, measured at the patient's head.

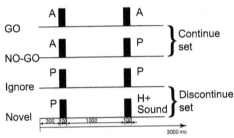

Figure 3.2 Schematic representation of the two-stimulus GO/NO-GO task. From top to bottom: time dynamics of stimuli in four categories of trials. Abbreviations: A, P, H stimuli are "Animals", "Plants", and "Humans". GO trials are when A—A stimuli require the subject to press a button. NO-GO trials are A—P stimuli, which require suppression of a prepared action. GO and NO-GO trials represent "Continue set" in which subjects have to prepare for action after the first stimulus presentation (A). Ignore trials are stimuli pairs beginning with a P, which require no preparation for action. Novel trials are pairs requiring no action, with presentation of a novel sound as the second stimuli. Ignore and Novel trials represent "Discontinue set", in which subjects do not need to prepare for action after the first stimulus presentation. Time intervals are depicted at the bottom.

The trials consisted of presentations of paired stimuli with inter-stimulus intervals of 1 s. Duration of stimuli was 100 ms. Four categories of trials were used (see Figure 3.2): A—A, A—P, P—P, and P—(H + Sound).

The trials were grouped into four blocks with 100 trials each. In each block a unique set of five A, five P, and five H stimuli were selected. Each block consisted of a pseudo-random presentation of 100 pairs of stimuli with equal probability for each stimulus category and for each trial category. Participants practiced the task before the recording started. Subjects rested for a few minutes after each 200 trials. Subjects sat upright in a comfortable chair looking at a computer screen. The task was to press a button with the right hand to all A—A pairs as fast as possible, and to withhold button pressing to other pairs A—P, P—P, P—(H + Sound) (Figure 3.2).

According to the task design, two preparatory sets were distinguished in the trials (Figure 3.2). They are: "Continue set", in which A is presented as the first stimulus and the subject is supposed to prepare to respond; and the "Discontinue set", in which P is presented as the first stimulus and the subject does not need to prepare to respond. In a "Continue set" A—A pairs will be referred to as "GO trials", A—P pairs as "NO-GO trials". In a "Discontinue set" P—P pairs will be referred to as "Ignore trials" and P—(H + Sound) pairs as "Novel trials" (see Figure 3.2).

The subject responses were recorded in a separate channel on the amplifier. Averages for response latency and response time variance across trials were calculated for each subject individually. Omission errors (failure to respond in GO trials) and commission errors (failure to suppress a response to NO-GO trials) were also computed for each subject separately.

In gathering data EEG was recorded from 19 scalp sites, bandpass filtered between 0.53 and 50 Hz and digitized at a rate of 250 samples per second per channel. The electrodes were applied according to the International 10−20 system. The EEG was recorded referentially to linked ears, allowing computational re-referencing of the data (re-montaging). For decomposing ERPs into independent components, the EEG computationally was re-referenced to the common average montage. EOG was recorded from two electrodes placed above and below the right eye. All electrode impedances were below 5 Ohms.

To standardize data collection procedures across the four laboratories, the same protocol was used: (1) EEG was recorded with a 19-channel electroencephalographic PC-controlled system, the "Mitsar-201" (CE 0537) manufactured by Mitsar, Ltd (www.mitsar-medical.com); (2) electrodes were applied using caps manufactured by Electro-cap International, Inc. (www.electro-cap.com/caps.htm); (3) the tin recessed electrodes contacted the scalp using ECI ELECTRO-GEL; (4) stimuli were presented on similar 17 inch computer screens which were positioned 1.5 meters in front of the subjects and occupied the same range of the visual field (3.8°); (5) images of stimuli as well as the stimuli presentation protocols were standardized; (6) all trials were presented using "Psytask", a computer code written by one of the authors (VAP); (7) subjects were recruited according to the same inclusion/exclusion criteria (see paragraph "Subjects" above).

Eye Movement Correction

Eyeblink artifacts were corrected by zeroing the activation curves of individual ICA components corresponding to eye blinks using methods similar to those described in Jung et al. (2000) and Vigário (1997). Comparison of this method with an EOG regression technique is described by Tereshchenko, Ponomarev, Kropotov, and Müller (2009). In addition, epochs with excessive amplitude of filtered EEG and/or excessive faster and/or slower frequency activity were automatically marked and excluded from further analysis. The epoch exclusion thresholds were set as follow: (1) 100 μV for non-filtered EEG; (2) 50 μV for slow waves in the 0−1 Hz band; and (3) 35 μV for fast waves filtered in the band 20−35 Hz.

METHODOLOGY OF DECOMPOSITION OF COLLECTION OF ERPs INTO INDEPENDENT COMPONENTS

The goal of independent component analysis (ICA) is to utilize the differences in scalp distribution between different generators of ERP activity to separate the corresponding activation time courses (Makeig, Bell, Jung, & Sejnowski, 1996). Components are constructed by optimizing the mutual independence of all activation time curves, leading to a natural and intuitive definition of an ERP component as a stable potential distribution which cannot be further decomposed into independently activated sources.

In the present study ICA was performed on the full ERP scalp location × time-series matrix. ERPs were constructed in response to the second (S2) stimuli in a time interval −100 and +1000 ms after the second (S2) stimulus presentation. The ICA of the ERPs was made separately for Continue sets and Discontinue sets The number of training points was computed as follows: Number of subjects (297) × Number of categories of trials (2) (GO/NO-GO for Continue set, Novel/Ignore for Discontinue set) × Number of 4 ms time intervals (250 samples/s × 1.1) = 163,350. This number is much larger than that required to obtain good quality decomposition: $20 \times 19^2 = 7220$ (Onton & Makeig, 2006).

Assumptions that underlie the application of ICA to individual ERPs are as follow: (1) summation of the electric currents induced by separate generators is linear at the scalp electrodes; (2) spatial distribution of components' generators remains fixed across time; (3) generators of spatially separated components vary independently from each other across subjects (Makeig et al., 1996; Onton & Makeig, 2006).

Briefly, the method implemented is as follows: The input data are the collection of individual ERPs arranged in a matrix P of 19 channels (rows) by T time points (columns) in which T is a product of N (number of subjects) and number of time intervals in the epoch of analysis for the two task conditions. The ICA finds an "unmixing" matrix (U) that gives the matrix S of the sources (ICs) when multiplied by the original data matrix (P),

$$S = UP$$

where S and P are $19 \times T$ matrices and U is 19×19 matrix. $S(t)$ are maximally independent. In our work matrix U is found by means of the

Infomax algorithm, which is an iteration procedure that maximizes the mutual information between S.

According to the linear algebra,

$$P = U^{-1}S,$$

where U^{-1} is the inverse matrix of U (also called mixing matrix), and the ith column of the mixing matrix represents the topography of i-independent component; S_i represents time course of the i-independent component. The ICA method (Makeig et al., 1996) was implemented in the analysis software written by one of the authors (VAP). The topographies and activation time courses of the components were tested against the corresponding results obtained by means of "InforMax" software in EEGLAB, a freely available interactive Matlab toolbox for processing continuous and event-related electrophysiological data (http://sccn.ucsd.edu/eeglab).

The topographies of the independent components are presented as topographic maps, while time courses of the components (also called "activation time courses") are presented as graphics with time corresponding to the x-axis. In this paper the "power" of the components is characterized by a variance $VAR_i = \sum\sum(U_{ij}^{-1}S_{ik})^2/(N_{samp}N_{chan})$ where $N_{samp} = $ number of time points and $N_{chan} = $ number of channels. The topographies are divided by the square root of the variance of the corresponding components, while the normalized activation curves are multiplied by the square root of the variance.

METHODOLOGY OF DECOMPOSITION OF INDIVIDUAL ERPs INTO INDEPENDENT COMPONENTS

The essence of neurometrics is a comparison of individual EEG parameters with normative data. In our approach there is a need for decomposing an individual's ERPs into independent components by means of the spatial filters extracted for the collection of "normal" ERPs. It is done as follows: The ith independent source S_i can be found as

$$S_i = U_{zi}P,$$

where U_{zi} is matrix U in which all rows are zeroed except the ith row.

According to linear algebra,

$$P_i = U^{-1}S_i = U^{-1}U_{zi}P.$$

In our work, we used this filter for decomposing individual ERP difference waves into the independent components.

The sLORETA (standardized low resolution tomography) imaging approach was used for locating the generators of the ICA components extracted in this study (ICs). The free software is provided by the Key Institute for Brain—Mind Research in Zurich, Switzerland (www.uzh.ch/keyinst/loreta.htm). For theoretical issues of this method see Pascual-Marqui (2002).

Amplitudes of the components were computed for each condition and each subject separately. Student's t-test was used for assessing statistical significance of deviation of the ICs from the baseline, as well as for assessing statistical significance of the difference between conditions. To assess the strength of a component in one condition (for example, NO-GO) in comparison to another condition (for example, GO) the effect size was calculated as $d = M_1 - M_2/SD$ where $M1$ and $M2$ are mean values of the component in conditions 1 and 2, and SD is the pooled standard deviation (Cohen, 1988).

Using the above-mentioned technology, we are able to decompose individual ERPs into distinct components. Comparison with the database can be easily made by computing z-scores for each time interval and for each component separately.

INDEPENDENT COMPONENTS IN GO/NO-GO TASK

From 19 components separated by ICA those that corresponded to horizontal and vertical eye movements were excluded from further analysis. Among the remaining components only those with highest values of variance (altogether constituting more than 90% of the signal variance) were analyzed. To estimate the reliability of the ICA decomposition we used a split-half method. All subjects participating in the study were separated into two groups, either odd or even, according to the number at which they appeared in the database. This separation gives an equivalent age and gender distribution in both groups. ICA was applied to the array of ERPs computed to the second stimulus for the two subject groups, as well as for the Continue and Discontinue task conditions. Topographies and time courses of the resultant ICs were compared with each other. The measure of similarity of components is given by two correlation coefficients obtained separately for topographies and time courses.

Visual inspection of the extracted components shows that some ICs computed for Continue and Discontinue sets are quite similar. The components that do not differ between the two preparatory sets are presented in Figure 3.3.

In our two-stimulus paradigm design, the second paired stimuli have one thing in common: they all include brief presentations of visual stimuli. So, if our null hypothesis is correct, and the ICA enables us to decompose ERPs into functionally meaningful components, then there must be components that are common to Continue and Discontinue sets, and that reflect stages of visual information flow. We indeed were able to separate at least three set-invariant components which (according to their time course and localization) reflect sequential stages of visual information processing in the occipital—temporal—parietal networks.

One of the components was localized in the occipital lobe and consisted of a sequence of positive (with peak latency of 100 ms), negative (150 ms) and positive (240 ms) fluctuations resembling previous findings of the visual N1 wave (see, for example, Hillyard & Anllo-Vento, 1998; Näätänen, 1992; Paz-Caballero & García-Austt, 1992).

The other two visual components were localized over the temporal-parietal junction in the left and right hemispheres and consisted of a sequence of positive (with peak latency of 120 ms), negative (170 ms), and positive (240 ms) fluctuations. These two ICs appear to correspond to bilateral occipito-temporally distributed N170 waves described in numerous studies on ERP correlates of object processing (Itier & Taylor, 2004). The N170 wave is reliably larger for faces than to any object category tested (Itier & Taylor, 2004a,b). Although the exact neuronal generators of this wave are still debated, this wave may reflect structural visual encoding (Rossion et al., 2003).

Our recent study with stroke patients who experienced hemispatial neglect in the visual field contralateral to the area of damage (Kropotov, Brunner, in preparation) showed severe impairment of the P 240 fluctuation of the component. This fact enables us to suggest that the above-mentioned components generated in the left and right temporal-parietal junctions are associated with detecting salience of the visual stimulus.

The remaining independent components are set dependent and are analyzed separately for each preparatory set. In order to associate the components with some functional meaning GO and NO-GO conditions were contrasted for the Continue set, while Novel and Ignore conditions were contrasted for the Discontinue set.

The components that are specific for Continue set are presented in Figure 3.4. According to sLORETA they are localized to the middle

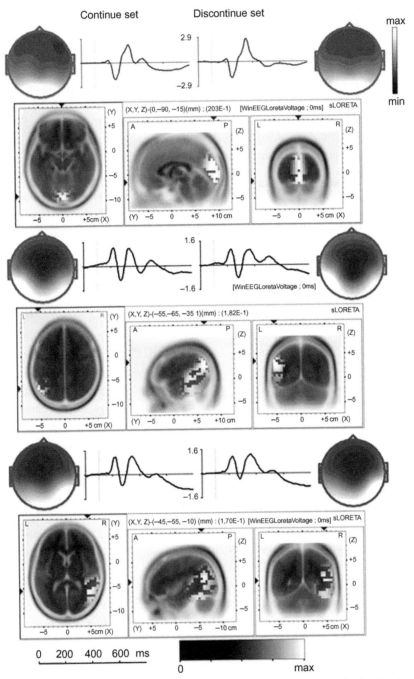

Figure 3.3 Occipitally and temporally generated components are similar for Continue and Discontinue sets. At the left is the topography and on the right the time course of the components. Below each pair of graphs is the sLORETA imaging of the component.

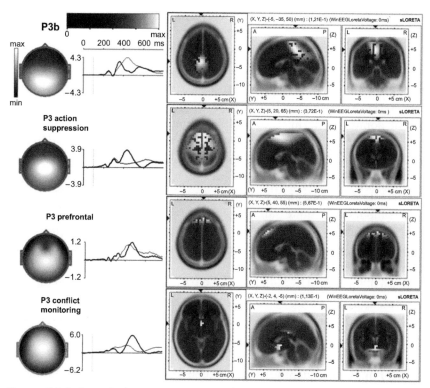

Figure 3.4 Independent components specifically generated in Continue set — Executive components. From left to right: topography, time course separately for GO (thin line) and NO-GO (thick line) conditions, and sLORETA imaging.

parietal cortex, supplementary motor cortex, frontal eye fields of the frontal lobe, and the anterior part of the cingulate cortex.

Our ICA data show that the P300 GO wave (elicited in response to GO cues) consists of at least two ICs with similar peak latencies (around 340—350 ms). The largest IC is a parietally distributed positive component, and the smallest is a frontally generated component. According to sLORETA the large component is generated in Brodmann areas 5 and 7 of the parietal cortex, while the smaller component is generated over the BA 8.

The parietal P300 component has similar time course for GO and NO-GO conditions up to 280 ms and deviates substantially at 340 ms with effect size of 1.5. The frontal P300 component was observed with almost the same amplitude but with slightly different latencies for GO and NO-GO conditions. It appeared that the parietal (BA 5 and 7) and frontal

(BA 8) areas were activated by both GO and NO-GO cues during at least the first 280 ms.

These ERP data fit well with recent fMRI (functional magnetic resonance imaging) studies showing that visual images of task-relevant stimuli are topographically represented both in parietal and frontal cortical areas (for a recent review see Silver & Kastner, 2009). The parietal P300 component dominates during a 300–400 ms time window in GO condition in comparison to NO-GO condition. The peak latency (around 340 ms) and topography (parietal distribution) of this component fit the corresponding parameters of a conventional P3b wave which is elicited in oddball paradigms in response to rare targets (for review see Polich, 2007). This component is quite similar to the parietal component extracted by ICA on an array of individual ERPs computed for healthy subjects and schizophrenic patients performing a one stimulus GO/NO-GO task (Olbrich et al., 2005).

Several functional meanings of the P3b components were suggested (for recent reviews see Polich, 2007). The most influential of them relates the component to the updating of working memory (Donchin, 1981). However, this was loosely defined at the psychological level, and was not associated with a neurophysiological circuit or cellular mechanism. Consequently it was criticized (Verleger, 1988). In intracranial recordings (Clarke, Halgren, & Chauvel, 1999; Kropotov & Ponomarev, 1991) the P3b-like waves were found in various cortical and subcortical structures, indicating a widespread distribution of the P3b component.

Analysis of independent components in our work shows that the late positive wave to NO-GO cues includes two ICs. The first component has a central distribution with peak latency of 340 ms, which is 60 ms shorter than the mean latency of response, and it is completely absent in response to GO cues. According to sLORETA imaging, this component is generated over the premotor cortex (Brodmann area 6). This component appears to correspond to subdurally recorded potentials found over pre-supplementary motor cortex in GO/NO-GO tasks in epileptic patients in response to NO-GO cues (Ikeda et al., 1999). The involvement of this part of the cortex in motor inhibition was demonstrated by the fact that direct stimulation of the pre-supplementary motor cortex in epileptic patients inhibited ongoing, habitual motor actions (Ikeda, Lüders, Burgess, & Shibasaki, 1993). A recent meta-analysis of fMRI studies in GO/NO-GO tasks demonstrates that the Brodmann area 6 is one of the most commonly activated areas of the cortex (Simmonds, Pekar, & Mostofsky, 2008), thus supporting the involvement of this area in response selection and response inhibition. We associate the centrally distributed P340 NO-GO-related IC separated in our study with inhibition of a prepared motor action in response to NO-GO cues.

The second NO-GO-related IC identified in the study has a more frontal distribution in comparison to the P340 motor suppression component. This second component peaks at 400 ms, corresponding to the mean latency of response to GO cues. It should be stressed here that, when contrasted to GO cues, this component exhibits a strong negative peak at 270 ms. This negative part of the IC may be associated with the NO-GO N270 component commonly found as a difference between ERPs to NO-GO and GO cues and coined as the N2 NO-GO (Bekker, Kenemans, & Verbaten, 2005; Pfefferbaum, Ford, Weller, & Kopell, 1985). This N2 NO-GO peaks before a virtual response, it has been associated with response inhibition (Jodo & Kayama, 1992) and conflict monitoring (Nieuwenhuis, Yeung, van den Wildenberg, & Ridderinkhof, 2003). The wave has been inconsistently localized in various cortical areas including the anterior cingulate cortex (Bekker et al., 2005), the inferior prefrontal and left premotor areas (Kiefer, Marzinzik, Weisbrod, Scherg, & Spitzer, 1998), the medial posterior cortex (Nieuwenhuis et al., 2003), and the right lateral orbitofrontal areas (Bokura, Yamaguchi, & Kobayashi, 2001). Our sLORETA imaging supports source localization of the component in the anterior cingulate cortex.

Taking in account involvement of the anterior cingulate cortex in a hypothetical conflict monitoring operation (Botvinick, 2007; Schall, Stuphorn, & Brown, 2002; van Veen & Carter, 2002), we associate the P400 frontal-central IC selected in our work with conflict monitoring. Indeed, in the two-stimulus paradigm used here the subject develops a behavioral model: to press a button in response to two "animals" (A–A). When the second stimulus is a "plant" appearing after first "animal" (NO-GO condition), this stimulus does not fit the behavioral model (a conflict), and this conflict seems to activate neurons in the anterior cingulate cortex that monitor this conflict situation.

The components that are specific for the Discontinue set are presented in Figure 3.5. They include a component generated in the primary auditory cortex. It has a negative part with a latency of 120 ms which corresponds to the conventional auditory N1 component which has been found in numerous studies previously (for review see Näätänen, 1992).

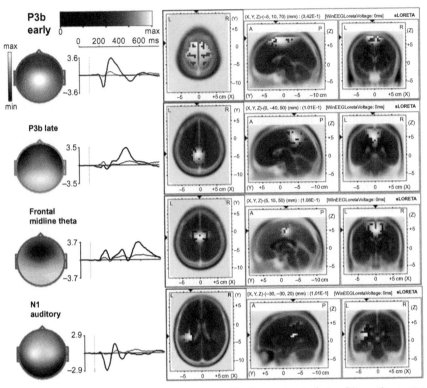

Figure 3.5 Independent components specifically generated in Discontinue set novelty-related components. From left to right: topography, time course separately for Ignore (thin line) and Novel (thick line) conditions, and sLORETA imaging.

The second novelty component has a central distribution with a positive fluctuation peaking at 220 ms, corresponding to the novelty component found in previous studies by using conventional current density mapping (Escera et al., 1998), by principal component analysis (Dien, Spencer, & Donchin, 2003), and by IC analysis performed on single-trial EEG epochs (Debener et al., 2005).

Two models were suggested to explain the functional meaning of the novelty P3a: an attention-switching model (Escera, Yago, & Alho, 2001) and a response inhibition model (Goldstein et al., 2002). In the attention-switching model the novelty P3 reflects involuntary switching of attention to deviant events that distract the subject from a primary task. In the response inhibition model, it is assumed that the detection of a deviant event leads to context updating and, after proper identification of the stimulus, to suppression of response that was activated by the deviance detection. In our work using sLORETA imaging, this component is generated in the premotor cortical area, which supports the response inhibition model. Indeed the topography of this component is similar to the topography of the P3 suppression component separated from the collection of NO-GO and GO ERPs (see discussion of executive components above).

The third component has a parietal distribution with a positive wave peaking at 360 ms. It fits quite well with the topography and time course of the parietally distributed component (P3b) observed in our present work in response to GO and NO-GO cues. The late parietal part of the electrical brain response to novel stimuli was reported in previous studies (Escera et al., 1998, 2001).

Our work confirmed the previous attempts at separating novelty-related components and enabled us to dissociate a new component. This component was found to be generated in the mid-cingulate cortex and consists of a burst of theta waves with a frequency of 6.25 Hz. The frequency and location of this theta burst corresponds to the parameters of the "frontal midline theta" rhythm (Inanaga, 1998). The functional meaning of the frontal midline theta rhythm in humans is not clear, however some evidence associates it with an orienting response (Dietl, Dirlich, Vogl, Lechner, & Strian, 1999) and with allocation of cognitive resources by an attentional system (Sauseng, Hoppe, Klimesch, Gerloff, & Hummel, 2007). It should be noted here that application of principal component analysis enabled some authors (Dien et al., 2003) to localize the novelty P3 in the anterior cingulate cortex.

APPLICATION OF ERP/ICA METHODOLOGY FOR ADHD – RESPONSE INHIBITION

We use the above-mentioned methodology for analysis of ERP data in an ADHD population when compared to norms. According to Russel Barkley, the core of the disorder is impairment of response inhibition (Barkley, 1997). If this hypothesis is correct, then we should see a decrease of the independent component associated with action suppression in an ADHD population. Here we present the results of our study with a group of ADHD children of ages 8 to 12. We compared independent components presented above between this group and a group of healthy subjects of the same age taken from the HBI database. We found that two out of 11 independent components were significantly reduced in the ADHD population, with relative large effect size (Figure 3.6). The first of these

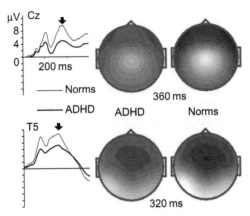

Figure 3.6 Reduction of central and left temporal independent components in ADHD. Number of ADHD patients is 94, number of control subjects, 69. Top: time courses and topographies of independent components obtained on 19 channel ERPs by spatial filtration. Thick line: ADHD; thin line: healthy subjects.

two components (Figure 3.6, top) appears to be associated with action suppression (see discussion above regarding the executive components) whereas the second component is associated with detecting salience of the stimulus (see discussion of the sensory components).

Note that ERP components were obtained by spatial filtration described above (see methodology of decomposition of individual ERPs into independent components). That means that any individual ERPs can be decomposed into independent components and any individual component can be statistically compared to normative data. The results of such comparison are presented in the scattergram in Figure 3.7.

The scattergram maps each individual's ERP independent components (circles − normal, triangles − ADHD) into the two-dimensional space with indexes of action inhibition and salience of the stimulus depicted at the x- and y-axis correspondingly. Two groups of the ADHD population can be separated: those with decrease of the action suppression component (might be associated with impulsive/hyperkinetic type of ADHD) and those with decrease of the salience detection component (might be associated with inattention type of ADHD).

ERPs AS INDEXES OF NEUROFEEDBACK EFFICACY

In a critique raised by Loo and Barkley it is stated that neurofeedback studies do not report pre- and post-qEEG differences since the EEG is

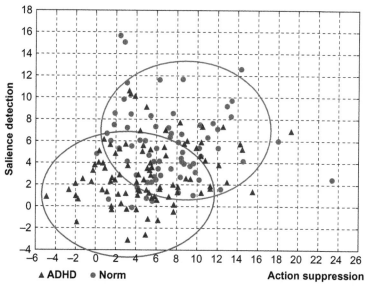

Figure 3.7 Scattergram of action suppression vs. working memory components in ADHD (triangles) and healthy subjects (circles). X-axis: amplitude of the action suppression component averaged over 100–700 ms time interval. Y-axis: amplitude of the working memory component averaged over 50–500 ms time interval.

the basis of treatment in neurofeedback (Loo & Barkley, 2005). One explanation of a few reports in the literature regarding post-pre spectra differences resides in a large variance of EEG spectra in theta, alpha, and beta frequency bands. There are several endophenotypes of EEG spectra in the normal and ADHD populations (Johnstone, Gunkelman, & Lunt, 2005). This heterogeneity leads to a large variance of EEG power taken for any frequency band. Consequently, changes induced by neurofeedback training usually are smaller than this inter-individual variance which makes the task of proving statistical pre-post QEEG difference rather difficult but not impossible providing an appropriate study design was selected (see Chapter 15 in this book).

However, ERPs parameters are more sensitive to neurofeedback training. In contrast to EEG spectra they reflect stages of information flow in the brain. When continuous performance tasks (such as GO/NO-GO) are implemented, ERPs are shown to be reliable markers of the executive system of the brain.

In our recent study (Kropotov et al., 2005) we used relative beta as a neurofeedback parameter for modulation behavior of ADHD children. The neurofeedback parameter was defined as a ratio of EEG power in a beta frequency band (15—18 Hz) and EEG power in the remainder of the EEG band, i.e., in 4—14 Hz and 19—30 Hz frequency bands. The EEG was recorded bipolar from C3 and Fz electrodes in the standard 10—20 system. A typical training session included 20 minutes of relative beta training. The biofeedback procedure consisted of the following computations: power spectrum was calculated for a 1-second epoch every 250 ms using Fast Fourier Transformation. Visual feedback was provided by a bar against a background on a computer screen. The height of the bar followed the dynamics of the biofeedback parameter. The participant's task was to keep the bar above a threshold determined at the pre-training 2 minute interval.

In addition to the simple visual feedback, a so-called video mode was used. In this mode, the biofeedback parameter controlled the level of a noise generated by a separate electronic unit called a Jammer (the unit was designed specifically for this purpose in our laboratory). The amplitude of the noise was maximal if the biofeedback parameter was minimal, and decreased gradually up to zero while the parameter approached a threshold. The noise was mixed with the video-signal of a video-player and was fed to a TV-set. Thus the patient actually also controlled the quality of the picture on the screen by his/her brainwaves, i.e., when the biofeedback parameter was higher than the threshold, the picture on the screen was clear, otherwise the TV picture was blurred by the noise.

Usually during the first five to eight sessions, patients performed training in the simple visual mode with the bar to be able to get a feeling for the procedure. Then training in the video mode started. The patient was instructed about the rationale of the procedure, as well as about the dependence of the biofeedback signal on the brain activity and attention. Before the procedure, the patient tried to relax, decrease muscular tension, and maintain regular diaphragmatic breath. The patient was asked to assess his or her own internal state and feelings when the biofeedback parameter surpassed the threshold and to reproduce this state. Different patients used different strategies with a common denominator of concentrating on a particular external object. The number of training sessions for each patient depended on several factors such as age, type of ADHD, learning curves, and parent reports, and varied from 15 to 22 (mean 17). The termination criteria were: (1) stabilization of training performance during the last three to five sessions, and (2) stabilization of patient's behavior according to parents' reports. Sessions were administrated two to five times per week for 5—8 weeks. The dynamics of the biofeedback parameter (training curve) was obtained for each patient and for each session.

It should be noted that not all patients were able to reliably elevate the relative beta activity even after 10–20 sessions. The quality of patient's performance, i.e., the ability of a patient to increase the neurofeedback parameter during training periods, was assessed. We considered the training session to be successful if a patient was able to increase the biofeedback parameter during training periods in more than 25% of sessions in comparison to resting periods. Patients were referred to as "good performers" if they were successful in more than 60% of sessions. Seventy-one patients (82.5%) were assigned to the "good" performance group. Those patients who had less than 60% successful training sessions were referred to as "bad performers". Fifteen patients (17.5%) were assigned to the "bad" performance group. This group was considered as a control group in the following data analysis.

To test functioning of the executive system, ERPs in the auditory two-stimulus GO/NO-GO task were recorded before and after all sessions of neurofeedback. ERPs to NO-GO cues superimposed on each other in "before" and "after" recordings are presented in Figure 3.8a. One can see enhancement of the positive component at the frontal leads after 20 sessions of the relative beta training.

The grand average ERPs differences and their maps computed by subtraction of the ERPs made before any interventions from those made after 20 sessions of the relative beta neurofeedback are presented in Figure 3.8b,c. A statistically significant increase of ERPs in response to NO-GO cues was found in the group of good performers, but not in the group of bad performers (not shown in Figure 3.8). It should be noted that the relative beta training did not change early (with latencies of 80–180 ms) components of ERPs, but induced significant enhancement of later positive components. Thus, our data indicate that this type of relative beta training does not effect auditory information processing in the human brain, while significantly changing the functioning of the executive system reflected in later ERP components.

Theoretically, our protocol differs from conventional protocols, because elevation of the biofeedback parameter in our study could be achieved by increasing beta power, and/or by decreasing theta as well as alpha power. However, as the results of our study indicate, the application of this relative beta protocol turns out to be as effective as conventional protocols. Indeed, 80% of our patients were able to significantly increase their neurofeedback

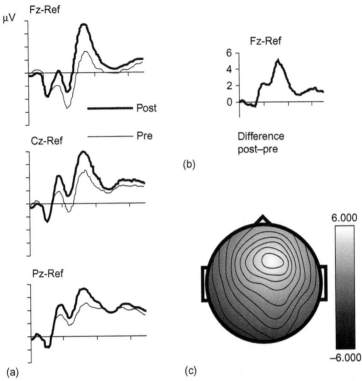

Figure 3.8 ERPs in the two-stimulus auditory GO/NO-GO task recorded before and after 20 sessions of relative beta training. (a) Grand average ERPs in response to NO-GO stimuli in the two-stimulus auditory GO/NO-GO test for the group of good performers before and after 20 sessions of the relative beta training. Thin line: ERPs taken before training; thick line: ERPs taken after 20 sessions of training. (b) ERPs differences induced by 20 sessions of neurofeedback in the group of good performers. (c) Map of the ERP changes induced by 20 sessions of neurofeedback. *(Adapted from Kropotov et al., 2005.)*

parameters in more than 60% of sessions. Moreover, according to parents' assessment by the SNAP-IV, neurofeedback significantly improved behavior as reflected in changes of inattention and impulsivity.

ERPs AS INDEX OF tDCS EFFECT

tDCS — transcranial direct current stimulation — is a technique of neuromodulation that applies direct current (i.e., a flow of electric charge that does not change direction and value) to the brain by means of electrodes placed on the head. Only 10% of the electric current passes through the cortex. However, this current seems to be enough to induce substantial changes in excitability of cortical neurons. Experiments indicate that anodal stimulation (at least as applied to electrodes located above the motor cortex) increases excitability of neurons while the cathodal stimulation has an opposite effect (Nitsche & Paulus, 2000).

The first report of ERP changes during tDCS in humans was made by a group from the University of Goettingen, Germany (Antal, Kincses, Nitsche, Bartfai, & Paulus, 2004). They found that cathodal polarization induced a mild facilitatory after-effect on P100 whereas anodal polarization induced no after-effect. Later, a group from University of Rome "La Sapienza" (Italy) found that tDCS at 1 mA induced changes in ERPs that persist after polarization ends. tDCS was applied through surface electrodes placed over the occipital scalp (polarizing) and over the anterior or posterior neck-base (Accornero, Li Voti, La Riccia, & Gregori, 2007). tDCS was applied at two durations, 3 and 10 min and both polarities. Visual evoked potentials were obtained with black-and-white pattern-reversal checkerboards (two cycles per degree), at two levels of contrast. To avoid habituation owing to a constant checkerboard-reversal rate, patterns were reversed at a frequency of 2 Hz $\pm 20\%$.

In this study anodal polarization reduced VEP-P100 amplitude whereas cathodal polarization significantly increased amplitude; but both polarities left latency statistically unchanged (Figure 3.9). These changes persisted for some minutes after polarization ended depending on the duration of tDCS and on the contrast level of visual stimuli, with lower contrast exhibiting higher effect.

In a pilot study with ERPs obtained in a GO/NO-GO task we attempted to find effects of anodal polarization on cognitive ERPs components. The anodal stimulation was 0.2–0.4 mA with 20 min duration. ERPs in the two-stimulus GO/NO-GO task described above were recorded before and after tDCS. In order to obtain reliable ERPs in each subject, 200 trials were presented in each condition. Seven healthy subjects (students from St Petersburg State University) participated in this pilot study. Some results are shown in Figure 3.10. As one can see, anodal stimulation at the area located between Pz, P3, and Cz induced changes in the N2 component, likely produced by altering excitability of neurons in the cingulate cortex.

We can conclude that in contrast to spontaneous EEG reflecting neuronal mechanisms of cortical self-regulation, ERPs are associated with stages of information flow within the cortex. ICA provides a powerful

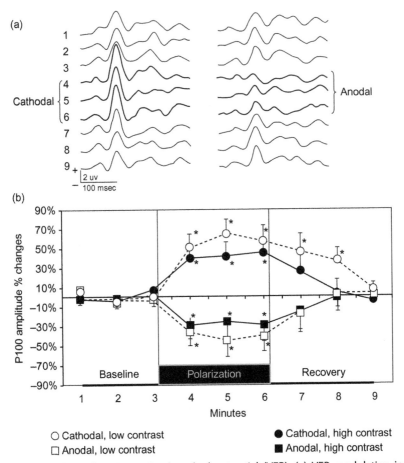

Figure 3.9 Effect of tDCS on visual evoked potential (VEP). (a) VEP modulation in a representative subject: each trace is an average of 60 visual stimuli sampled sequentially a minute. tDCS was applied for 3 minutes. (b) Grand average VEP P100 amplitude modulation induced by tDCS. *(Adapted from Accornero et al., 2007.)*

tool for decomposing ERPs into functionally meaningful components. The independent components of the two-stimulus GO/NO-GO are generated in distinct cortical areas and show different time dynamics. These components index different psychological operations in sensory systems (such as detecting salience of the visual stimulus) and the executive system of the brain (such as action suppression and conflict monitoring). Two of those components (salience and action suppression components) significantly differ between ADHD and healthy populations. They can be considered as endophenotypes (biological markers) of ADHD. The

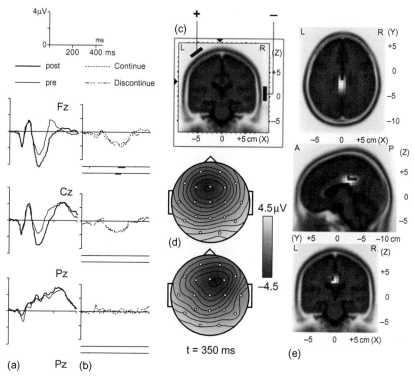

Figure 3.10 ERP to the first stimulus in the two-stimulus GO/NO-GO paradigm. ERPs were recorded before (thin line) and after (thick line) 20 minutes of tDCS. Electrodes were placed between Pz, P3, and Cz for anode and on the right mastoid for cathode. (a) ERPs in common reference montage to the first stimulus (Continue condition) before (pre, thin line) and after (post, thick line). (b) ERP differences (post−pre) for both Continue and Discontinue conditions. (c) Schematic presentation of electrode placement. (d) Maps of ERP differences (post−pre) taken at 350 ms after the first stimulus for Continue and Discontinue conditions. (e) sLORETA image of generators of the tDCS effect.

independent components of ERPs can be used as a diagnostic tool for defining functional impairment in a particular patient's brain as well as for defining effects of tDCS and neurofeedback in healthy subjects and patients.

REFERENCES

Accornero, N., Li Voti, P., La Riccia, M., & Gregori, B. (2007). Visual evoked potentials modulation during direct current cortical polarization. *Experimental Brain Research, 178*(2), 261−266.

Antal, A., Kincses, T. Z., Nitsche, M. A., Bartfai, O., & Paulus, W. (2004). Excitability changes induced in the human primary visual cortex by transcranial direct current stimulation: Direct electrophysiological evidence. *Investigative Ophthalmology and Visual Science*, 45(2), 702–707.

Arns, M., de Ridder, S., Strehl, U., Breteler, M., & Coenen, A. (2009). Efficacy of neurofeedback treatment in ADHD: The effects on inattention, impulsivity and hyperactivity: A meta-analysis. *Clinical EEG and Neuroscience*, 40(3), 180–189.

Barkley, R. A. (1997). Behavioral inhibition, sustained attention, and executive functions: Constructing a unifying theory of ADHD. *Psychological Bulletin*, 121, 65–94.

Bekker, E. M., Kenemans, J. L., & Verbaten, M. N. (2005). Source analysis of the N2 in a cued Go/NoGo task. *Brain Research: Cognitive Brain Research*, 22, 221–231.

Bokura, H., Yamaguchi, S., & Kobayashi, S. (2001). Electrophysiological correlates for response inhibition in a Go/NoGo task. *Clinical Neurophysiology*, 112, 2224–2232.

Botvinick, M. M. (2007). Conflict monitoring and decision making: Reconciling two perspectives on anterior cingulate function. *Cognitive Affective & Behavioral Neuroscience*, 7(4), 356–366.

Bugli, C., & Lambert, P. (2007). Comparison between principal component analysis and independent component analysis in electroencephalograms modeling. *Biometrical Journal*, 49(2), 312–327.

Clarke, J. M., Halgren, E., & Chauvel, P. (1999). Intracranial ERPs in humans during a lateralized visual oddball task: II. Temporal, parietal, and frontal recordings. *Clinical Neurophysiology*, 110(7), 1226–1244.

Cohen, J. (1988). *Statistical power analysis for the behavioral sciences* (2nd ed.). Hillsdale, NJ: Lawrence Erlbaum.

Congedo, M., Gouy-Pailler, C., & Jutten, C. (2008). On the blind source separation of human electroencephalogram by approximate joint diagonalization of second order statistics. *Clinical Neurophysiology*, 119(12), 2677–2686.

Curtin, LL. (1984). The Yerkes–Dodson law. *Nursing Management*, 15(5), 7–8.

Debener, S., Makeig, S., Delorme, A., & Engel, A. K. (2005). What is novel in the novelty oddball paradigm? Functional significance of the novelty P3 event-related potential as revealed by independent component analysis. *Brain Research: Cognitive Brain Research*, 22(3), 309–321.

Dien, J., Spencer, K. M., & Donchin, E. (2003). Localization of the event-related potential novelty response as defined by principal components analysis. *Brain Research: Cognitive Brain Research*, 17(3), 637–650.

Dietl, T., Dirlich, G., Vogl, L., Lechner, C., & Strian, F. (1999). Orienting response and frontal midline theta activity: A somatosensory spectral perturbation study. *Clinical Neurophysiology*, 110(7), 1204–1209.

Donchin, E. (1981). Surprise! Surprise! *Psychophysiology*, 18(5), 493–513.

Donchin, E., Miller, G. A., & Farwell, L. A. (1986). The endogenous components of the event-related potential – a diagnostic tool? *Progress in Brain Research*, 70, 87–102.

Duncan, C. C., Barry, R. J., Connolly, J. F., Fischer, C., Michie, P. T., Näätänen, R., et al. (2009). Event-related potentials in clinical research: Guidelines for eliciting, recording, and quantifying mismatch negativity, P300, and N400. *Clinical Neurophysiology*, 120(11), 1883–1908.

Escera, C., Alho, K., Winkler, I., & Näätänen, R. (1998). Neural mechanisms of involuntary attention to acoustic novelty and change. *Journal of Cognitive Neuroscience*, 10(5), 590–604.

Escera, C., Yago, E., & Alho, K. (2001). Electrical responses reveal the temporal dynamics of brain events during involuntary attention switching. *Europe Journal of Neuroscience*, 14, 877–883.

Goldstein, A., Spencer, K. M., & Donchin, E. (2002). The influence of stimulus deviance and novelty on the P300 and novelty P3. *Psychophysiology*, *39*, 781−790.

Gordon, E., Cooper, N., Rennie, C., Hermens, D., & Williams, L. M. (2005). Integrative neuroscience: The role of a standardized database. *Clinical EEG and Neuroscience*, *36*(2), 64−75.

Gottesman, I. I., & Gould, T. D. (2003). The endophenotype concept in psychiatry: Etymology and strategic intentions. *American Journal of Psychiatry*, *160*(4), 636−645.

Hillyard, S. A., & Anllo-Vento, L. (1998). Event-related brain potentials in the study of visual selective attention. *Proceedings of the National Academy of Sciences of thee U S A*, *95*(3), 781−787.

Ikeda, A., Lüders, H. O., Burgess, R. C., & Shibasaki, H. (1993). Movement-related potentials associated with single and repetitive movements recorded from human supplementary motor area. *Electroencephalography and Clinical Neurophysiology*, *89*(4), 269−277.

Ikeda, A., Yazawa, S., Kunieda, T., Ohara, S., Terada, K., Mikuni, N., et al. (1999). Cognitive motor control in human pre-supplementary motor area studied by subdural recording of discrimination/selection-related potentials. *Brain*, *122*, 915−931.

Inanaga, K. (1998). Frontal midline theta rhythm and mental activity. *Psychiatry and Clinical Neurosciences*, *52*(6), 555−566.

Itier, R. J., & Taylor, M. J. (2004a). N170 or N1? Spatiotemporal differences between object and face processing using ERPs. *Cerebral Cortex*, *14*, 132−142.

Itier, R. J., & Taylor, M. J. (2004b). Source analysis of the N170 to faces and objects. *Neuroreport*, *15*(8), 1261−1265.

James, C. J., & Hesse, C. W. (2005). Independent component analysis for biomedical signals. *Physiological Measurement*, *26*(1), R15−39.

Jodo, E., & Kayama, Y. (1992). Relation of a negative ERP component to response inhibition in a Go/No-Go task. *Electroencephalography and Clinical Neurophysiology*, *82*, 477−482.

John, E. Roy (1977). *Neurometrics: Clinical applications of quantitative electrophysiology.* Hillsdale, NJ: Lawrence Erlbaum Associates.

John, E. Roy (1990). Principles of neurometrics. *American Journal of EEG Technology*, *30*, 251−266.

Johnstone, J., Gunkelman, J., & Lunt, J. (2005). Clinical database development: Characterization of EEG phenotypes. *Clinical EEG and Neuroscience*, *36*, 99−107.

Jung, T. P., Makeig, S., Humphries, C., Lee, T. W., McKeown, M. J., Iragui, V., et al. (2000). Removing electroencephalographic artifacts by blind source separation. *Psychophysiology*, *37*(2), 163−178.

Kiefer, M., Marzinzik, F., Weisbrod, M., Scherg, M., & Spitzer, M. (1998). The time course of brain activations during response inhibition: Evidence from event-related potentials in a Go/No Go task. *NeuroReport*, *9*, 765−770.

Kropotov, J. D. (2009). *Quantitative EEG, event related potentials and neurotherapy* San Diego, CA: Academic Press, Elsevier.

Kropotov, J. D., Grin-Yatsenko, V. A., Ponomarev, V. A., Chutko, L. S., Yakovenko, E. A., & Nikishena, I. S. (2005). ERPs correlates of EEG relative beta training in ADHD children. *International Journal of Psychophysiology*, *55*(1), 23−34.

Kropotov, J. D., & Ponomarev, V. A. (1991). Subcortical neuronal correlates of component P300 in man. *Electroencephalography and Clinical Neurophysiology*, *78*, 40−49.

Liu, J., Kiehl, K. A., Pearlson, G., Perrone-Bizzozero, N. I., Eichele, T., & Calhoun, V. D. (2009). Genetic determinants of target and novelty-related event-related potentials in the auditory oddball response. *Neuroimage*, *46*(3), 809−816.

Loo, S. K., & Barkley, R. A. (2005). Clinical utility of EEG in attention deficit hyperactivity disorder. *Applied Neuropsychology*, *12*(2), 64−76.

Makeig, S., Bell, A. J., Jung, T. -P., & Sejnowski, T. J. (1996). Independent component analysis of electroencephalographic data. *Advances in Neural Information Processing Systems, 8*, 145–151.

Makeig, S., Delorme, A., Westerfield, M., Jung, T. P., Townsend, J., Courchesne, E., et al. (2004). Electroencephalographic brain dynamics following manually responded visual targets. *PLoS Biology, 2*(6), 747–762.

Makeig, S., Westerfield, M., Jung, T. P., Covington, J., Townsend, J., Sejnowski, T. J., et al. (1999). Functionally independent components of the late positive event-related potential during visual spatial attention. *Journal of Neuroscience, 19*, 2665–2680.

Makeig, S., Westerfield, M., Jung, T. P., Enghoff, S., Townsend, J., Courchesne, E., et al. (2002). Dynamic brain sources of visual evoked responses. *Science, 295*, 690–694.

Mehta, J., Jerger, S., Jerger, J., & Martin, J. (2009). Electrophysiological correlates of word comprehension: Event-related potential (ERP) and independent component analysis (ICA). *International Journal of Audiology, 48*(1), 1–11.

Näätänen, R. (1992). *Attention and brain function.* Hillsdale, NJ: Lawrence Erlbaum Associates.

Nieuwenhuis, S., Yeung, N., van den Wildenberg, W. K., & Ridderinkhof, W. W. (2003). Electrophysiological correlates of anterior cingulate function in a Go/No-Go task: Effects of response conflict and trial type frequency. *Cognitive Affective & Behavioral Neuroscience, 3*, 17–26.

Nitsche, M. A., & Paulus, W. (2000). Excitability changes induced in the human motor cortex by weak transcranial direct current stimulation. *Journal of Physiology, 527*, 633–639.

Olbrich, H. M., Maes, H., Valerius, G., Langosch, J. M., & Feige, B. (2005). Event-related potential correlates selectively reflect cognitive dysfunction in schizophrenics. *Journal of Neural Transmission, 112*(2), 283–295.

Onton, J., & Makeig, S. (2006). Information-based modeling of event-related brain dynamics. *Progress in Brain Research, 159*, 99–120.

Pascual-Marqui, R. D. (2002). Standardized low-resolution brain electromagnetic tomography (sLORETA): Technical details. *Methods and Findings in Experimental Clinical Pharmacology, 24*(Suppl D), 5–12.

Paz-Caballero, M. D., & García-Austt, E. (1992). ERP components related to stimulus selection processes. *Electroencephalography and Clinical Neurophysiology, 82*(5), 369–376.

Pfefferbaum, A., Ford, J. M., Weller, B. J., & Kopell, B. S. (1985). ERPs to response production and inhibition. *Electroencephalography and Clinical Neurophysiology, 60*, 423–434.

Polich, J. (2007). Updating P300: An integrative theory of P3a and P3b. *Journal of Clinical Neurophysiology, 118*(10), 2128–2148.

Prichep, L. S., John, E. R., Ferris, S. H., Reisberg, B., Almas, M., Alper, K., et al. (1994). Quantitative EEG correlates of cognitive deterioration in the elderly. *Neurobiology and Aging, 15*(1), 85–90.

Rossion, B., Caldara, R., Seghier, M., Schuller, A. M., Lazeyras, F., & Mayer, E. (2003). A network of occipito-temporal face-sensitive areas besides the right middle fusiform gyrus is necessary for normal face processing. *Brain, 126*, 2381–2395.

Sauseng, P., Hoppe, J., Klimesch, W., Gerloff, C., & Hummel, F. C. (2007). Dissociation of sustained attention from central executive functions: Local activity and interregional connectivity in the theta range. *European Journal of Neuroscience, 25*(2), 587–593.

Schall, J. D., Stuphorn, V., & Brown, J. W. (2002). Monitoring and control of action by the frontal lobes. *Neuron, 36*(2), 309–322.

Silver, M. A., & Kastner, S. (2009). Topographic maps in human frontal and parietal cortex. *Trends in Cognitive Science, 13*, 488–495.

Simmonds, D. J., Pekar, J. J., & Mostofsky, S. H. (2008). Meta-analysis of Go/No-go tasks demonstrating that fMRI activation associated with response inhibition is task-dependent. *Neuropsychologia, 46*(1), 224−232.

Tereshchenko, E. P., Ponomarev, V. A., Kropotov, J. D., & Müller, A. (2009). Comparative efficiencies of different methods for removing blink artifacts in analyzing quantitative electroencephalogram and event-related potentials. *Human Physiology, 35*(2), 241−247.

Thatcher, R. W., Moore, N., John, E. R., Duffy, F., Hughes, J. R., & Krieger, M. (1999). qEEG and traumatic brain injury: Rebuttal of the American Academy of Neurology 1997 report by the EEG and Clinical Neuroscience Society. *Clinical Electroencephalography, 30*(3), 94−98.

van Veen, V., & Carter, C. S. (2002). The anterior cingulate as a conflict monitor: fMRI and ERP studies. *Physiology & Behavior, 77*(4-5), 477−482.

Verleger, R. (1988). Event related potentials and cognition: A critique of context updating hypothesis and alternative interpretation of P3. *Behavioral Brain Science, 11*, 343−427.

Vigário, R. N. (1997). Extraction of ocular artefacts from EEG using independent component analysis. *Electroencephalography and Clinical Neurophysiology, 103*(3), 395−404.

Zeman, P. M., Till, B. C., Livingston, N. J., Tanaka, J. W., & Driessen, P. F. (2007). Independent component analysis and clustering improve signal-to-noise ratio for statistical analysis of event-related potentials. *Clinical Neurophysiology, 118*(12), 2591−2604.

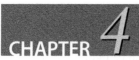

CHAPTER 4

EEG Vigilance and Phenotypes in Neuropsychiatry: Implications for Intervention

Martijn Arns[1], Jay Gunkelman[2], Sebastian Olbrich[3],
Christian Sander[3], and Ulrich Hegerl[3]

[1]Research Institute Brainclinics, Nijmegen, and Utrecht University, Department of Experimental Psychology, Utrecht, The Netherlands
[2]Q-Pro Worldwide, Crockett, California, USA
[3]University of Leipzig, Leipzig, Germany

Contents

INTRODUCTION

Since the discovery of EEG by Hans Berger in 1929 (Berger, 1929) much research has been dedicated to measuring EEG under different conditions as well as measuring EEG in a variety of disorders ranging from neurological to

Neurofeedback and Neuromodulation Techniques and Applications
DOI: 10.1016/B978-0-12-382235-2.00004-4

psychiatric disorders. In the early years EEG was mainly inspected visually until equipment became available that made possible Fourier analysis on EEG data to extract the spectral content of a signal. This eventually enabled the field of quantitative EEG (qEEG) as we know it today. In the simplest form one speaks of qEEG when the EEG is submitted to spectral analysis (Niedermeyer & Da Silva, 2004). In this respect some prefer to speak of "normative EEG" to clarify that the EEG should not only be submitted to spectral analysis but also compared to a control group and/or normative database (Kaiser, personal communication).

The group led by Ross Adey at the UCLA Brain Research Institute in the period 1961–1974 pioneered the first developments of qEEG. They were the first to use digital computers in the analysis of EEG with the production of brain maps and developed the first normative library of brain maps. See Figure 4.1 for photos of the first equipment developed to measure EEG in outer space and during driving. As part of the Space

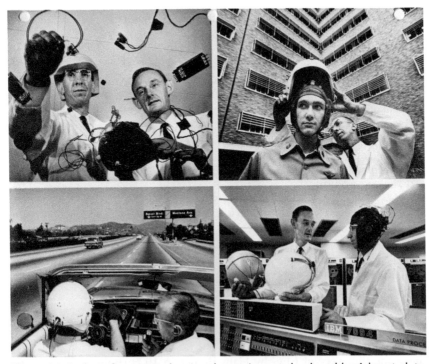

Figure 4.1 A photo from 1963 showing the equipment developed by Adey et al. to measure EEG in space. Ross Adey – who pioneered qEEG – is on the right in the top-left picture. *(Courtesy of the Computer History Museum.)*

Biology Laboratory they studied the effects of outer space and space travel on the brain, to determine whether prolonged space flight would be possible for the human body. As part of this NASA program Graham and Dietlein were the first to coin the term "normative EEG" (Kaiser, personal communication; Graham & Dietlein, 1965).

In the last 20 years, due to the increasing availability of affordable computer equipment, the field of qEEG has expanded even further and has become available for clinicians. Along with this, several different normative databases have also been developed and are available to most clinicians. Examples of such databases are Neuroguide (Thatcher), Brain Resource International Brain Database (Gordon), Neurometrics (John et al., 1992), SKIL (Sterman), NeuroRep (Hudspeth) and Eureka3 (NovaTech). For a description and comparison of these databases also see Johnstone et al. (Johnstone, Gunkelman, & Lunt, 2005).

In this chapter, where we speak of qEEG we focus on normative EEG, or qEEG data that are compared to a control group or normative database. Furthermore, in this chapter we will limit the application of qEEG to neuropsychiatric conditions and will not focus on more strictly neurological applications that fall beyond the scope of the chapter. Where we report on EEG power measures we will only report on absolute EEG unless stated otherwise. Relative EEG power measures often obscure findings making it unclear what is actually going on in the EEG, e.g., if the total absolute alpha power is decreased, it could show up as an increased "relative" beta and theta power.

Personalized Medicine: "Prognostics" Rather than "Diagnostics"

Current conventional treatment methods in psychiatry are based on behavioral interventions and medication ("systemic" approach). Recent large-scale studies increasingly often are showing the limitations of these conventional treatments (both behavioral and drug treatment) in psychiatry. The largest trial to date in over 3000 depressive patients investigating treatment effects in depression (the STAR⋆D trial) demonstrated limited clinical efficacy of antidepressants and cognitive behavior therapy (CBT) in the treatment of depression with remission rates of 36.8% per single treatment and 33% treatment resistance after four cumulative treatments (Rush et al., 2006). Some methodological issues potentially limit the generalizability of these results, such as a selection bias (the fact that most participants in this trial had no health insurance), lack of a placebo control, and not checking lithium levels. However, these and other studies

(Keller et al., 2000; Kirsch et al., 2008) do demonstrate there is a need for improved efficacy in depression treatment. A similar initiative investigating the effects of different treatment approaches in attention deficit hyperactivity disorder (ADHD) (the NIMH-MTA trial) also clearly showed a lack of long-term effects for stimulant medication, multicomponent behavior therapy, and multimodal treatment (Molina et al., 2009). Furthermore, in general, response rates to stimulant medication in ADHD are estimated to be 70% (see Hermens, Rowe, Gordon, & Williams, 2006 for an overview). New drug developments in psychiatry are not demonstrating major breakthroughs, but rather "refinements", i.e. showing fewer side effects, but not a drastically improved efficacy rate. Recently it was also announced that two major pharmaceutical companies (GSK and AstraZeneca) will no longer develop psychiatric medications (Nierenberg, 2010). So what do these developments mean?

These developments suggest something might be wrong with the current approach to psychiatric treatments. Rather than blaming this on the industry, it seems more likely that something is wrong with our definitions of psychiatric disorders and hence the DSM-IV. Brain surgeons who want to remove a tumor from the brain first make sure they exactly pinpoint the location of this tumor by employing brain-imaging techniques. Of course they do not simply rely on behavior to undertake such surgery. So why do we still mainly use behavior in psychiatry to guide our treatments? Engaging in a direct interaction with the brain (e.g., medication, neurofeedback, rTMS) requires knowledge about the current status of the brain. A new development along these lines is the development of Personalized Medicine. In this area the goal is to prescribe *the right treatment, for the right person at the right time* as opposed to the current one-size-fits-all treatments. Genotypic and phenotypic information or "Biomarkers" lie at the basis of Personalized Medicine. Usually in this context genetic markers are considered that can predict effects of medication, such as the classical example of herceptin. Herceptin is a drug used for breast cancer treatment, but only for patients showing an over-expression for a specific protein better known as human epidermal growth factor receptor 2 (HER2) (Piccart-Gebhart et al., 2005). This drug only works well with this specific sub-group of patients, who are easily distinguished by a genetic test where HER2 is considered the biomarker. Given there is no psychiatric disorder that is completely genetically determined (Hyman, 2007), a strictly genetic approach to Personalized Medicine for psychiatry seems therefore less plausible.

In this context Gordon (2007) proposed the term "neuromarker", and Johnstone et al. (2005) the term "EEG phenotype'" as examples of biomarkers. In another context EEG-vigilance regulation has also been proposed as a state-dependent trait (Hegerl, Olbrich, Schönknecht, & Sander, 2008). The underlying idea behind these concepts is that neuroimaging data such as EEG, fMRI, PET scans etc. can be considered stable phenotypes incorporating both the effects of nature and nurture. This potentially makes such markers ideal candidates as biomarkers, which could predict treatment outcome for treatments such as antidepressants or stimulants, but also for other treatments such as neurofeedback. These developments, currently subsumed under the umbrella term "Personalized Medicine", are not completely new. The quest for biomarkers to predict treatment outcome has a long history. For example, Satterfield et al. (Satterfield, Cantwell, Saul, Lesser, & Podosin, 1973; Satterfield, Lesser, & Podosin, 1971) were the first to investigate the potential use of EEG in predicting treatment outcome to stimulant medication, and Roth, Kay, Shaw, & Green (1957) investigated barbiturate-induced EEG changes (delta increase) and found this predicted to some degree the long-term outcome (3–6 months) to ECT in depression. In this development the focus is hence more on "prognostics" rather than "diagnostics". In this chapter we will review the history of EEG and qEEG findings in ADHD and depression and their limitations for this Personalized Medicine approach. Thereafter, we will present two more "theoretically" driven models, which have recently been investigated in more detail and show promise for the further development of EEG-based Personalized Medicine.

HISTORY OF EEG RESEARCH IN ADHD AND DEPRESSION
ADHD

Considerable research has been carried out investigating the neurophysiology of ADHD. The first report describing EEG findings in "behavior problem children" stems from 1938 (Jasper, Solomon, & Bradley, 1938). In those early days Jasper et al. (1938) already described an EEG pattern we now call the Frontal Slow EEG: "There were occasionally two or three waves also in the central or frontal regions at frequencies below what is considered the normal alpha range, that is, at frequencies of 5–6/sec ..." (Jasper et al., 1938, p. 644). The most predominant feature in the group of children resembling most closely the current diagnosis of

ADHD (hyperactive, impulsive, highly variable) were the occurrence of slow waves from one or more regions and an "abnormal EEG" in 83% of the cases. Most older studies investigating the EEG in Minimal Cerebral Dysfunction (MCD) or Minimal Brain Damage (MBD) (the earlier diagnosis for ADHD) reported incidences of around 50% "abnormal EEG" as compared to control groups showing, on average, 15% abnormal EEGs (for an overview see: Capute, Niedermeyer, & Richardson, 1968; Hughes, DeLeo, & Melyn, 2000; Stevens, Sachdev, & Milstein, 1968). However, it is to be noted that Stevens et al. (1968) earlier stated that the presence or absence of an "abnormal EEG" alone is of little value in predicting clinical or etiological features.

Capute et al. (1968) reported that the most common "abnormality" in MBD was excessive bilateral posterior slowing, which is similar to a slowed alpha peak frequency. In this regard it is also interesting to note that Cohn & Nardini (1958) described an EEG pattern of bi-occipital slow activity, which they related to aggressive clinical behavior. They stated that this activity "is sometimes sensitive, in a way similar to that of the occipital alpha output, to opening and closing the eyelids ... has a distribution that corresponds grossly to that of the occipital alpha activity." This suggests they also observed a slowed alpha peak frequency (APF) rather than a true slow occipital rhythm. Stevens et al. (1968) correlated different EEG abnormalities to behavioral profiles and found that slowing of EEG frequencies (occipital) was related to hyperactivity, difficulty with labeling and poor figure–ground discrimination. Furthermore, no clear behavioral syndrome was associated with predominant, frontal EEG abnormalities, suggesting that core problems such as hyperactivity are more related to a slowed alpha peak frequency rather than to frontal excess slow activity.

Paroxysmal EEG Abnormalities

Part of the above mentioned "abnormal EEG findings" consist of the so-called "paroxysmal" or "epileptiform discharges". The estimated incidences of paroxysmal EEG in some ADHD groups were around 12–13% (Capute et al., 1968; Satterfield et al., 1973) to approximately 30% (Hughes et al., 2000), which are high as compared to 1–2% in normal populations (Goodwin, 1947; Richter, Zimmerman, Raichle, & Liske, 1971). Note that these people did not suffer from epilepsy, but simply exhibited a paroxysmal EEG in the absence of seizures. The exact implications of such EEG activity in subjects without overt signs of epilepsy are not very well understood and many neurologists will see no need to treat these subjects as epileptics. In a very large study among jet fighter pilots, Lennox-Buchthal, Buchthal, and Rosenfalck (1960) classified 6.4% as "marked and paroxysmally abnormal". Moreover, they found that pilots with such EEGs were three times more likely to have their plane crashed due to pilot error, indicating that even though these people are not "epileptic" their brains are "not normal" and hence the presence of paroxysmal EEG continues to be an exclusion criterion for becoming a pilot. This at least suggests such an EEG pattern might have implications for behavior; however, more research is required to investigate that.

The Era of Computerized EEG Analysis

With the introduction of qEEG and computerized EEG analysis many more studies have been carried out investigating the neurophysiology of ADHD. The introduction of computerized EEG made EEG analysis much easier since many analyses could be performed in an automated fashion.

"Excess Theta" and "Theta/Beta Ratio"

The most consistent findings reported in the literature are those of increased absolute power in theta (Bresnahan, Anderson, & Barry, 1999; Chabot & Serfontein, 1996; Clarke, Barry, McCarthy, & Selikowitz, 1998;[1] Clarke, Barry, McCarthy, & Selikowitz, 2001c; DeFrance, Smith, Schweitzer, Ginsberg, & Sands, 1996; Janzen, Graap, Stephanson, Marshall, & Fitzsimmons, 1995; Lazzaro et al., 1999; Lazzaro et al., 1998; Mann, Lubar, Zimmerman, Miller, & Muenchen, 1992; Matsuura et al., 1993), and sometimes increased absolute delta EEG power (Bresnahan et al., 1999; Clarke et al., 2001c; Kuperman, Johnson, Arndt, Lindgren, & Wolraich, 1996; Matsuura et al., 1993).

Lubar in 1991 laid the foundation for the concept of the theta/beta power ratio as a measure that could discriminate "normal" children from children with ADD, learning disorders and ADHD (Lubar, 1991). This measure was investigated further by many others, with the clearest replication from Monastra et al. (1999) who demonstrated in a multicenter study in 482 subjects and a single electrode location (Cz) they could classify with an accuracy of 88% children with ADHD based on the theta/beta power ratio. Since these initial findings by Lubar many groups have further investigated the EEG in ADHD, mainly using computerized power

---

[1] Clarke et al., 1998 and Clarke et al. (2001c) excluded an "excess beta group" from their analysis, which means that they excluded about 20% of children with ADHD thereby potentially biasing their results.

spectral EEG analysis (FFT) and coherence. Furthermore, Boutros, Fraenkel, & Feingold (2005), using a meta-analysis incorporating more than 1100 subjects with ADHD/ADD, concluded that increased theta activity in ADHD is a robust enough finding to warrant further development as a diagnostic test or biomarker for ADHD, with data suggesting that relative theta power is an even stronger predictor.

In contrast to the results described in the previous section, almost none of the recent studies reports on alpha peak frequency, but only on spectral power measures in ADHD, whereas from this old research clear relations have been reported between the slowing of this APF and behavioral measures such as hyperactivity (Stevens et al., 1968). As indicated by Steriade, Gloor, Linás, Lopes de Silva, and Mesulam (1990), theta may be a slowing down of alpha activity, suggesting that perhaps the often-reported excess theta consists of both a slowed alpha peak frequency and real excess slow activity. In Figure 4.2, this is illustrated in detail. This

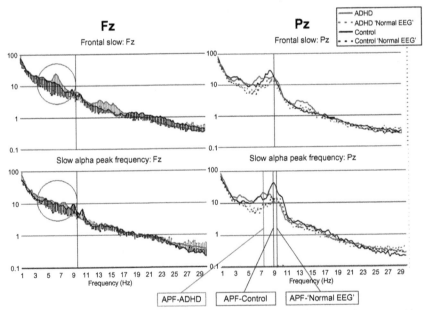

Figure 4.2 *(See Color Plate Section)* This figure clearly shows that the sub-group with a slowed alpha peak frequency (bottom), present parietally, also show elevated "theta EEG power" at frontal sites. However, this is not true "frontal slow", but simply the effect of the slowed alpha peak frequency. This demonstrates that a raised theta/beta ratio at least also includes the slow APF sub-group, which neurophysiologically is a different group, as demonstrated later with respect to treatment outcome to stimulant medication. *(From Arns, Gunkelman, Breteler, & Spronk (2008); reproduced with permission.)*

figure shows the spectral content of ADHD children and data from a control group for both frontal (Fz) and parietal (Pz) locations. The dotted lines reflect the groups with a "normal EEG" and the solid lines show the spectral power of the sub-groups with a "Frontal Slow" (top) or "Slowed Alpha Peak Frequency" (bottom). As can be seen, the spectral content for the frontal slow group is increased in the theta frequency range, mainly at Fz, as would be expected. However, the ADHD group with the slowed APF at Pz showed an average APF of 7.5 Hz. In the frontal locations this also shows up as an "increased theta EEG power" whereas this obviously is due to the excessive slowing of the APF.

In another study by Lansbergen, Arns, van Dongen-Boomsma, Spronk, & Buitelaar (in press) this was further tested. They calculated the theta/beta ratio in a group 49 ADHD children and 49 matched controls using both fixed frequency bands and also using individualized EEG frequency bands based on the approach suggested by Klimesch (1999). In this study a significantly deviating theta/beta ratio was only found for the "fixed" EEG frequency bands, but there was no significant difference when the individualized EEG frequency bands were employed, further demonstrating that most of the above-reported studies have indeed been picking up both real elevated theta, but also patients with a slow APF which are two neurophysiologically very different groups. Therefore, although the theta/beta ratio and the "excess theta" can discriminate a group of children with ADHD very well from healthy controls, this measure is probably *not a specific* measure since they incorporate different sub-types of ADHD. So from a Personalized Medicine approach this is not optimal, since it is expected that these sub-types respond differentially to medication as well, which will be clearly demonstrated later.

Increased or Decreased Beta?

The literature is less consistent about the decreased absolute beta in ADHD (Callaway, Halliday, & Naylor, 1983; Dykman, Ackerman, Oglesby, & Holcomb, 1982; Mann et al., 1992; Matsuura et al., 1993). This was not found in several other studies (Barry, Clarke, Johnstone, & Brown, 2009; Clarke et al., 2001c; Lazzaro et al., 1999; Lazzaro et al., 1998) and was found actually to be increased in one study (Kuperman et al., 1996). Furthermore, some studies have also reported a specific sub-group in ADHD with excess beta ranging from 13% (Chabot, Merkin, Wood, Davenport, & Serfontein, 1996) to 20% (Clarke et al., 1998; Clarke, Barry, McCarthy & Selikowitz, 2001b), and most prevalent in males with ADHD. Clarke et al. (2001a) also reported that about 10% of the excess beta group showed beta spindles, and Arns et al. reported that 16% had beta spindles (Arns et al., 2008). In summary, several studies point to the existence of an ADHD sub-group with excess beta.

In general, minor differences have been found in studies between the DSM-IV TR (DSM) ADHD and ADD diagnosis, mainly showing a less severe pattern of deviation in the ADD group as compared to the ADHD group (Barry, Clarke & Johnstone, 2003; Chabot et al., 1996).

EEG as a Prognostic Tool: Treatment Prediction in ADHD

Satterfield and colleagues (1971, 1973) were the first to investigate the potential use of EEG in predicting treatment outcome to stimulant medication. They found that children with excess slow wave activity and large amplitude evoked potentials were more likely to respond to stimulant medication (Satterfield et al., 1971) or more generally that abnormal EEG findings could be considered a predictor for positive treatment outcome (Satterfield et al., 1973). Chabot et al. (Chabot, diMichele, Prichep, & John, 2001; Chabot, Orgill, Crawford, Harris, & Serfontein, 1999) found that ADHD and ADD children with excess relative alpha or beta power were likely to show behavioral improvement, whereas the relative excess theta group showed a lower response and a higher probability of a negative response to medication. Their group exhibiting this "excess theta" was described as: "generalized excess of theta absolute and relative power, *decreased alpha mean frequency,* and frontal theta hypercoherence (emphasis added)". Note the mention of decreased alpha mean frequency, suggesting that in fact they were looking at a combined group of excess theta and slowed APF.

In contrast, Clarke, Barry, McCarthy, & Selikowitz (2002a, 2002b) and Suffin and Emory (1995) showed that in ADHD and ADD good responders to stimulant medication were characterized by increased theta and theta/beta ratios. Clarke et al. (2003), however, showed that an excess beta group also responded well to stimulants, in agreement with Chabot et al. (1999). They noted, however, that there were few EEG normalizations. In line with this, Hermens et al. (2005) showed that increased beta was related to better treatment outcome in ADHD.

As pointed out earlier and demonstrated in Figure 4.2, Arns et al. (2008) separated a frontal slow wave group from a slowed alpha peak frequency group, but most importantly demonstrated that only the frontal slow group responded to stimulant medication, whereas the slowed alpha

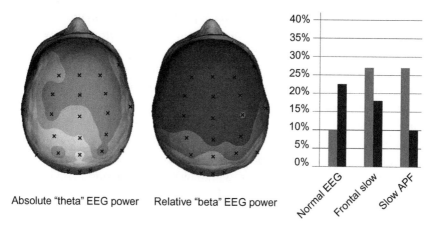

Absolute "theta" EEG power   Relative "beta" EEG power

Figure 4.3 *(See Color Plate Section)* The averaged brain activity of 275 ADHD patients compared to a matched control group. The figure left shows the increased theta (p <0.0001) and right the decreased relative beta power (p <0.0001). Note the fronto-central localization. The graph on the right shows that when inspecting the individual data sets only 25% of children with ADHD (red) indeed exhibit "real frontal slow" or frontal theta. Finally, about the same percentage exhibit a slow APF pattern, which after filtering will show up as "theta" but in fact is alpha, as explained below.

peak frequency group did not respond (Arns et al., 2008). These results further demonstrate that many of the previous studies reporting on frontal theta have mixed up frontal slow and slowed alpha peak frequency groups, as illustrated in Figure 4.3. Furthermore, this finding also helps explain the above contradictory findings between Chabot et al. (1999, 2001) versus the results from Clarke et al. (2002a, 2002b) and Suffin and Emory (1995).

Depression

In 1973 d'Elia & Perris were the first to investigate parietal alpha power asymmetry in depression (psychotic depression in this case) and reported that the left to right ratio correlated to the depression score both before and after ECT (d'Elia & Perris, 1973). Furthermore, the treatment effects of ECT were mainly reflected in left hemisphere changes.

In 1983 a group led by Davidson started publishing pioneering work on frontal alpha asymmetry in depression. They reported a relative hyperactivation of the right frontal cortex which was not found for the parietal cortex (Schaffer, Davidson, & Saron, 1983). In their 1990 paper Henriques and Davidson laid a further foundation for the concept of frontal alpha asymmetry in depression, where they consider "approach" and "withdrawal" as the essential basis for this asymmetry: "The approach system facilitates appetitive behavior and generates certain forms of positive affect. The withdrawal system facilitates the withdrawal of an organism from sources of aversive stimulation and generates certain forms of negative affect ..." (Davidson, 1998). These two systems have been conceptualized as relatively orthogonal. They interpreted the decreased left-sided frontal activation as a deficit in the approach system, and hence subjects with this condition are more prone to certain negative affective states and depressive disorders, given a certain level of environmental stress. On the other hand, they suggested that the right-sided frontal activation is related to withdrawal related emotion and psychopathology such as anxiety disorders (Henriques & Davidson, 1990). Support for the Approach–Withdrawal model comes from many correlational studies (for an overview see Davidson, 1998) but also from some studies such as those involving manipulation of frontal EEG asymmetry by neurofeedback (Allen, Harmon-Jones, & Cavender, 2001; Baehr, Rosenfeld, & Baehr, 1997). Besides these frontal deficits they also reported a decreased right-parietal activation found in both previously and currently depressed patients. They related this to selective spatial cognitive deficits which are reported to accompany depression and which might also explain some of the symptoms in affective disorders that require the decoding of non-verbal, expressive behavior (Henriques & Davidson, 1990).

In the often-cited Henriques and Davidson paper researchers used data from 15 depressed subjects and 13 controls (Henriques & Davidson, 1991). They reported significant differences in alpha asymmetry between depressive patients and controls, with medium p-values (p = 0.2; 0.3). As can be clearly seen in Figure 4.4, they reported that only 2/13 normals (15%) deviated significantly from the depressive asymmetry scores and only 1/15 depressives (7%) deviated significantly from the normal asymmetry scores (based on a Cz montage). Therefore, there is more overlap between groups than there are differences – also see figure 4 in Henriques & Davidson, (1990), showing the individual data. This clearly demonstrates that these data are unusable for diagnostic and/or prognostic purposes, which is also acknowledged by Davidson (Davidson, 1998) in contrast to the "over-interpretation" of this finding in many qEEG and neurofeedback practices.

Measures of frontal asymmetry in depressed patients are only moderately stable over time (Debener et al., 2000; Tomarken, Davidson, Wheeler, & Kinney, 1992), leading the Davidson group to average frontal alpha asymmetry measures over at least two occasions (separated by weeks) in their more

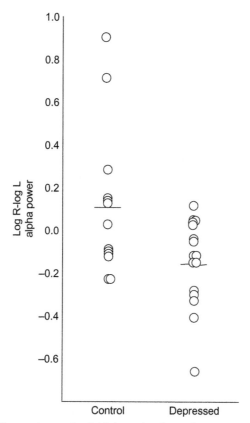

Figure 4.4 This figure shows the initial results from the Henriques and Davidson paper (1990) demonstrating the differences in "frontal alpha asymmetry" between healthy controls and depressed subjects. Note the large overlap between these two groups. They reported that 2/15 normals and 1/15 depressive differed significantly from the other group. These findings demonstrate that alpha asymmetry is not likely to be of clinical use when applied to individual patients, but only useful in group-averaged data. *(From Henriques & Davidson, 1990; reproduced with permission.)*

recent work (Davidson, 1998). Furthermore, eyes-open and eyes-closed data are also averaged (weighted average) in order to obtain more stable estimates of EEG asymmetry (Henriques & Davidson, 1991). The finding that this measure is only moderately stable over time has led some authors to question the "stable trait" status of alpha asymmetry (Debener et al., 2000).

Most studies investigating the frontal alpha asymmetry did not find any correlation between alpha asymmetry and measures of mood such as depression severity (Debener et al., 2000; Henriques & Davidson, 1991).

A deviating alpha asymmetry is also found in previously depressed patients no longer meeting criteria for depression (Henriques & Davidson, 1990), suggesting that frontal alpha asymmetry could be considered a stable trait rather than a state-marker for depression. (Or, more specifically as Davidson phrased it: "that individual differences in prefrontal asymmetry are most appropriately viewed as diatheses that bias a person's affective style, and then in turn modulate an individual's vulnerability to develop depression ..." [Davidson, 1998].) On the other hand, some have suggested that resting frontal alpha asymmetry reflects the joint contribution of a trait that is superimposed on state-like factors (Tomarken et al., 1992). This was supported empirically by Hagemann, Naumann, & Thayer (2001), who found that about 60% of the variance was explained by a latent trait and about 40% was due to state-like fluctuations. Allen, Urry, Hitt, & Coan (2004) showed that about 60% of the variance in alpha asymmetry is stable across time, despite substantial clinical improvements over time. Finally, several studies have demonstrated that alpha asymmetry was also influenced by differences in cranial and brain parenchymal asymmetries in bone thickness (Myslobodsky, Bar-Ziv, van Praag, & Glicksohn, 1989) and different EEG montages (Hagemann et al., 2001; Hagemann, Naumann, Becker, Maier & Bartussek, 1998; Reid, Duke, & Allen, 1998), whereas, Henriques and Davidson (1990) found the effects to be consistent across different referencing procedures. In an excellent review of methodological problems with frontal alpha asymmetry measures by Hagemann (2004) many other confounding factors are discussed, such as the effect of situational factors (e.g., sex of the experimenter in relation to the sex of the subject, montages, etc.) and for a review of structural skull deviations and their potential of confounding frontal alpha asymmetry variables, see Myslobodsky, Coppola, & Weinberger (1991).

Alpha power is traditionally seen as an occipital-parietal EEG rhythm, and is most often maximal at these locations. As Hagemann et al. (2001) suggest, the above-mentioned contradictory validity ratings also may be explained in terms of signal-to-noise ratios. Since alpha activity is not maximal at frontal sites and sometimes there is little to no alpha at those sites, the signal of interest — alpha — can be too low to result into a reliable measurement of alpha asymmetry. Finally, EEG vigilance could also play a role in some of the contradictory findings since studies measuring short EEG segments (2–3 min) more often find alpha asymmetry as compared to studies measuring longer EEG segments (e.g., 8 minutes) (Davidson, 1998; Reid et al., 1998).

EEG as a Prognostic Tool: Treatment Prediction in Depression

One of the first attempts at using the EEG as a prognostic tool in depression stems from 1957. Roth et al. (1957) investigated barbiturate-induced EEG changes (delta increase) and found this predicted to some degree the long-term outcome (3–6 months) of ECT in depression. In 2001 Bruder et al. investigated the use of alpha asymmetry and dichotic listening tasks to predict treatment outcomes to SSRIs (selective serotonin reuptake inhibitors) and found that non-responders showed more right-frontal activation as compared to responders which seemed to be a gender specific effect (for females only). Few, if any other studies have been reported on the prognostic use of alpha asymmetry in depression. Other authors have used EEG-derived measures such as EEG cordance (Leuchter et al., 2009) and ERP-derived measures (loudness intensity dependence [LDAEP]) (Hegerl, Gallinat & Juckel, 2001) to predict treatment outcome to antidepressants; however these are beyond the scope of this chapter. In general, there are no reliable EEG-based predictors that can predict treatment outcome to antidepressants based on pre-treatment EEG and most likely for this purpose an integrative approach is required using data from multiple domains such as EEG, ERP, neuropsychology, and genetics as a recent pilot-study demonstrated (Spronk, Arns, Barnett, Cooper, & Gordon, 2010).

A relatively new treatment approach for depression, which is largely based on the frontal asymmetry hypothesis, is rTMS or repetitive transcranial magnetic stimulation. This treatment usually focuses on "stimulating" the left frontal cortex or "inhibiting" the right frontal cortex. For a full overview of details also see Chapter 10 by Spronk, Arns, and Fitzgerald in this volume.

Conclusion: Averaged Group Data vs. Individual Client Data

As has been clearly shown above, both the excess theta and the theta/beta ratio in ADHD and the frontal alpha asymmetry in depression, show a good correspondence to their respective DSM diagnosis, i.e., in *groups* of patients with the disorder these markers are usually found. However, it was also clearly shown that these measures have limited use for individualized or personalized approaches when the goal is to personalize treatment given their (a) non-specificity ("theta" EEG power comprised of two distinct sub-types, namely slow APF and frontal slow) or their (b) under-representation on the individual level (only 1 in 15 depressives differing significantly on their frontal alpha asymmetry as compared to a control group).

Influence of Vigilance/Arousal

In the above sections on the theta/beta ratio and alpha asymmetry there is another aspect, not yet addressed, which deserves more attention. Many studies use different lengths of EEG recordings. In the ADHD studies the recording lengths for EEG data vary between 2 minutes to over 20 minutes. All studies from the group of Adam Clarke (Clarke et al., 1998; Clarke et al., 2001a, 2001b, 2001d; Clarke et al., 2002a, 2002b), for example, have collected 20 minutes of eyes-closed EEG and selected a 1-minute EEG from these 20 minutes for final analysis (Clarke, personal communication). The studies by Chabot also consisted of 20–30 minutes eyes-closed EEG, whereas others have shorter recording times only during eyes-open (e.g. Bresnahan et al., 1999; Lazzaro et al., 1998, 1999).

Furthermore, for frontal alpha asymmetry it was reported that studies measuring short EEG segments (2–3 min) more often find the expected alpha asymmetry as compared to studies measuring longer EEG segments (e.g. 8 min) (Davidson, 1998; Reid et al., 1998). Bruder et al. (2001) stated:

> One possibility is that hemispheric asymmetry differences between fluoxetine responders and non-responders may depend upon level of arousal. Eyes closed during resting EEG is the least arousing condition, whereas eyes open leads to an increase in arousal and dichotic listening requires active task performance ...

thus hinting at a potential role of vigilance.

In all these studies the "EEG dynamics" have not been investigated, but accumulated EEG power across a full record has been used. Therefore, we will now address the EEG Vigilance model (Bente, 1964) in more detail to demonstrate potential value of studying EEG dynamics during eyes closed conditions. This might help explain some of the contradictory findings, and, perhaps above all, provide a more coherent and personalized framework for the discovery and interpretation of EEG findings with prognostic value.

EEG AND qEEG: MODELS AND THEORY

In the following sections we will explain in more detail the EEG Vigilance model, which is a theory-driven approach, and one that has been around since the first reports by Dieter Bente (1964). It has roots in the writings of Loomis, Harvey, and Hobart (1937) and was modified by Roth (1961).

After that we will address a more recently published and employed qEEG model, namely the EEG Phenotype model by Johnstone, Gunkelman, & Lunt (2005).

EEG VIGILANCE MODEL

The regulation of vigilance and its flexible adaptation to internal and environmental needs are of fundamental importance for all higher organisms. Vigilance has to be adapted to the respective environmental situation, ensuring a high vigilance level in situations of danger and a reduced vigilance level during times of recreation. However, the interplay between environment and vigilance regulation also works the other way around: The environment actively created by a person can also depend on vigilance regulation. If the capacity of the brain to maintain a high vigilance level is reduced, a person will normally feel sleepy and thus seek an environment with low external stimulation and a chance to sleep. However, under certain circumstances such an unstable vigilance regulation can also induce a compensatory behavioral pattern termed here as vigilance autostabilization behavior. Hyperactivity, sensation-seeking, and other behavioral patterns create a highly stimulating environment. The resulting increase in external stimulation counteracts the impending vigilance decline and leads to a stabilization of vigilance. An everyday example would be the hyperactive, "high-spirited" behavior of overtired children. Related to this, mania has been described as sensation-seeking gone out of control. By contrast, in times of a tonically high vigilance level, a person might avoid additional external stimulation and withdraw as an autoregulatory behavior. The proposed concept of vigilance autostabilization behavior is related to earlier theories of brain function (Bente, 1964; Ulrich & Frick, 1986; Wundt, 1874), personality (Eysenck, 1990) and sensation-seeking (Zuckerman, 1985).

EEG-Vigilance Algorithm — "VIGALL"

In parallel to the transition from active wakefulness to deep sleep the human brain takes on different global functional states. These functional states are reflected in the spectral composition and topography of the electroencephalogram (EEG) and have been termed vigilance stages. These states correspond to different levels of alertness at the behavioral level. Several stages can be separated during the transition from tense to relaxed wakefulness and further on to drowsiness until sleep onset.

In 1937, Loomis et al. (later modified by Roth (1961), Bente et al. (1964), and others [e.g., Klimesch, 1999; Ulrich & Frick, 1986]) proposed classifications for vigilance stages occurring during transition from active wakefulness to sleep onset. They are based on the following EEG phenomena during eyes-closed, which have been confirmed by research:

- Posterior alpha mostly seen after eye-closing with a frequency of 8–12 Hz and an occipital focus. This oscillation has been referred to as "idling rhythm" (Niedermeyer, 1997) because it marks a state of relaxed wakefulness, corresponding to vigilance stage A1 according to Bente (1964) and Loomis (1937).
- Alpha power anteriorization occurs increasingly after several minutes of relaxed wakefulness. Alpha peak frequency shows a slight decrease. This phenomenon is reported to occur during transition to drowsiness (Broughton & Hasan, 1995; Connemann et al., 2005; De Gennaro, Ferrara, Curcio, & Cristiani, 2001; De Gennaro et al., 2004; De Gennaro et al., 2005; Pivik & Harman, 1995) and corresponds to vigilance stage A2 and A3 (Bente, 1964; Loomis et al., 1937).
- Low voltage EEG is increasingly observed during lower vigilance stages. The alpha rhythm disappears (alpha drop-out) and beta power increases (De Gennaro, Ferrara & Bertini, 2001; Merica & Fortune, 2004; Tanaka, Hayashi, & Hori, 1996, 1997). This EEG pattern corresponds to vigilance stage B1 (Roth, 1961). The EEG in this state is similar to the EEG during intense mental activity and eyes-open condition.
- Increased delta and theta activity is observed in parallel with increasing subjective drowsiness (Strijkstra, Beersma, Drayer, Halbesma, & Daan, 2003; Tanaka et al., 1996, 1997), corresponding to vigilance stages B2 and B3 (Roth, 1961).
- The occurrence of K-complexes and sleep spindles mark the beginning of definite sleep (Cash et al., 2009; De Gennaro & Ferrara, 2003; Tanaka et al., 1997).

Based on these EEG features a computer-based algorithm has been created for separating different EEG-vigilance stages (Figure 4.5) for consecutive EEG segments. The first version of the algorithm "VIGALL" (Vigilance Algorithm Leipzig) was based upon the Fast Fourier-derived power of the four main EEG frequency bands alpha, beta, delta, and theta during 2-second segments of continuous EEG data at different sites. An improved second version of the algorithm now takes into account the intra-cortical source power (derived by low resolution tomography, LORETA) of

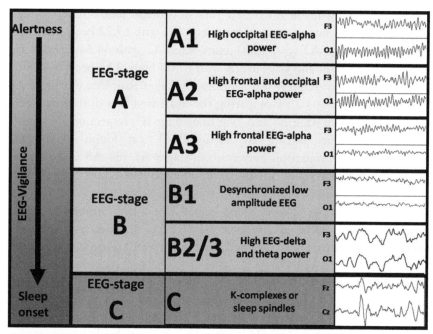

Figure 4.5 EEG-vigilance stages on the continuum from high to low vigilance levels (left column). The main criteria of the EEG-vigilance classification algorithm are given for six distinct EEG-vigilance stages (middle columns). Examples of native two-second EEG curves are presented in the right column.

different regions of interest (ROIs). The segment length is technically not restricted to a minimum duration because the power is computed by complex demodulation instead of Fourier transformation with its reciprocal relationship between segment length and usable frequency resolution.

Validation of EEG Vigilance

EEG Vigilance and the Autonomous Nervous System

Further evidence for the validity of the EEG-vigilance concept comes from results of studies concerning the functional level of the autonomic nervous system (ANS). Its two counteracting parts, the sympathetic and the parasympathetic branch, regulate homeostatic processes for adapting the organism to actual needs, e.g. increased blood flow and sweating during a fight-or-flight reaction in case of danger (increased sympathetic tone) or decreased breathing frequency and increased metabolic activity during the resting phase (increased parasympathetic tone). It was found that average heart rates decreased from stage A1 with 67.22 beats per minute (bpm) to stage A2 with 65.31 bpm, stage A3 with 64.54 bpm, stage B1 with 63.28 bpm and stage B2/3 with 61.06 bpm. The heart beat rate related to vigilance stage A was significantly larger than that during stage B (T $=$ 2.90, p $<$0.02). Comparing the heart beat rate during the sub-stages of "vigilance stage A" and "vigilance stage B", respectively, a significantly higher rate during B1 versus B2/3 was found (T $=$ 2.92, p $<$0.02). The comparison between sub-stages A1 and A3 failed to be significant after correction for the three multiple t-tests, but there was a trend towards a higher heart beat rate during vigilance stage A1 versus A3 (T $=$ 2.38, p $<$0.04). These results suggest that a decrease of the global functional brain levels, as assessable by VIGALL goes in parallel with decreased sympathetic and increased parasympathetic activity.

Switching Between Different EEG-Vigilance Stages

The EEG-vigilance algorithm and the underlying concept imply that decline of vigilance during rest follows a certain order from high to low vigilance stages. Hence it would be expected that switches between neighboring stages occur more often than switches to more distant stages. The analysis of 15 resting EEGs (Olbrich et al., 2009) showed that the real transition probabilities (rTP) of all switches between vigilance stages differed indeed from the expected transition probabilities (eTP) (see Figure 4.6). Switches between neighboring stages occurred significantly more often than a random process would reveal. These findings underline that the vigilance stage sequences during rest follow a certain order and give further validity to the EEG-vigilance algorithm VIGALL.

EEG-Vigilance Regulation in Psychiatric Disorders

As described earlier, changes in vigilance are also related to behavior. A decrease in vigilance or an "unstable" vigilance regulation can lead to two different behaviors: (1) the organism decides to go to sleep and the vigilance reverts to sleep stages or, (2) the organism exhibits "autostabilization behavior" to counter-regulate their vigilance level such as hyperactivity and sensation-seeking behavior. Figure 4.7 depicts this process in more detail. A physiological or "normal" vigilance regulation decreases over time. However, there are two deviating patterns of vigilance regulation – as can be seen in the figure – namely the "rigid regulation" and the "labile regulation". The first example of rigid regulation is characterized

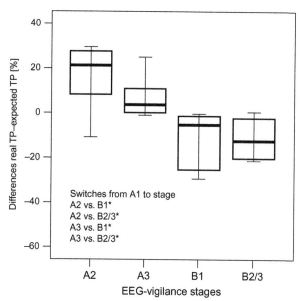

Figure 4.6 The differences between real (rTP) and expected (eTP) transition probabilities for stage A1 were significantly higher for switches to stages A2 and A3 than for switches to stages B1 and B2/3. This indicates that vigilance decline is a more or less homogeneous process with switches between neighboring EEG-vigilance stages occurring more often than switches between distant vigilance stages. *(After Olbrich et al., 2009.)*

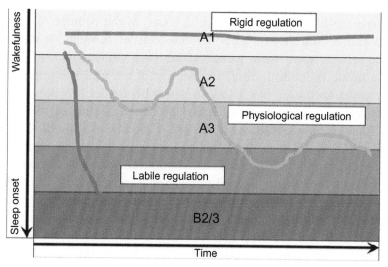

Figure 4.7 The different modes of vigilance regulation, namely the rigid regulation, a physiological or "normal" regulation, and a labile vigilance regulation.

by an inability to downregulate one's vigilance level and such individuals might avoid additional external stimulation and withdraw themselves as autoregulatory behavior. This is a behavioral pattern that is also often seen in depression. In contrast to this, individuals characterized by a labile regulation have an inability to maintain their vigilance level and/or exhibit unstable vigilance regulation. This type of vigilance regulation could induce a vigilance autostabilization behavior characterized by hyperactivity, sensation-seeking, and other behavioral patterns to create a highly stimulating environment. The resulting increase in external stimulation counteracts the impending vigilance decline and leads to a stabilization of vigilance. An everyday example would be the hyperactive, "high-spirited" behavior of overtired children. This behavioral pattern matches the behavior also seen in ADHD and mania.

Mania and Depression

Manic patients do not appear to be sleepy or tired. When evaluating EEG recordings of such patients, one would expect to find signs of a cortical hyperarousal. However, when studied under resting conditions with eyes closed, acutely manic patients consistently show rapid declines in vigilance within the first minute of EEG recording (Bschor, Müller-Oerlinghausen & Ulrich, 2001; Ulrich, 1994; Van Sweden, 1986); a sub-group (19%) even shows signs of micro sleeps (defined as abrupt intrusion of sleep spindles) within the first 10 seconds (Small, Milstein, & Medlock, 1997). This finding generally has been neglected in theories on the pathophysiology of mania and is difficult to incorporate into current concepts. It does not appear to be a mere consequence of the sleep deficits often occurring within manic episodes. Instead, a causal role of the vigilance impairment in the pathomechanism of mania is suggested by the fact that sleep deficits can trigger or worsen hypomanic and/or manic syndromes in patients with bipolar disorders (Barbini, Bertelli, Colombo & Smeraldi, 1996; Wehr, 1992). Some symptoms of mania can be interpreted as autoregulatory reactions of the organism aimed to counteract the vigilance instability by increasing the level of external stimulation (Hegerl et al., 2008). While this might lead to vigilance stabilization, in many cases a vicious circle is initiated since this behavioral syndrome and the associated lack of sleepiness may aggravate the sleep deficit as well as the instability of vigilance regulation resulting in a vicious circle. According to this concept, most publications on treatment of mania using vigilance stabilizing agents such as psychostimulants reported an improvement within one or two hours of

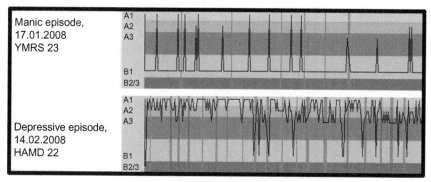

Figure 4.8 Time course of EEG-vigilance stages for consecutive 2-second segments of a 10-minute resting EEG in a patient with bipolar affective disorder during a manic episode (top: Young Mania Rating Scale 23) and during depression (bottom: Hamilton Depression Score 22). Labile vigilance regulation is found during the manic state while during depression the vigilance level does not drop to low vigilance stages. Vertical lines mark segments with artifacts.

first dose (Beckmann & Heinemann, 1976; Brown & Mueller, 1979; Bschor et al., 2001).

In contrast to the unstable vigilance regulation in mania, a hyperstable vigilance regulation may be observed during depressive episodes (Ulrich, 1994). This goes in parallel with a difficulty falling asleep, an inner restlessness, and a hyperactivity of the hypothalamic–pituitary–adrenal axis often found in depressed patients. One could hypothesize that depressive symptomatology with sensation avoidance and withdrawal may serve an autoregulatory function to counteract a hyperstable vigilance regulation. Also see Figure 4.8 for a case example of a bipolar patient recorded in his manic episode (top) and depressive episode (bottom) and the obtained EEG-vigilance stages. This example clearly shows that − within subject − a labile vigilance regulation is associated with the manic phase, whereas a rigid vigilance regulation is associated with the depressive phase of the disorder.

Vigilance Regulation in Attention Deficit Hyperactivity Disorder (ADHD)

Support for an unstable vigilance regulation in ADHD is provided by the fact that this disorder is associated with sleepiness and shortened mean sleep latency in the Multiple Sleep Latency Test, a finding that is not explained by differences in preceding nocturnal sleep (Golan, Shahar, Ravid, & Pillar, 2004). Furthermore, there is convincing empirical evidence that

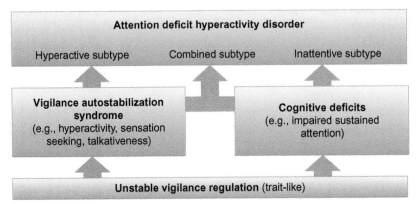

Figure 4.9 Overview of the relation between an unstable vigilance regulation and the behavioral symptoms of ADHD. *(Adapted from Hegerl, Sander, Olbrich, & Schoenknecht, 2009.)*

disorders affecting sleep quality (e.g. restless legs syndrome, periodic limb movement syndrome) are associated with pediatric ADHD or increased ADHD severity (e.g. Chervin et al., 2002). Also, ADHD-like behavior can be induced in children by sleep restriction (Fallone, Acebo, Arnedt, Seifer, & Carskadon, 2001; Golan et al., 2004) and improved by reducing sleep deficits (Dahl, Pelham, & Wierson, 1991).

Taken together, these data suggest that a labile vigilance regulation is a pathogenetic factor in ADHD. Some symptoms of ADHD can be seen as a direct result of the unstable vigilance regulation (deficits in sustained attention, distractibility), while other symptoms (e.g. hyperactivity, "sensation-seeking") can be interpreted as vigilance stabilizing syndrome, as is summarized in Figure 4.9. Therefore, the well-documented effectiveness of psychostimulants in pediatric ADHD (Pliszka, 2007) could be explained by their vigilance stabilizing property.

In another study Sander et al. (2010), using the same data as Arns et al. (2008), directly investigated EEG-vigilance regulation in children with ADHD, and its relationship to treatment outcome after stimulant medication. In Figure 4.10 the amount of time spent per vigilance stage is plotted.

As hypothesized, the results show that ADHD patients spent significantly less time in A1-stages than controls, and compared to controls tended to remain longer in A2-stages, suggesting children with ADHD indeed showed lower EEG vigilance. Comparable results were found when age was included as a covariate. Furthermore, when comparing the percentage rate of stage-switches (corrected for switches into, between, and out of segments

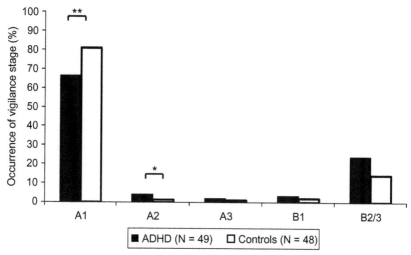

Figure 4.10 Percentage occurrence of vigilance stages A1, A2, and B2/3 in ADHD-patients (black) compared to healthy controls (white) during 2 minutes of resting EEG with closed eyes. The ADHD patients showed more A2 and less A1 stages, suggesting an unstable or labile vigilance regulation. *(After Sander et al., 2010.)*

containing artifacts), ADHD patients were shown to switch between different vigilance stages more often than controls (ADHD: 26.02%; Controls: 19.09%), indicating a less stable vigilance regulation in ADHD.

Subjects were also classified according to their "predominant EEG vigilance stage" over the entire recording period. Thirty-eight subjects in the ADHD group (77.6%) and 43 subjects in the control group (89.6%) were classified as "A1-type", 10 ADHD patients (20.4%) and 4 controls (8.3%) as "B2/3-type", and 1 subject from both groups was classified as "B1-type". Although the trends were in the expected direction (higher percentage of ADHD children with lower EEG vigilance), no significant differences between the ADHD and control group were found. The relationship between the "predominant EEG vigilance stage" and treatment outcome after stimulant medication was investigated as can be seen in Figure 4.11. The "low vigilance" group consisted of the ADHD children with predominantly B stages in their EEG whereas the "high vigilance" group consisted of the ADHD children with predominantly A stages in the EEG. The "low vigilance" group achieved worse pre-treatment results as compared to the "high vigilance" group on all continuous performance test (CPT) scores (slower mean reaction time with less standard deviation, more false positives, false negatives, and total errors) and, after

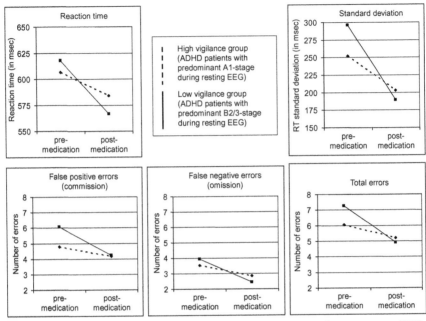

Figure 4.11 Results of the ADHD group on the continuous performance test (CPT). Subjects performed the CPT in non-medicated state (pre-treatment) and after at least 4 weeks of medication with stimulants (methylphenidate, dexamphetamine). Shown separately are the results of those ADHD patients whose resting EEG showed signs of an unstable vigilance (low vigilance group, N = 10), resulting in a greater proportion of time spent in lower vigilance stages, compared to those ADHD patients who exhibited predominantly higher A1-stages during the 2 minutes of resting EEG (high vigilance group, N = 30). *(After Sander et al., 2010.)*

stimulant medication, improved most on all scores, resulting in better post-treatment performance as compared to the "high vigilance" group (see Figure 4.11). However, repeated measurement ANOVAs showed a main effect of time (pre- vs. post-treatment) for all CPT results besides the reaction times, but no significant main effect of vigilance group. For total errors, there was a tendency for a vigilance × time interaction.

In this study it was confirmed that ADHD patients spent less time in stages of higher vigilance (A1) and demonstrated more fluctuations in vigilance levels, seen as a higher number of stage switches. In general, those ADHD patients who at baseline demonstrated more signs of an unstable vigilance achieved numerically worse results on the CPT during the baseline condition. After 4 weeks of medication with methylphenidate or dexamphetamine they tended to improve better than patients who had demonstrated a higher vigilance level at baseline. The fact that these differences did not reach statistical significance, suggests that the study might have been underpowered concerning this aspect. However, findings suggest that EEG vigilance level is related to initial performance on the CPT, and tends to also predict treatment outcome numerically on most measures.

One important limitation of this study was the brevity of the available EEG data. In usual practice, EEG-vigilance classification is based on recordings of 10 minutes or longer, since differences in vigilance regulation manifest themselves only after sufficient time. By analyzing vigilance during 2 minutes of resting EEG only slight differences could be detected between ADHD patients and healthy controls. Assuming that ADHD patients do generally present with trait-like vigilance instability, one has to argue that it may have been easier to distinguish patients with more or less severe vigilance instability if longer EEG recordings had been available.

EEG PHENOTYPE MODEL

Classifying disorders as being "subtypes" of specific disorders where the subtypes match the various EEG patterns seen in the disorder is a seductive exercise. Though the clustering of EEG patterns together as subtypes may expand our understanding of client response to therapy, it still remains attached to diagnosis based on the *Diagnostic and Statistical Manual of Mental Disorders* (DSM), which is based not on physiology, but on behavior. Unfortunately, DSM classification frequently does not predict therapeutic response by individuals within the DSM grouping (as was explained above in the Personalized Medicine section).

Endophenotypes are an intermediate step between genetics and behavior, which represent the expression or lack of expression of the genetics. In 2005 the second author (J.G.) and associates submitted a paper proposing a set of EEG patterns as "phenotypes" where the genetic links were known, and as "candidate phenotypes" where the linkage to genetics remained unknown (Johnstone et al., 2005). These proposed EEG-based phenotypes are semi-stable states of neurophysiological function, and can be identified from the raw EEG waveforms.

The authors proposed a framework that permitted researchers and clinicians to describe much of the observed EEG variance with a small number of categories of phenotypical divergence. These groupings are not identical to the DSM groupings, and they are observed to cut across the DSM categories. Unlike the DSM, these phenotypes were observed to predict an individual's response to both neurofeedback and medication approaches to therapy.

Past research involving statistical analysis of electroencephalography (EEG) has documented groupings of EEG/qEEG features within psychiatric populations (John, Prichep, & Almas, 1992). And, extensive experience with clinical EEGs and QEEG across the last four decades has shown that a limited set of EEG patterns characterize the majority of the variance seen in the EEG. The proposed phenotype approach to EEG/qEEG groupings considers phenotypes as an intermediate step between genetics and behaviors, involving expression of both genetic and environmental factors. They are seen as reliable indices of brain function which can help predict response to therapy, whether with medications or with neuromodulation techniques such as neurofeedback.

Any single phenotype may be seen in a wide variety of DSM groupings, from post-traumatic encephalopathy, to affective- and attentional-related DSM groupings, like depression or ADHD. The very concept of an EEG pattern's being a "subtype" of a specific disorder seems fatally flawed due to the lack of specificity of any of these patterns for any single DSM classification (as was demonstrated above in the examples of excess theta, theta/beta ratio, and frontal alpha asymmetry). It is our opinion that transcending the limited perspective of the DSM through the use of the EEG phenotypes will result in improved outcomes. Of course, this will need to be validated by results of research and clinical practice.

The literature on medication response prediction suggests that a phenotypic perspective may help enhance efficacy when prescribing medication, as seen in the work by Suffin & Emory (1995), showing attentional and affective disorders to respond better to medication related to their EEG pattern than to behavior. Improved outcomes may also be seen in neurofeedback, as demonstrated in the clinical outcome improvement reported by Wright and Gunkelman (1998) when they added the EEG phenotype approach to guide neurofeedback.

EEG patterns known to be genetically linked provide a databased start for a proposed initial list of EEG phenotypic patterns. The low-voltage fast pattern was shown to have genetic correlates in a recently published study of the EEG in alcoholism (Enoch, White, Harris, Rohrbaugh, & Goldman, 2002), and by others who have identified the genetic link to gene 4's regulation over gamma amino butyric acid (GABA-A) receptors (Bierut et al., 2002) and the serotonergic HTR3B gene (Ducci et al., 2009). Furthermore, a clear relationship was recently reported between the COMT gene and alpha peak frequency, where the Val/Val genotype showed a 1.4 Hz slower APF as compared to the Met/Met group (Bodenmann et al., 2009).

Another genetically linked EEG pattern was identified in idiopathic epilepsy (Haug et al., 2003). The paroxysmal epileptiform bursts seen in the EEG in these clinical cases may occasionally exceed 400–600 microvolts, with spikes and slow components emerging from a relatively normal background EEG. In a paper surveying genetic factors in epilepsy, Kaneko, Iwasa, Okada, and Hirose (2002) showed that the most common human genetic epilepsies display a complex pattern of inheritance and that the identities of the specific genes are largely unknown, despite recent advances in genetics. They showed the genetic markers associated with certain types of epilepsy, including those with neurodegenerative characteristics and some familial idiopathic epilepsies (Haug et al., 2003). A similar pattern is seen in a group of subjects with benign childhood epilepsy with centro-temporal spikes, found in a small number of cases with de novo terminal deletions of a portion of chromosome 1q. This suggests that this chromosomal location could be a potential site for a candidate gene (Vaughn, Greenwood, Aylsworth, & Tennison, 1996).

The listing in Table 4.1 of the candidate phenotype patterns is presented for the reader's convenience, though a reading of the original 2005 article (Johnstone et al., 2005) is advised for more detail regarding implications for neurofeedback or medication response prediction.

One critical point must be remembered when viewing the listing: *the various phenotypes may coexist.* The various combinations and permutations of the phenotypes are too numerous to be handled completely in this limited chapter presentation. Thus, this list should not be construed as a replacement for professional assistance in designing a neurofeedback intervention or in prescribing medication, nor in any way can this be used to fully characterize an individual's EEG/qEEG.

Inter-rater Reliability

In Arns et al. (2008) the inter-rater reliability for rating the EEG phenotypes between two raters (MA & JG) were investigated in children with ADHD and a matched control group. The inter-rater reliabilities were found to be generally high, as can be seen in Table 4.2. This suggests that these EEG phenotypes can be reliably identified by two well-trained raters, with most Kappa values around 0.90 or better. However, persistent

Table 4.1 A summary of the EEG phenotypes

Low-voltage fast:	Low-voltage EEG with relative beta dominating
Epileptiform:	Transient spike/wave, sharp waves, paroxysmal EEG
Diffuse slow activity:	Increased delta and theta (1–7 Hz) with or without slower alpha
Focal abnormalities:	Focal slow activity or focal lack of EEG power
Mixed fast and slow:	Increased slower activity, lack of organized alpha, increased beta
Frontal lobe hypoperfusion:	Frontal theta, slow alpha, or alpha activity
Frontal asymmetries:	Frontal asymmetry (generally measured at F3, F4)
Excess temporal lobe alpha:	Increased temporal alpha activity (Kappa)
Faster alpha variants:	Alpha peak frequency greater than 11–12 Hz parietally
Spindling excessive beta:	Rhythmic beta with a spindle morphology (beware of medication effects, especially benzodiazepines)
Persistent eyes–open alpha:	Alpha does not attenuate by at least 50% with eyes open as compared to eyes closed

Table 4.2 Number of subjects in the different EEG phenotype groups and the inter-rater reliabilities for the different EEG phenotypes

	ADHD (N)	Controls (N)	Inter-rater reliability
"Normal EEG"	5	11	Kappa: 0.90; p <0.000
Frontal slow	13	9	Kappa: 0.94; p <0.000
Low APF	13	5	Kappa: 0.90; p <0.000
Frontal beta spindles	8	10	Kappa: 0.97; p <0.000
Low voltage	6	1	Kappa: 0.93; p <0.000
Frontal alpha	8	4	Kappa: 0.47; p <0.000
Persistent alpha EO	7	5	Kappa: 0.64; p <0.000
Temporal alpha	5	6	Kappa: 0.89; p <0.000
High APF	3	5	Kappa: 0.94; p <0.000

eyes-open alpha and frontal alpha phenotypes had lower inter-rater reliability. Table 4.2 shows the number of subjects per EEG phenotype subgroup, together with the exact Kappa values. For ADHD the phenotype ratings were not blind to diagnosis, which could have affected the ratings. However, given the small differences between the ADHD and control group in prevalence of EEG phenotypes, this most likely did not have a dramatic effect. For the depression EEG phenotype data the rating was performed blinded to diagnosis and similar effects are found, suggesting that blinding probably did not affect the ratings.

Prevalence of EEG Phenotypes in ADHD and Depression

Figure 4.12 shows the prevalence of the different EEG phenotypes in ADHD (top) and depression (bottom) and in matched normal controls. The depression data are unpublished and are from a group of 113 unmedicated Depressed patients and 121 matched controls and the ADHD data are from Arns et al. (2008). Note that these EEG phenotypes deviate slightly from the originally published phenotypes and that the presence of mu rhythm was also included, whereas this was not part of the original EEG phenotypes and this is in principal considered a normal variant type EEG.

The ADHD group tended to show a higher occurrence of frontal slow, slow APF, and low voltage EEG as compared to the control group. However, the Mann–Whitney test found a significant difference only between the ADHD and control group for the low APF (p = 0.038; Z = −2.076) and a near significant difference for the low voltage EEG (p = 0.051; Z = −1.951). The difference for frontal slow was not significant (p = 0.335). This lack of effect is probably due to the low subject numbers per sub-group.

For depression, the Mann–Whitney test results showed that only the prevalence for frontal alpha (p = 0.017; Z = −2.385) and mu at C4 (p = 0.020; Z = −1.707) were significant between groups. Furthermore, One-Way ANOVA revealed no difference for age. There also was a significant difference in frontal alpha peak frequency (p = 0.025; F = 5.089; DF = 1, 214) between the depressed (9.62 Hz) and non-depressed groups (9.27 Hz), which was not different for Pz (p = 0.632; F = 0.231; DF = 1, 225), indicating the depressed clients had a faster APF at frontal sites.

It is an interesting finding that the prevalence of the different EEG phenotypes is comparable for the ADHD, depression, and control groups, demonstrating that, in principle there are no large fundamental and qualitative differences in the brain activity of these disorders. However, as was already shown in Figure 4.2, the expression of a given EEG phenotype is more deviant for the ADHD group as compared to the control group, indicating the differences have to be sought in the quantitative deviation *within* a respective phenotype, i.e. it is not the "eye color" but the intensity

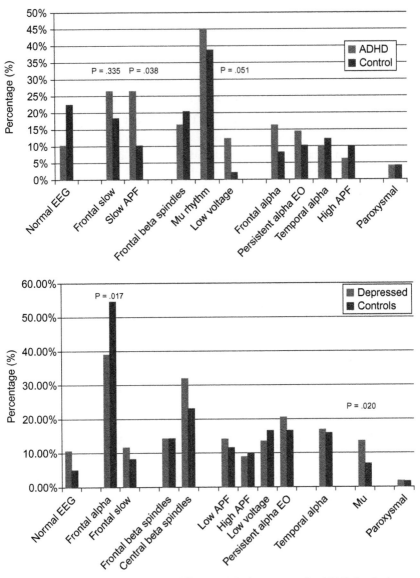

Figure 4.12 The occurrence of the different EEG phenotypes for ADHD (top), depression (bottom) and matched control groups (black). Note the higher occurrence of frontal slow, slow alpha peak frequency, and low voltage EEG in the ADHD group. For depression note the lower prevalence of frontal alpha and the higher prevalence of mu rhythm. Also note that the control group has similar prevalences of most of the EEG phenotypes and for all groups between 2 and 4% display a paroxysmal EEG.

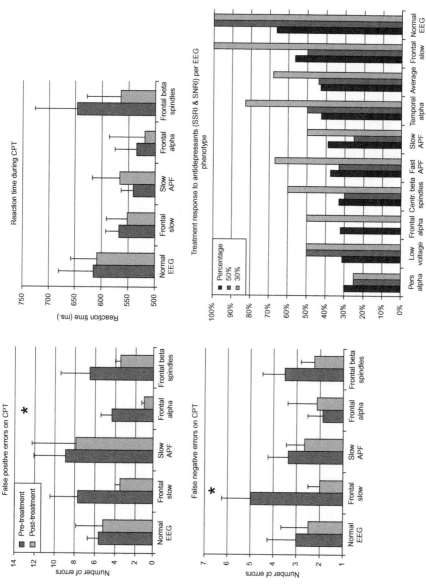

Figure 4.13 Pre-treatment and post-treatment performance for the ADHD (CPT measures: left) and depression (HAM-D measures: right) for EEG phenotypes (ADHD: N = 45; depression N = 27). (* p <0.05). (ADHD figures from Arns et al., 2008.)

of the eye color that makes the distinction between normal and pathological. Furthermore, as was also demonstrated in Arns et al. (2008), and shown in Figure 4.13, these phenotypes do predict treatment outcome to stimulant medication in ADHD. The group with frontal slow EEG and the group with frontal alpha both responded to stimulant medication, whereas the other groups did not. The frontal slow group also performed worst initially suggesting a relation between their frontal slow EEG and inattention during intake. Importantly, these data also clearly demonstrate that the slowed APF group does not respond to stimulant medication, thereby further emphasizing the need to separate the slow APF from the frontal slow group (as noted above in the theta/beta ratio discussion).

In regard to depression, only a limited sub-sample of 27 subjects' post-treatment HAM-D scores were available. These data are currently published in the *Journal of Affective Disorders* (Spronk et al., 2010) and data suggest for this group an integrative approach employing neuropsychological data, genetic data, and ERP data predicted treatment outcome best. In Figure 4.13 the EEG phenotypes showing the largest decrease in HAM-D scores due to antidepressant medication are shown. Although results have to be treated with caution due to very low subject numbers, these data suggest that the frontal alpha phenotype (a reasonably large sub-group of N = 10) does not predict treatment outcome well (in contrast to what would be expected based on work of Suffin & Emory [1995] and others).

EEG PHENOTYPE VS. EEG VIGILANCE: TOWARDS A COHERENT MODEL?

In this chapter we have reviewed the history of EEG findings in ADHD and depression and presented some new data employing the EEG Vigilance model and the EEG Phenotype model. We have pointed out that some of the older concepts such as excess theta, theta/beta ratio, and frontal alpha asymmetry have many limitations such as low specificity and low predictive validity and hence their use in predicting treatment outcome or guiding treatment is limited. Both the EEG Vigilance approach and EEG Phenotype approach have shown some promise in predicting treatment outcome, but have also shown some limitations. Below we discuss the presented data in a somewhat more detailed way and strive to incorporate these results in a more coherent framework with Personalized Medicine as the goal in mind.

Similarities Between EEG Phenotypes and EEG Vigilance

From the previous two sections it should be clear that there are similarities among the qualitatively different EEG phenotypes on one hand and the EEG vigilance stages on the other hand. In the EEG Vigilance model, several "phenotypes" are seen as involving state changes related to vigilance, such as the frontal alpha being similar to vigilance stage A3, or the frontal slow similar to vigilance stage B3. At first sight, this appears to be contradictory; phenotypes are by definition regarded as stable − trait like − biomarkers, which should not be susceptible to state changes. However, the EEG Vigilance model has shown that several of these EEG phenotypes can occur within the same subject as time progresses with corresponding probabilities of switching from stage A1 to stage A2 vigilance. On the other hand Hegerl also proposed EEG-vigilance regulation as a *state-dependent trait* (Hegerl et al., 2008), suggesting the EEG Vigilance approach is not just state-related. Given these similarities in these models we propose that the "EEG phenotype" in this respect can be interpreted as the "predominant vigilance" state of a given person. Below we will demonstrate this further based on the data presented in the previous sections.

In the EEG Phenotype studies, what was classified as a "normal EEG" was in reality an EEG that could not be classified in any of the EEG phenotypes, often consisting of regular and well-developed parieto-occipital alpha, or stage A1 in EEG Vigilance terms.

ADHD

ADHD was characterized by an increased incidence of frontal slow (not significant) and low voltage EEG. Furthermore, there was a tendency for increased frontal alpha and decreased "normal EEG" in ADHD. These results are all in line with the EEG Vigilance results, suggesting a labile vigilance regulation (frontal slow = B3; low voltage = B1; frontal alpha = A3) and normal controls demonstrated higher EEG vigilance (more "normal" EEG = A1). Furthermore, the EEG phenotypes characterized by this "lower vigilance" level (frontal slow = B3 and frontal alpha = A3) also were the only groups responding to stimulant medication.

Depression

Depression was characterized by a lower occurrence of the frontal alpha EEG phenotype and a higher occurrence of a "normal" EEG (not significant) suggesting less A3 and more A1 EEG-vigilance stages. These results hence support a rigid vigilance regulation in depression (Ulrich, 1994). This goes in parallel with a difficulty falling asleep, an inner restlessness, and a hyperactivity of the hypothalamic–pituitary–adrenal axis often found in depressed patients. In line with the EEG vigilance and the auto-stabilization concept it is understandable that depressive symptomatology with sensation avoidance and withdrawal may have the autoregulatory function to counteract the hyperstable vigilance regulation.

Unique Contributions of Both Methods

The unique contribution from the EEG Phenotype model is the identification of a slow APF group, which was shown to be a group that does not respond to stimulant medication. In the EEG Vigilance model APF does not play a role. As a matter of fact the algorithm "personalizes" EEG frequency bands based on the individual APF, thereby ensuring the individual APF does not contaminate the data. Therefore, in ADHD there is a large sub-group of children with a slow APF, who do not respond well to treatment with stimulant medication. Their symptomatology cannot be explained by a labile vigilance regulation and autostabilization behavior. Therefore, it is important that future studies investigate what treatments are best suited for treating this sub-group of ADHD. Neurofeedback in the treatment of ADHD has shown great promise (Arns et al., 2009) but at this moment it is not known if children with a slow APF are also among the children who respond well to neurofeed-back. Several studies have employed rTMS at or above the APF with good results in schizophrenia (Jin et al., 2006), in healthy people to improve cognitive function (Klimesch, Sauseng, & Gerloff, 2003) but without an improved effect in depression (Arns, Spronk, & Fitzgerald, 2010). It is obvious that more research is required to find appropriate treatment for patients with a slowed APF.

Some specific EEG phenotypes have not been covered extensively in this chapter, but do deserve further study. For example the beta-spindle or beta excess sub-group — which has been observed in ADHD (Arns et al., 2008; Chabot et al., 1996; Clarke et al., 1998; Clarke et al., 2001b) — rarely has been investigated. And, in depression research cited earlier, it was shown that a very large proportion of the depressive patients ($>30\%$) exhibited beta spindles at Cz and these also tended to respond unfavorably to antidepressant medication (see Figure 4.13). Finally, from many studies it has become clear that a small sub-group with paroxysmal EEG is found in both patient populations as well as control groups. Although these cannot be considered as status epilepticus, there is some evidence suggesting this brain pattern has behavioral implications (Lennox-Buchtal et al., 1960) and may require a different treatment approach such as anticonvulsants or SMR/SCP neurofeedback.

Whereas the EEG phenotype approach is based on visual inspection of the EEG and hence subject to interpretation, the biggest advantage of the EEG Vigilance approach is that it is a quantified approach using a computer algorithm, and hence may be considered more objective. However, there are no reliable norms or cut-off scores available yet to classify EEG vigilance stages into "normal" or "deviating" values. Furthermore, with the EEG Vigilance approach it is very hard to distinguish the true B1 (alpha drop-out, low-voltage beta stage) stage from a desynchronized EEG due to cognitive processing.

At this time there is no single framework, theory or approach that can be used to interpret all EEG and qEEG findings. In this chapter we attempted to explain a small part of the large spectrum of related findings, and provide a theoretical framework based on the Vigilance model, and its relationship to EEG and behaviors. Obviously, much more research is required to understand the role of psychophysiology (EEG, ERPs) in the future of Personalized Medicine.

ACKNOWLEDGMENTS

We wish to acknowledge the data used from the Brain Resource International Database (BRID), Werner van den Bergh for fruitful discussions on this topic, and Pim Drinkenburg and Leon Kenemans for the great collaboration, which will hopefully evolve the concepts of Personalized Medicine further.

REFERENCES

Allen, J. J., Harmon-Jones, E., & Cavender, J. H. (2001). Manipulation of frontal EEG asymmetry through biofeedback alters self-reported emotional responses and facial EMG. *Psychophysiology, 38*(4), 685–693.

Allen, J. J., Urry, H. L., Hitt, S. K., & Coan, J. A. (2004). The stability of resting frontal electroencephalographic asymmetry in depression. *Psychophysiology, 41*(2), 269–280.

Arns, M., de Ridder, S., Strehl, U., Breteler, M., & Coenen, A. (2009). Efficacy of neurofeedback treatment in ADHD: The effects on inattention, impulsivity and hyperactivity: A meta-analysis. *Clinical EEG and Neuroscience: Official Journal of the EEG and Clinical Neuroscience Society (ENCS)*, *40*(3), 180–189.

Arns, M., Gunkelman, J., Breteler, M., & Spronk, D. (2008). EEG phenotypes predict treatment outcome to stimulants in children with ADHD. *Journal of Integrative Neuroscience*, *7*(3), 421–438.

Arns, M., Spronk, D., & Fitzgerald, P. B. (2010). Potential differential effects of 9 Hz rTMS and 10 Hz rTMS in the treatment of depression. *Brain Stimulation*, *3*, 124–126.

Baehr, E., Rosenfeld, J. P., & Baehr, R. (1997). The clinical use of an alpha asymmetry protocol in the neurofeedback treatment of depression: Two case studies. *Journal of Neurotherapy*, *2*(3), 10–23.

Barbini, B., Bertelli, S., Colombo, C., & Smeraldi, E. (1996). Sleep loss, a possible factor in augmenting manic episode. *Psychiatry Research*, *65*(2), 121–125.

Barry, R. J., Clarke, A. R., & Johnstone, S. J. (2003). A review of electrophysiology in attention-deficit/hyperactivity disorder: I. Qualitative and quantitative electroencephalography. *Clinical Neurophysiology*, *114*(2), 171–183.

Barry, R. J., Clarke, A. R., Johnstone, S. J., & Brown, C. R. (2009). EEG differences in children between eyes-closed and eyes-open resting conditions. *Clinical Neurophysiology*, *120*(10), 1806–1811.

Beckmann, H., & Heinemann, H. (1976). Proceedings: D-Amphetamine in manic syndrome (authors trans.). *Arzneimittel-Forschung*, *26*(6), 1185–1186.

Bente, D. (1964). *Die insuffizienz des vigilitatstonus*. Thesis, Habilitationsschrift, Erlangen.

Berger, H. (1929). Uber das Elektrenkephalogramm des Menschen. *Archiv für Psychiatrie und Nervenkranlcheiten*, *87*, 527–570.

Bierut, L. J., Saccone, N. L., Rice, J. P., Goate, A., Foroud, T., Edenberg, H., et al. (2002). Defining alcohol-related phenotypes in humans. The collaborative study on the genetics of alcoholism. *Alcohol Research and Health*, *26*(3), 208–213.

Bodenmann, S., Rusterholz, T., Dürr, R., Stoll, C., Bachmann, V., Geissler, E., et al. (2009). The functional val158met polymorphism of COMT predicts interindividual differences in brain alpha oscillations in young men. *Journal of Neuroscience*, *29*(35), 10 855–10 862.

Boutros, N., Fraenkel, L., & Feingold, A. (2005). A four-step approach for developing diagnostic tests in psychiatry: EEG in ADHD as a test case. *Journal of Neuropsychiatry and Clinical Neurosciences*, *17*(4), 455–464.

Bresnahan, S. M., Anderson, J. W., & Barry, R. J. (1999). Age-related changes in quantitative EEG in attention-deficit/hyperactivity disorder. *Biological Psychiatry*, *46*(12), 1690–1697.

Broughton, R., & Hasan, J. (1995). Quantitative topographic electroencephalographic mapping during drowsiness and sleep onset. *Journal of Clinical Neurophysiology: Official Publication of the American Electroencephalographic Society*, *12*(4), 372–386.

Brown, W. A., & Mueller, B. (1979). Alleviation of manic symptoms with catecholamine agonists. *American Journal of Psychiatry*, *136*(2), 230–231.

Bruder, G. E., Stewart, J. W., Tenke, C. E., McGrath, P. J., Leite, P., Bhattacharya, N., et al. (2001). Electroencephalographic and perceptual asymmetry differences between responders and nonresponders to an SSRI antidepressant. *Biological Psychiatry*, *49*(5), 416–425.

Bschor, T., Müller-Oerlinghausen, B., & Ulrich, G. (2001). Decreased level of EEG-vigilance in acute mania as a possible predictor for a rapid effect of methylphenidate: A case study. *Clinical EEG (Electroencephalography)*, *32*(1), 36–39.

Callaway, E., Halliday, R., & Naylor, H. (1983). Hyperactive children's event-related potentials fail to support underarousal and maturational-lag theories. *Archives of General Psychiatry*, *40*(11), 1243–1248.

Capute, A. J., Niedermeyer, E. F. L., & Richardson, F. (1968). The electroencephalogram in children with minimal cerebral dysfunction. *Pediatrics, 41*(6), 1104.

Cash, S. S., Halgren, E., Dehghani, N., Rossetti, A. O., Thesen, T., Wang, C., et al. (2009). The human k-complex represents an isolated cortical down-state. *Science (New York, NY), 324*(5930), 1084–1087.

Chabot, R. J., di Michele, F., Prichep, L., & John, E. R. (2001). The clinical role of computerized EEG in the evaluation and treatment of learning and attention disorders in children and adolescents. *Journal of Neuropsychiatry and Clinical Neurosciences, 13*(2), 171–186.

Chabot, R. J., Merkin, H., Wood, L. M., Davenport, T. L., & Serfontein, G. (1996). Sensitivity and specificity of qEEG in children with attention deficit or specific developmental learning disorders. *Clinical EEG (Electroencephalography), 27*(1), 26–34.

Chabot, R. J., Orgill, A. A., Crawford, G., Harris, M. J., & Serfontein, G. (1999). Behavioral and electrophysiologic predictors of treatment response to stimulants in children with attention disorders. *Journal of Child Neurology, 14*(6), 343.

Chabot, R. J., & Serfontein, G. (1996). Quantitative electroencephalographic profiles of children with attention deficit disorder. *Biological Psychiatry, 40*(10), 951–963.

Chervin, R. D., Archbold, K. H., Dillon, J. E., Pituch, K. J., Panahi, P., Dahl, R. E., et al. (2002). Associations between symptoms of inattention, hyperactivity, restless legs, and periodic leg movements. *Sleep, 25*(2), 213–218.

Clarke, A. R., Barry, R. J., McCarthy, R., & Selikowitz, M. (1998). EEG analysis in attention-deficit/hyperactivity disorder: A comparative study of two subtypes. *Psychiatry Research, 81*(1), 19–29.

Clarke, A. R., Barry, R. J., McCarthy, R., & Selikowitz, M. (2001a). Age and sex effects in the EEG: Differences in two subtypes of attention-deficit/hyperactivity disorder. *Clinical Neurophysiology: Official Journal of the International Federation of Clinical Neurophysiology, 112* (5), 815–826.

Clarke, A. R., Barry, R. J., McCarthy, R., & Selikowitz, M. (2001b). EEG-defined subtypes of children with attention-deficit/hyperactivity disorder. *Clinical Neurophysiology, 112*(11), 2098–2105.

Clarke, A. R., Barry, R. J., McCarthy, R., & Selikowitz, M. (2001c). Electroencephalogram differences in two subtypes of attention-deficit/hyperactivity disorder. *Psychophysiology, 38*(02), 212–221.

Clarke, A. R., Barry, R. J., McCarthy, R., & Selikowitz, M. (2001d). Excess beta activity in children with attention-deficit/hyperactivity disorder: An atypical electrophysiological group. *Psychiatry Research, 103*(2-3), 205–218.

Clarke, A. R., Barry, R. J., McCarthy, R., & Selikowitz, M. (2002a). Children with attention-deficit/hyperactivity disorder and comorbid oppositional defiant disorder: An EEG analysis. *Psychiatry Research, 111*(2-3), 181–190.

Clarke, A. R., Barry, R. J., McCarthy, R., & Selikowitz, M. (2002b). EEG analysis of children with attention-deficit/hyperactivity disorder and comorbid reading disabilities. *Journal of Learning Disabilities, 35*(3), 276.

Clarke, A. R., Barry, R. J., McCarthy, R., Selikowitz, M., Clarke, D. C., & Croft, R. J. (2003). EEG activity in girls with attention-deficit/hyperactivity disorder. *Clinical Neurophysiology: Official Journal of the International Federation of Clinical Neurophysiology, 114*(2), 319–328.

Cohn, R., & Nardini, J. E. (1958). The correlation of bilateral occipital slow activity in the human EEG with certain disorders of behavior. *American Journal of Psychiatry, 115* (1), 44–54.

Connemann, B. J., Mann, K., Lange-Asschenfeldt, C., Ruchsow, M., Schreckenberger, M., Bartenstein, P., et al. (2005). Anterior limbic alpha-like activity: A low resolution electromagnetic tomography study with lorazepam challenge. *Clinical Neurophysiology: Official Journal of the International Federation of Clinical Neurophysiology*, *116*(4), 886–894.

Dahl, R. E., Pelham, W. E., & Wierson, M. (1991). The role of sleep disturbances in attention deficit disorder symptoms: A case study. *Journal of Pediatric Psychology*, *16*(2), 229–239.

Davidson, R. J. (1998). Anterior electrophysiological asymmetries, emotion, and depression: Conceptual and methodological conundrums. *Psychophysiology*, *35*(5), 607–614.

Debener, S., Beauducel, A., Nessler, D., Brocke, B., Heilemann, H., & Kayser, J. (2000). Is resting anterior EEG alpha asymmetry a trait marker for depression? Findings for healthy adults and clinically depressed patients. *Neuropsychobiology*, *41*(1), 31–37.

DeFrance, J. F., Smith, S., Schweitzer, F. C., Ginsberg, L., & Sands, S. (1996). Topographical analyses of attention disorders of childhood. *International Journal of Neuroscience*, *87*(1-2), 41–61.

d'Elia, G., & Perris, C. (1973). Cerebral functional dominance and depression. An analysis of EEG amplitude in depressed patients. *Acta Psychiatrica Scandinavica*, *49*(3), 191.

Ducci, F., Enoch, M. A., Yuan, Q., Shen, P. H., White, K. V., Hodgkinson, C., et al. (2009). HTR3B is associated with alcoholism with antisocial behavior and alpha EEG power – an intermediate phenotype for alcoholism and co-morbid behaviors. *Alcohol*, *43*(1), 73–84.

Dykman, R. A., Ackerman, P. T., Oglesby, D. M., & Holcomb, P. J. (1982). Autonomic responsivity during visual search of hyperactive and reading-disabled children. *Pavlovian Journal of Biological Science*, *17*(3), 150–157.

Enoch, M. A., White, K. V., Harris, C. R., Rohrbaugh, J. W., & Goldman, D. (2002). The relationship between two intermediate phenotypes for alcoholism: Low voltage alpha EEG and low P300 ERP amplitude. *Journal of Studies on Alcohol*, *63*(5), 509–517.

Eysenck, H. J. (1990). Biological dimensions of personality. In L. A. Pervin (Ed.), *Handbook of personality: Theory and research* (pp. 244–276). New York: Guilford.

Fallone, G., Acebo, C., Arnedt, J. T., Seifer, R., & Carskadon, M. A. (2001). Effects of acute sleep restriction on behavior, sustained attention, and response inhibition in children. *Perceptual and Motor Skills*, *93*(1), 213–229.

De Gennaro, L., & Ferrara, M. (2003). Sleep spindles: An overview. *Sleep Medicine Reviews*, 7(5), 423–440.

De Gennaro, L., Ferrara, M., & Bertini, M. (2001). The boundary between wakefulness and sleep: Quantitative electroencephalographic changes during the sleep onset period. *Neuroscience*, *107*(1), 1–11.

De Gennaro, L., Ferrara, M., Curcio, G., & Cristiani, R. (2001). Antero-posterior EEG changes during the wakefulness–sleep transition. *Clinical Neurophysiology: Official Journal of the International Federation of Clinical Neurophysiology*, *112*(10), 1901–1911.

De Gennaro, L., Vecchio, F., Ferrara, M., Curcio, G., Rossini, P. M., & Babiloni, C. (2004). Changes in fronto-posterior functional coupling at sleep onset in humans. *Journal of Sleep Research*, *13*(3), 209–217.

De Gennaro, L., Vecchio, F., Ferrara, M., Curcio, G., Rossini, P. M., & Babiloni, C. (2005). Antero-posterior functional coupling at sleep onset: Changes as a function of increased sleep pressure. *Brain Research Bulletin*, *65*(2), 133–140.

Golan, N., Shahar, E., Ravid, S., & Pillar, G (2004). Sleep disorders and daytime sleepiness in children with attention-deficit/hyperactivity disorder. *Sleep*, *27*(2), 261–266.

Goodwin, J. E. (1947). The significance of alpha variants in the EEG, and their relationship to an epileptiform syndrome. *American Journal of Psychiatry*, *104*(6), 369–379.

Gordon, E. (2007). Integrating genomics and neuromarkers for the era of brain-related Personalized Medicine. *Personalized Medicine*, *4*(2), 201–215.

Graham, M. A., & Dietlein, L. F. (1965). Technical details of data acquisition for normative EEG reference library. Analysis of central nervous system and cardiovascular data using computer methods. *NASA SP, 72*, 433.

Hagemann, D. (2004). Individual differences in anterior EEG asymmetry: Methodological problems and solutions. *Biological Psychology, 67*(1-2), 157–182.

Hagemann, D., Naumann, E., Becker, G., Maier, S., & Bartussek, D. (1998). Frontal brain asymmetry and affective style: A conceptual replication. *Psychophysiology, 35*(4), 372–388.

Hagemann, D., Naumann, E., & Thayer, J. F. (2001). The quest for the EEG reference revisited: A glance from brain asymmetry research. *Psychophysiology, 38*(5), 847–857.

Haug, K., Warnstedt, M., Alekov, A. K., Sander, T., Ramírez, A., Poser, B., et al. (2003). Mutations in CLCN2 encoding a voltage-gated chloride channel are associated with idiopathic generalized epilepsies. *Nature Genetics, 33*(4), 527–532.

Hegerl, U., Gallinat, J., & Juckel, G. (2001). Event-related potentials. Do they reflect central serotonergic neurotransmission and do they predict clinical response to serotonin agonists? *Journal of Affective Disorders, 62*(1-2), 93–100.

Hegerl, U., Olbrich, S., Schönknecht, P., & Sander, C. (2008). Manic behavior as an autoregulatory attempt to stabilize vigilance. *Der Nervenarzt, 79*(11), 1283–1284, 1286-1290.

Hegerl, U., Sander, C., Olbrich, S., & Schoenknecht, P. (2009). Are psychostimulants a treatment option in mania? *Pharmacopsychiatry, 42*(5), 169–174.

Hegerl, U., Stein, M., Mulert, C., Mergl, R., Olbrich, S., Dichgans, E., et al. (2008). EEG-Vigilance differences between patients with borderline personality disorder, patients with obsessive-compulsive disorder and healthy controls. *European Archives of Psychiatry and Clinical Neuroscience, 258*(3), 137–143.

Henriques, J. B., & Davidson, R. J. (1990). Regional brain electrical asymmetries discriminate between previously depressed and healthy control subjects. *Journal of Abnormal Psychology, 99*(1), 22–31.

Henriques, J. B., & Davidson, R. J. (1991). Left frontal hypoactivation in depression. *Journal of Abnormal Psychology, 100*(4), 535–545.

Hermens, D. F., Cooper, N. J., Kohn, M., Clarke, S., & Gordon, E. (2005). Predicting stimulant medication response in ADHD: Evidence from an integrated profile of neuropsychological, psychophysiological and clinical factors. *Journal of Integrative Neuroscience, 4*(1), 107–121.

Hermens, D. F., Rowe, D. L., Gordon, E., & Williams, L. M. (2006). Integrative neuroscience approach to predict ADHD stimulant response. *Expert Review of Neurotherapeutics, 6*(5), 753–763.

Hughes, J. R., DeLeo, A. J., & Melyn, M. A. (2000). The electroencephalogram in attention deficit-hyperactivity disorder: Emphasis on epileptiform discharges. *Epilepsy & Behavior: E&B, 1*(4), 271–277.

Hyman, S. E. (2007). Can neuroscience be integrated into the DSM-V? *Nature Reviews Neuroscience, 8*(9), 725–732.

Janzen, T., Graap, K., Stephanson, S., Marshall, W., & Fitzsimmons, G. (1995). Differences in baseline EEG measures for ADD and normally achieving preadolescent males. *Biofeedback and Self-Regulation, 20*(1), 65–82.

Jasper, H. H., Solomon, P., & Bradley, C. (1938). Electroencephalographic analyses of behavior problem children. *American Journal of Psychiatry, 95*(3), 641.

Jin, Y., Potkin, S. G., Kemp, A. S., Huerta, S. T., Alva, G., Thai, T. M., et al. (2006). Therapeutic effects of individualized alpha frequency transcranial magnetic stimulation (alpha TMS) on the negative symptoms of schizophrenia. *Schizophrenia Bulletin, 32*(3), 556–561.

John, E. R., Prichep, L. S., & Almas, M. (1992). Subtyping of psychiatric patients by cluster analysis of QEEG. *Brain Topography, 4*(4), 321–326.

Johnstone, J., Gunkelman, J., & Lunt, J. (2005). Clinical database development: Characterization of EEG phenotypes. *Clinical EEG and Neuroscience: Official Journal of the EEG and Clinical Neuroscience Society (ENCS), 36*(2), 99–107.

Kaneko, S., Iwasa, H., Okada, M., & Hirose, S. (2002). Autosomal dominant nocturnal frontal lobe epilepsy (ADNFLE). *Ryoikibetsu Shokogun Shirizu, 37 Pt 6*, 315–317.

Keller, M. B., McCullough, J. P., Klein, D. N., Arnow, B., Dunner, D. L., Gelenberg, A. J., et al. (2000). A comparison of nefazodone, the cognitive behavioral-analysis system of psychotherapy, and their combination for the treatment of chronic depression. *New England Journal of Medicine, 342*(20), 1462–1470.

Kirsch, I., Deacon, B. J., Huedo-Medina, T. B., Scoboria, A., Moore, T. J., & Johnson, B. T. (2008). Initial severity and antidepressant benefits: A meta-analysis of data submitted to the food and drug administration. *PLoS Medicine, 5*(2), e45.

Klimesch, W. (1999). EEG alpha and theta oscillations reflect cognitive and memory performance: A review and analysis. *Brain Research Brain Research Reviews, 29*(2-3), 169–195.

Klimesch, W., Sauseng, P., & Gerloff, C. (2003). Short Communication: Enhancing cognitive performance with repetitive transcranial magnetic stimulation at human individual alpha frequency. *European Journal of Neuroscience, 17*, 1129–1133.

Kuperman, S., Johnson, B., Arndt, S., Lindgren, S., & Wolraich, M. (1996). Quantitative EEG differences in a nonclinical sample of children with ADHD and undifferentiated ADD. *Journal of the American Academy of Child and Adolescent Psychiatry, 35*(8), 1009–1017.

Lansbergen, M., Arns, M., van Dongen-Boomsma, M., Spronk, D., & Buitelaar, J. K. (in press). The increase in theta/beta ratio on resting state EEG in boys with attention-deficit/hyperactivity disorder is medicated by slow alpha peak frequency. *Progress in Neuro-Psychopharmacology and Biological Psychiatry.*

Lazzaro, I., Gordon, E., Li, W., Lim, C. L., Plahn, M., Whitmont, S., et al. (1999). Simultaneous EEG and EDA measures in adolescent attention deficit hyperactivity disorder. *International Journal of Psychophysiology: Official Journal of the International Organization of Psychophysiology, 34*(2), 123–134.

Lazzaro, I., Gordon, E., Whitmont, S., Plahn, M., Li, W., Clarke, S., et al. (1998). Quantified EEG activity in adolescent attention deficit hyperactivity disorder. *Clinical EEG (Electroencephalography), 29*(1), 37–42.

Lennox-Buchthal, M., Buchthal, F., & Rosenfalck, P. (1960). Correlation of electroencephalographic findings with crash rate of military jet pilots. *Epilepsia, 1*, 366–372.

Leuchter, A. F., Cook, I. A., Marangell, L. B., Gilmer, W. S., Burgoyne, K. S., Howland, R. H., et al. (2009). Comparative effectiveness of biomarkers and clinical indicators for predicting outcomes of SSRI treatment in major depressive disorder: Results of the BRITE-MD study. *Psychiatry Research, 169*(2), 124–131.

Loomis, A. L., Harvey, E. N., & Hobart, G. A. (1937). Cerebral states during sleep as studied by human brain potentials. *Jouranl of Experimental Psychology, 21*, 127–144.

Lubar, J. F. (1991). Discourse on the development of EEG diagnostics and biofeedback for attention-deficit/hyperactivity disorders. *Applied Psychophysiology and Biofeedback, 16*(3), 201–225.

Mann, C. A., Lubar, J. F., Zimmerman, A. W., Miller, C. A., & Muenchen, R. A. (1992). Quantitative analysis of EEG in boys with attention-deficit-hyperactivity disorder: Controlled study with clinical implications. *Pediatric Neurology, 8*(1), 30–36.

Matsuura, M., Okubo, Y., Toru, M., Kojima, T., He, Y., Hou, Y., et al. (1993). A cross-national EEG study of children with emotional and behavioral problems: A

WHO collaborative study in the Western Pacific region. *Biological Psychiatry, 34*(1-2), 59–65.

Merica, H., & Fortune, R. D. (2004). State transitions between wake and sleep, and within the ultradian cycle, with focus on the link to neuronal activity. *Sleep Medicine Reviews, 8*(6), 473–485.

Molina, B. S., Hinshaw, S. P., Swanson, J. M., Arnold, L. E., Vitiello, B., Jensen, P. S., et al. (2009). The MTA at 8 years: Prospective follow-up of children treated for combined-type ADHD in a multisite study. *Journal of the American Academy of Child and Adolescent Psychiatry, 48*(5), 484–500.

Monastra, V. J., Lubar, J. F., Linden, M., VanDeusen, P., Green, G., Wing, W., et al. (1999). Assessing attention deficit hyperactivity disorder via quantitative electroencephalography: An initial validation study. *Neuropsychology, 13*(3), 424–433.

Myslobodsky, M. S., Bar-Ziv, J., van Praag, H., & Glicksohn, J. (1989). Bilateral alpha distribution and anatomic brain asymmetries. *Brain Topography, 1*(4), 229–235.

Myslobodsky, M. S., Coppola, R., & Weinberger, D. R. (1991). EEG laterality in the era of structural brain imaging. *Brain Topography, 3*(3), 381–390.

Niedermeyer, E. (1997). Alpha rhythms as physiological and abnormal phenomena. *International Journal of Psychophysiology: Official Journal of the International Organization of Psychophysiology, 26*(1-3), 31–49.

Niedermeyer, E., & Da Silva, F. H. L. (2004). *Electroencephalography: Basic principles, clinical applications, and related fields*. Philadelphia, PA: Lippincott Williams & Wilkins.

Nierenberg, A. A. (2010). The perfect storm: CNS drug development in trouble. *CNS Spectrums, 15*(5), 282–283.

Olbrich, S., Mulert, C., Karch, S., Trenner, M., Leicht, G., Pogarell, O., et al. (2009). EEG-Vigilance and BOLD effect during simultaneous EEG/fMRI measurement. *Neuroimage, 45*(2), 319–332.

Piccart-Gebhart, M. J., Procter, M., Leyland-Jones, B., Goldhirsch, A., Untch, M., Smith, I., et al. (2005). Trastuzumab after adjuvant chemotherapy in her2-positive breast cancer. *New England Journal of Medicine, 353*(16), 1659–1672.

Pivik, R. T., & Harman, K. (1995). A reconceptualization of EEG alpha activity as an index of arousal during sleep: All alpha activity is not equal. *Journal of Sleep Research, 4*(3), 131–137.

Pliszka, S. R. (2007). Pharmacologic treatment of attention-deficit/hyperactivity disorder: Efficacy, safety and mechanisms of action. *Neuropsychology Review, 17*(1), 61–72.

Reid, S. A., Duke, L. M., & Allen, J. J. (1998). Resting frontal electroencephalographic asymmetry in depression: Inconsistencies suggest the need to identify mediating factors. *Psychophysiology, 35*(4), 389–404.

Richter, P. L., Zimmerman, E. A., Raichle, M. E., & Liske, E. (1971). Electroencephalograms of 2,947 united states air force academy cadets (1965-1969). *Aerospace Medicine, 42*(9), 1011–1014.

Roth, B. (1961). The clinical and theoretical importance of EEG rhythms corresponding to states of lowered vigilance. *Electroencephalography and Clinical Neurophysiology, 13,* 395–399.

Roth, M., Kay, D. W., Shaw, J., & Green, J. (1957). Prognosis and pentothal induced electroencephalographic changes in electro-convulsive treatment; an approach to the problem of regulation of convulsive therapy. *Electroencephalography and Clinical Neurophysiology, 9*(2), 225–237.

Rush, A. J., Trivedi, M. H., Wisniewski, S. R., Nierenberg, A. A., Stewart, J. W., Warden, D., et al. (2006). Acute and longer-term outcomes in depressed outpatients requiring one or several treatment steps: A STAR D report. *American Journal of Psychiatry, 163*(11), 1905–1917.

Sander, C., Arns, M., Olbrich, S., & Hegerl, U. (2010). EEG-Vigilance and response to stimulants in paediatric patients with attention deficit/hyperactivity disorder. *Clinical Neurophysiology, 121*(9), 1511–1518.

Satterfield, J. H., Cantwell, D. P., Saul, R. E., Lesser, L. I., & Podosin, R. L. (1973). Response to stimulant drug treatment in hyperactive children: Prediction from EEG and neurological findings. *Journal of Autism and Childhood Schizophrenia, 3*(1), 36–48.

Satterfield, J. H., Lesser, L. I., & Podosin, R. L. (1971). Evoked cortical potentials in hyperkinetic children. *California Medicine, 115*(3), 48.

Schaffer, C. E., Davidson, R. J., & Saron, C. (1983). Frontal and parietal electroencephalogram asymmetry in depressed and nondepressed subjects. *Biological Psychiatry, 18*(7), 753–762.

Small, J. G., Milstein, V., & Medlock, C. E. (1997). Clinical EEG findings in mania. *Clinical EEG (Electroencephalography), 28*(4), 229–235.

Spronk, D., Arns, M., Barnett, K. J., Cooper, N. J., & Gordon, E. (2010). An investigation of EEG, genetic and cognitive markers of treatment response to antidepressant medication in patients with major depressive disorder: A pilot study. *Journal of Affective Disorders*, doi:10.1016/j.jad.2010.06.021.

Steriade, M., Gloor, P., Llinás, R. R., Lopes de Silva, F. H., & Mesulam, M. M. (1990). Report of IFCN committee on basic mechanisms. Basic mechanisms of cerebral rhythmic activities. *Electroencephalography and Clinical Neurophysiology, 76*(6), 481–508.

Stevens, J. R., Sachdev, K., & Milstein, V. (1968). Behavior disorders of childhood and the electroencephalogram. *Archives of Neurology, 18*(2), 160.

Strijkstra, A. M., Beersma, D. G., Drayer, B., Halbesma, N., & Daan, S. (2003). Subjective sleepiness correlates negatively with global alpha (8-12 hz) and positively with central frontal theta (4–8 hz) frequencies in the human resting awake electroencephalogram. *Neuroscience Letters, 340*(1), 17–20.

Suffin, S. C., & Emory, W. H. (1995). Neurometric subgroups in attentional and affective disorders and their association with pharmacotherapeutic outcome. *Clinical EEG (Electroencephalography), 26*(2), 76–83.

Tanaka, H., Hayashi, M., & Hori, T. (1996). Statistical features of hypnagogic EEG measured by a new scoring system. *Sleep (New York, NY), 19*(9), 731–738.

Tanaka, H., Hayashi, M., & Hori, T. (1997). Topographical characteristics and principal component structure of the hypnagogic EEG. *Sleep, 20*(7), 523–534.

Tomarken, A. J., Davidson, R. J., Wheeler, R. E., & Kinney, L. (1992). Psychometric properties of resting anterior EEG asymmetry: Temporal stability and internal consistency. *Psychophysiology, 29*(5), 576–592.

Ulrich, G. (1994). *Psychiatrische Elektroenzephalographie* Jena: Gustav Fischer Verlag.

Ulrich, G., & Frick, K. (1986). A new quantitative approach to the assessment of stages of vigilance as defined by spatiotemporal EEG patterning. *Perceptual and Motor Skills, 62*(2), 567–576.

Van Sweden, B. (1986). Disturbed vigilance in mania. *Biological Psychiatry, 21*(3), 311–313.

Vaughn, B. V., Greenwood, R. S., Aylsworth, A. S., & Tennison, M. B. (1996). Similarities of EEG and seizures in del (1q) and benign rolandic epilepsy. *Pediatric Neurology, 15*(3), 261–264.

Wehr, T. A. (1992). Improvement of depression and triggering of mania by sleep deprivation. *JAMA, 267*(4), 548–551.

Wright, C. & Gunkelman, J. (1998). QEEG evaluation doubles the rate of clinical success. Series data and case studies. Austin, TX, Society for the Study of Neuronal Regulation, 6th Annual Conference.

Wundt, W. M. (1874). *Grundzüge der physiologischen Psychologie* Leipzig: W. Engelman.

Zuckerman, M. (1985). Sensation seeking, mania, and monoamines. *Neuropsychobiology,* *13*(3), 121–128.

PART Two

Endogenous Neuromodulation Strategies

CHAPTER 5

Neurofeedback with Children with Attention Deficit Hyperactivity Disorder: A Randomized Double-Blind Placebo-Controlled Study

Roger J. deBeus[1] and David A. Kaiser[2]
[1]Department of Psychiatry and Behavioral Sciences, Quillen College of Medicine, East Tennessee State University, Johnson City, Tennessee, USA
[2]Wavestate Inc., Marina Del Ray, California, USA

Contents

Neurofeedback and Neuromodulation Techniques and Applications
DOI: 10.1016/B978-0-12-382235-2.00005-6

INTRODUCTION

Attention deficit hyperactivity disorder (ADHD) is the most common childhood mental health disorder, with an estimated prevalence of 7% to 10% in boys and 3% in girls aged 4–11 years (Sgrok, Roberts, Grossman, & Barozzine, 2000). ADHD is characterized by inattention, distractibility, hyperactivity, or excessive impulsivity, symptoms that cause impairment in more than one setting and cannot be explained by another disorder such as brain injury, a mood disorder, or an anxiety disorder (American Psychiatric Association [DSM-IV-TR], 2000). As many as 4 out of 5 children diagnosed with this disorder continue to suffer from attention problems in adolescence and adulthood (Monastra, 2005).

Anatomically, in terms of brain organization, many of these children exhibit immature development of frontostriatal circuitry (Clarke, Barry, McCarthy, & Selikowitz, 2001) along with other structural and functional brain disturbances including the cerebellum and parietal cortices (Cherkasova & Hechtman, 2009). There are also physiological components to ADHD that have been measured using quantitative electroencephalograph (qEEG). An elevated theta-to-beta power ratio, where theta exceeds beta activity many times over, has been used as an index of attentional dysregulation for more than 20 years (Barry, Clarke, Johnstone, McCarthy, & Selikowitz, 2009; Lubar, 1991; Lubar & Lubar, 1984; Satterfield, Schell, Backs, & Hidaka, 1984). Many ADHD children show variations of excessive slow-wave and fast-wave activity over the frontal cortex (Clarke et al., 2001). Chabot & Serfontein (1996) identified ADHD children's qEEG profiles consisting of: (1) increased focal theta localized within frontal and/or midline regions 92% of the time; (2) increased alpha localized within posterior and/or midline regions 84.1% of the time; (3) increased beta occurred in 13.1% localized in frontal and/or posterior regions.

Established Treatments for ADHD

The best documented and most widely used treatment for ADHD is stimulant medication. These studies show a robust effect in group data, with placebo-controlled effect sizes (Cohen's d) from 0.7 to 1.5 on parent and teacher ratings of attention and behavior (Arnold, 2004). Unfortunately, the response rate at the individual patient level is often less than satisfactory. An example of this can be gleaned from the 579-subject NIMH Multimodal Treatment Study of Children with ADHD (the MTA, MTA

Cooperative Group, 1999). This study randomly assigned rigorously diagnosed children aged 7−9 to one of four treatment conditions: (1) intensive medication management (MedMgt); (2) intensive behavioral treatment (Beh); (3) combination of intensive medication and behavioral treatments (Comb); (4) community-care comparison (CC), 2/3 of whom obtained stimulant medication from their community physician. Swanson et al. (2001) re-analyzed the MTA data to determine the percentage with satisfactory (near-normal) outcome after 14 months of treatment. These authors reported the following success rates for each group: MedMgt (56%), Beh (34%), Comb (68%), CC (25%). Even with the combination treatment, not available in most communities, almost 1/3 in the MTA study and 3/4 in the community were still left with less than completely optimal results.

Side effects of methylphenidate (Ritalin), one of the most popular psychostimulants used to mask or reduce ADHD symptoms in children, are the following: loss or delay of height (Faraone, Biederman, Morley, & Spencer, 2008); diminished sleep (Galland, Tripp, & Taylor, 2009); appetite problems (Sonuga-Barke, Coghill, Wigal, DeBacker, & Swanson, 2009); increased risk of suicide in pre-adolescents, aged 11−14 years (McCarthy, Cranswick, Potts, Taylor, & Wong, 2009); nervousness, headaches, and tachycardia (Klein-Schwartz, 2002). Further, in a study examining medication adherence in a subset of the MTA study, parents' reports were not consistent with saliva assays in almost half of the cases (Pappadopulos et al., 2009), indicating that compliance was not consistent with what the parents were reporting. Findings also indicated that non-adherence produced greater deleterious effects in children in the MedMgt condition compared with those receiving both medication and behavioral treatment. The combination of less than optimal outcomes, side effects and parents' or caretakers' failures to give medications suggests that behavioral methods play an important role in the treatment of ADHD.

Behavioral treatments can also be effective at treating this disorder (e.g., Pelham & Fabiano, 2008; Reeves & Anthony, 2009). Behavioral treatments include instructional programs to assist parents and teachers in identifying and assisting children with attention problems, and training programs where children are taught to take responsibility for monitoring and managing their own behavior (DuPaul & Stoner, 2003). Nearly two years after MTA's behavioral treatment finished, there had been no loss in its effectiveness and the majority of children who received it were still unmedicated (Jensen et al., 2007).

Use of Neurofeedback for Management of ADHD

Neurofeedback (NF) refers to operant conditioning of electroencephalographic (EEG) rhythms: healthy, age-appropriate brainwave activity is rewarded with visual, auditory, or even tactile stimulation, and undesirable activity is ignored or punished (Sterman, 1996). Neurofeedback to reduce ADHD symptoms has been studied for nearly 35 years (Lubar & Bahler, 1976; Lubar & Shouse, 1976). As a person becomes successful in regulating his or her own brain electrical activity, improvements in cognition and behaviors usually follow (Nash, 2000).

Using an ABA single-case design, Lubar and Shouse (1976) determined that rewarding the sensorimotor rhythm (SMR; 12–14 Hz) decreased hyperactive symptoms in a hyperkinetic child, whereas inhibiting the same SMR rhythm led to increased hyperactivity. Since this report, more than 60 scientific publications by dozens of investigators have examined the effectiveness of using neurofeedback in lieu of or adjunct to behavioral and/or pharmacological interventions for this disorder. Studies have included observational case studies, controlled trials, and randomized controlled trials (RCT). Much of the research has focused on enhancing beta activity (12–21 Hz) and suppressing theta (4–8 Hz) (Lubar & Shouse, 1976; see Monastra, 2005 for a review), although recent research has included slow cortical potential (SCP) training (e.g., Heinrich, Gevensleben, Freisleder, Moll, & Rothenberger, 2004).

Observational studies have separated subjects on a variety of factors including NF treatment effects (Lubar & Shouse, 1976), identifying responders versus non-responders (Lubar, Swartwood, Swartwood, & O'Donnell, 1995; Kropotov et al., 2005), and differences between completers and non-completers of treatment (e.g., Heywood & Beale, 2003). Controlled studies, non-randomized and RCTs, have compared NF to a comparative group such as wait-list controls (Carmody, Radvanski, Wadhwani, Sabo, & Vergara, 2001 [RCT]; Heinrich et al., 2004; Lévesque, Beauregard, & Mensour, 2006 [RCT]); Linden, Habib, & Radojevic, 1996 [RCT]), stimulants (Fuchs, Birbaumer, Lutzenberger, Gruzelier, & Kaiser, 2003; Rossiter, 2004; Rossiter & LaVaque, 1995), group therapy (Doehnert, Brandeis, Straub, Steinhausen, & Drechsler, 2008 [RCT]; Drechsler et al., 2007 [RCT]), electromyographic biofeedback (Bakhshayesh, 2007 [RCT]), computerized attention or cognitive training (Gevensleben et al., 2009a [RCT]; Holtmann et al., 2009 [RCT]), or comprehensive clinical care consisting of medication, parent training, and school consultation (Monastra, Monastra, & George, 2002).

Collectively, these studies suggest that NF treatment reduces the cardinal symptoms of ADHD as noted by a multitude of outcomes. In some studies parents and teachers reported improved attention and decreased hyperactivity and impulsivity (e.g., Dreschler et al., 2007; Fuchs et al., 2003; Gevensleben et al., 2009a; Leins et al., 2007; Monastra et al., 2002). Some studies have shown improvements in cognitive variables such as attention as measured with continuous performance tests (e.g., Fuchs et al., 2003; Heinrich et al., 2004; Kaiser & Othmer, 2000; Monastra et al., 2002), and/or in IQ (e.g., Lubar et al., 1995; Thompson & Thompson, 1998). Alhambra, Fowler, and Alhambra (1995) demonstrated that a reduction or discontinuation of stimulant medications was feasible, while others showed equivalency of NF effects to those of stimulants (e.g., Fuchs et al., 2003; Rossiter & LaVaque, 1995). In some studies qEEG variables changed as a function of treatment (e.g., Gevensleben et al., 2009b; Kropotov et al., 2005; Lubar et al., 1995; Monastra et al., 2002), and participants were able to maintain EEG (SCP) changes six months (Strehl et al., 2006) and two years after treatment (Gani, Birbaumer, & Strehl, 2008). Finally, recent research has included functional magnetic resonance imaging (fMRI) indices of change resulting from NF, the "gold standard" in neuropsychiatric and related research. For example, Lévesque et al. (2006) demonstrated a normalization of key neural substrates of selective attention and response inhibition as noted in changes of the anterior cingulate cortex, caudate, and substantia nigra. In summarizing NF research relating to ADHD, Monastra (2005) noted that significant clinical improvement was reported in nearly 75% of the patients treated with NF. And a recent meta-analysis concluded that NF was an efficacious treatment of ADHD, with a large effect size for inattention and impulsivity and a medium effect size for hyperactivity (Arns, de Ridder, Strehl, Breteler, & Coenen, 2009).

Despite the clinical success NF has shown, it is still not a widely accepted treatment for ADHD children. It seems the medical community will not accept this technique unless even clearer and more objective evidence can be documented. To this end, NF research may benefit from the methodology common in pharmacological studies, incorporating randomized control group designs, such as a placebo condition (Holtmann & Stadler, 2006). Monastra (2005) summarized the main flaws found in extant NF studies in ADHD: lack of adequate controls, especially sham/placebo; failure to control for treatment preference bias; confounding of several different treatments; lack of diagnostic rigor; absence of blinding; lack of randomization.

The most notable study to date that has addressed such NF research shortcomings was conducted by Gevensleben and colleagues (2009a). Their study was an RCT with participants assigned to a NF (theta/beta combined with SCP training) or computerized attention skills program. The rate of positive response, as identified by 25% improvement in the total ADHD score completed by parents, was 52% for the NF group and 29% for the attention training group. In attempting to explain the relatively low response rate in the NF group, the authors noted possible confounds such as participants' expectations and effort, specificity of training effects, and non-blind design. While this study shows clinical effectiveness of NF compared to an active control group, there remain specific effects of NF that can be addressed with blinded, placebo-controlled designs involving RCT.

The current study addresses the absence of blinded, placebo-controlled, RCT research in the NF literature. A crossover design was implemented to help in enrollment and prevent attrition, giving each participant an equal chance of receiving NF and placebo. In an effort to include a representative clinical sample, children with primary ADHD and co-occurring diagnoses were permitted as well as those using only stimulant medication. Based on previous reports outlining the importance of considering participants who effectively "learn" NF, versus those who do not learn (Doehnert et al., 2008; Dreschler et al., 2007; Lubar et al., 1995; Lubar, 1997; Kropotov et al., 2005; Monastra et al., 2002; Strehl et al., 2006), we identified learners and non-learners using pre- and post-session EEG data. Our primary hypothesis was that participants in the NF intervention who learned to change their EEG would improve in functioning compared to the placebo condition. Functioning was measured with Conners' parent and teacher ratings of DSM-IV ADHD symptoms (Conners, 2002a, 2002b), and participant's performance on the IVA CPT (Integrated Visual and Auditory Continuous Performance Test: Response Control and Attention Quotients).

METHOD

Participants

Children were recruited from flyer advertisements, and from two elementary schools and two clinic settings. One school was a public school and the other a private school specializing in serving children with ADHD and/or learning disabilities. The first clinic was in a hospital setting and the second was a neuropsychology clinic housed at a medical school. The intervention was conducted at these four facilities. After meeting inclusion/exclusion criteria, participants and primary caregiver(s) signed informed consent. The study and informed consent were approved by the Institutional Review Boards of the respective agencies. Parent(s) gave signed written informed consents, and each child was required to assent to the study in order to participate.

Inclusion Criteria

Criteria for inclusion were: (1) age 7–11 years; (2) meet DSM-IV criteria for an ADHD diagnosis by: (a) having a parent endorse six of nine symptoms of ADHD in a single category of either Inattention or Hyperactivity or in both categories (Combined), and (b) having a licensed clinical psychologist confirm the diagnosis on the basis of a structured clinical interview and formal testing; (3) the child's prescribing doctor and parent(s) have agreed for any stimulant medication (e.g., Ritalin, Concerta, Dexedrine, or Adderall) to be removed for at least 48 hours prior to being evaluated during the initial diagnostic work-up, prior to testing mid-way through the study, and again at the time of final testing; (4) the child has been in residence with the same primary caretaker for the previous six months or longer; (5) the child's parent(s) or guardian(s) expressed a willingness to transport and escort the child to the intake procedure, all 40 sessions, and to pre-, mid-, and post-testing sessions.

Exclusion Criteria

Criteria on which children were excluded from the study were: (1) below average intellectual ability, as defined by an IQ score below 80; (2) a history of any previous or present serious mental illness other than ADHD (e.g., mood disorder, anxiety disorder, psychotic disorder) for which the child has taken medications other than stimulant medications prescribed for ADHD; (3) any history of neurological disease, including seizures or head injury with loss of consciousness; (4) any known chronic medical illness or condition; (5) the use of any daily medication that is likely to significantly affect the child's concentration, affect, and activity level (other than stimulant medication — e.g., Ritalin, Dexedrene, Concerta, Adderall).

Design

This study used a randomized double-blind crossover design, allowing participants to serve as their own controls. Phases of the study included diagnostic work-up, baseline assessment, 20 sessions, mid-assessment, 20 sessions, and post-assessment. Upon completion of the baseline assessment, participants were randomized to receive either neurofeedback or placebo conditions. Children were randomized into each of the groups by computer generated random numbers and assigned by an administrative assistant not involved with either the assessments or interventions. Each group participated in their assigned procedure for 10 weeks. After a one-week washout period, the participants were crossed over to receive the other condition. Sessions occurred at the average rate of two times per week. Children, parents, and teachers were not required to do any supplemental behavior management techniques for the study. The investigators, families, subjects, and teachers were blind to the randomization order throughout the study period. Evaluation of the effectiveness of blinding was not done (Margraf et al., 1991).

Treatments

Setup of Sessions

Participants in both conditions were exposed to identical setups. The interface consisted of playing off-the-shelf Sony PlayStation video racing games (rated E) chosen by the child. Each child had his or her own memory card so game progress could be saved. Three electrodes were positioned on the child's head: active lead at the frontal midline (FZ) site (International 10−20 System), with ground on the right ear and reference lead on the left ear. Sensor sites were abraded with NuPrep and EEG paste was used to secure the sensors to the head. Impedances were below 10 kOhms for each site. Children in both conditions were given the same instructions on how the game interface worked. Once the electrodes were placed and equipment powered on, each child played the videogame for about 30 minutes per session.

All technicians were trained and supervised by a BCIA EEG-certified licensed clinical psychologist. There were two technicians delivering the intervention to maintain blindness to conditions at each location. Technician A applied the sensors and helped the child as needed to stay focused on the playing the games. Simple reward statements were made to the child that included: "try to be calm," "you're doing great," "good job," etc. Technician A did not know the condition the child was in. Technician B controlled the computers capturing the EEG information, and did know what condition the child was in. The only communication permitted between Technician A and B was for A to inform B that the child was ready to start, and for B to

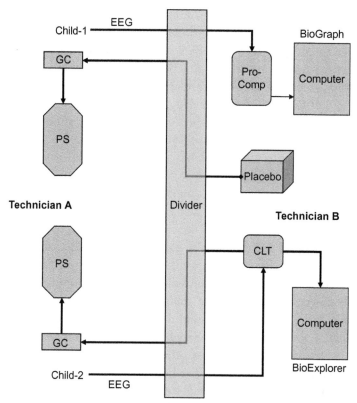

Figure 5.1 Session setup. Note: PS = Portable Sony PlayStation-1 with video screen; GC = game controller; EEG = electroencephalogram from child's head with sensor placed at FZ; Placebo = noncontingent feedback device; CLT = CyberLearning Technologies video game modulation unit; BioGraph software and ProComp amplifier from Thought Technology; BioExplorer software from CyberEvolution; Computers were Dell laptops.

inform A when the child had completed the session. The child and Technician A were separated by a divider from Technician B. See Figure 5.1 for a visual representation of the session setup.

Active Neurofeedback

The active neurofeedback condition used the neurofeedback training device developed by CyberLearning Technology, LLC (CLT). The technology behind the CLT neurofeedback device was tested and developed at NASA in research related to monitoring and training the engagement of pilots during flight deck operations, and has been further examined with

ADHD children (Palsson et al., 2001). The CLT neurofeedback device works through an interface that modulates the input to the video game controller based upon measured EEG activity. The trainee uses the game controller for normal game play functions. The sensitivity or responsiveness of the game controller is controlled by real-time EEG activity in two ways: speed of the race car and steering control. Normally, while playing a race car game, the player presses the 'X' button on the game controller to accelerate the car. With the CLT EEG interface, speed is controlled by a beta (12−20 Hz) to theta + alpha (4−12 Hz) ratio known as the Engagement Index (EI) developed at NASA. Lower ratios of engagement (more theta + alpha and less beta) cause the car to slow down or even stop, while higher ratios (less theta + alpha and more beta) allow the car to maintain full speed. Additionally the trainee received tactile feedback via the vibrator rumble function of the game controller. The rumble is typically activated when the car hits a wall, but in the CLT interface, this rumble function was disconnected from video game play and was connected as feedback based on sensorimotor rhythm (SMR: 12−15 Hz) amplitude thresholds. If the trainee's SMR amplitude was too low, the game controller vibrated as a warning. When the vibration continued non-stop for four seconds, steering control was lost. Steering control was regained when SMR amplitudes returned above threshold.

In summary, all active-treatment subjects received training to suppress slow wave theta + alpha (8−12 Hz) and enhance beta (12−20 Hz), including SMR (12−15 Hz) in the special way described above. Active sensor placement was the frontal midline (FZ) based on the International 10−20 System, with ground on the right ear and reference on the left ear. For each session, a 3-minute baseline was obtained for average EI ratio and SMR amplitudes to set thresholds. Thresholds were set at 70% reward for both the EI and SMR and were not changed during the session (i.e., no auto-thresholds were implemented). Additional equipment used was BioExplorer software (Version 1.0, CyberEvolution) to monitor integrity of the brainwave activity, and for later analysis of the data.

Placebo Neurofeedback

The placebo condition was identical to the active neurofeedback in all aspects: game choices, sensors placements, duration of sessions, and interaction with Technician A. The only difference was that there was a separate random feedback interface module controlled by Technician B. In order to mimic the effects of feedback on the EEG as in the active NF, the interface module had three buttons to control game feedback: (1) slowing down the speed of the car, (2) vibrating the hand controller, and (3) turning off steering control. Technician B followed a set schedule to press one of the three buttons for a predetermined length of time (1 to 5 seconds) once a minute during feedback. This non–contingent feedback occurred at the rate of 5%. Equipment used to monitor EEG for the placebo condition was ProComp + amplifiers and Biograph software (Version 3, Thought Technology).

Diagnostic Assessment

The diagnostic procedure consisted of a structured clinical interview, IQ, and achievement screening, and parent rating scales. For the structured clinical interview, the computerized Diagnostic Interview for Children and Adolescents-IV, Parent Version (DICA-IV: Reich, Leacock, & Shanfeld, 1997) was used to identify ADHD and other co–occurring disorders, and the diagnoses were confirmed by a licensed clinical psychologist. The ADHD diagnosis was further confirmed by using the Conners' Parent Rating Scales - Revised (CPRS-R: Conners, 2002a) DSM-IV ADHD Inattentive and Hyperactivity-Impulsive scales and requiring T-scores of 65 or higher on one or both scales.

Intellectual functioning (IQ) was estimated using the Wechsler Abbreviated Scale of Intelligence (WASI: Wechsler, 1999). It yields a Full-Scale IQ (FSIQ), Verbal IQ (VIQ), and Performance IQ (PIQ). Academic achievement was estimated with the Wechsler Individual Achievement Test — Abbreviated (WIAT-II-A: Psychological Corporation, 2001). The WIAT-II-A is a brief measure of academic skills in Word Reading, Spelling, and Numerical Operations.

Outcome Measures

Major assessments occurred at baseline, mid–assessment (after completion of first 20 sessions), and post–assessment (after the second 20 sessions). The primary outcome measure used was the DSM-IV ADHD Total scale of the Conners' teacher rating scales. This was because parents typically over-report responses to placebo in ADHD research (Grizenko et al., 2004).

Conners' Parent/Teacher Rating Scales-Revised: Long Version (CPRS-R:L/CTRS-R:L)

The CPRS-R:L and CTRS-R:L (Conners, 2002a, 2002b) are broadband rating scales of childhood psychopathology. Each item is rated on a four-point scale (not at all = 0, just a little = 1, pretty much = 2, and very much = 3). Raw scores for each scale are transformed by age and gender into T scores, with a mean of 50 and an SD of 10. The DSM-IV ADHD Inattentive (ADHDin), DSM-IV ADHD Hyperactive-Impulsive (ADHDhyp), and ADHD Total (ADHDtotal) scales for both parent and teacher were used as outcome measures. The teacher ADHD Total score was the primary outcome while the remaining scales were secondary outcomes. The CPRS-R:L and CTRS-R:L were given at baseline, mid- and post-assessment points.

The Integrated Visual and Auditory Continuous Performance Test (IVA)

The IVA (Turner & Sandford, 1995) is a computerized test that lasts approximately 13 minutes and presents 500 trials of the numbers 1 or 2 for 500 msec, with an interstimulus interval of 1500 msec. Numbers are presented through headphones and on a computer monitor in a pseudo-random pattern requiring the shifting of sets between the visual and auditory modalities. The subject is required to click the mouse only when he sees or hears a 1 and to inhibit clicking when he sees or hears a 2. During various segments of the IVA test, response sets change inviting more errors of commission, or impulsivity, and more errors of omission, or inattention. Raw scores for each scale are transformed by age into quotient scores, with a mean of 100 and SD of 15. The full scale Response Control Quotient (RCQ; commission), and full scale Attention Quotient (AQ; omission) scales were used as outcome measures. The IVA was administered at baseline, mid- and post-assessments.

Data Analysis

Based on previous findings indicating different response or learning rates to NF (Kropotov et al., 2005; Lubar et al., 1995; Monastra et al., 2002; Strehl et al., 2006), participants were first classified into learners and non-learners based on information from the active NF intervention. To do this, the Engagement Index (EI: beta/theta + alpha) at FZ from the first three sessions were averaged and compared to the average of the last three sessions. Participants with EI baseline-to-post increases (improved engagement) greater than one-half standard deviation from the average baseline EI were classified as learners and all others were classified as nonlearners (Norman, Sloan, & Wyrwich, 2003).

All outcome measures were converted to change scores (post-training minus pre-training) for analysis. Then the magnitudes of the effects of active NF to placebo were compared with two-tailed t-tests. Effect sizes (ES), Cohen's d, were calculated using change scores divided by the baseline pooled SD of that measure. Pearson product moment correlations were calculated to examine possible mechanisms of change regarding relationships between the primary outcome measure (CTRS-R ADHDtotal) and EI change scores. All statistical analyses were conducted using the Statistica analysis program (Version 9.1, StatSoft, 2010), and analyses were considered significant if p <0.05.

RESULTS
Sample Characteristics

A total of 92 children were recruited. Fifty-six were randomized into the study and three children (5%) did not complete the first 20 sessions. Forty-seven (84% of 56) children completed the NF intervention and 45 (80%) completed the placebo condition. However, only 42 children completed both conditions. Rate of dropout was not significant between the two conditions (χ2-test: p = 0.52). Participation attrition rates were 5% from baseline to mid-assessment, 20% from mid- to post-assessment, and 25% from baseline to completion. Missing data resulted from school or teacher changes, lack of compliance, or compromise of the blinded administration of sessions. These occurred at random and did not differ significantly between the two groups (χ2-test: p = 0.48). Final analyses were based on the 42 children who completed the entire study that was conducted from 2002 to 2004. See Table 5.1 for study sample characteristics.

NF Learners vs. Placebo

As described above, NF learners (NF-L) were identified by examining the active NF pre- and post-EEG session data for improved levels of engagement using the Engagement Index (EI: beta/theta + alpha). EI improvement was operationalized as an increase of one-half SD from pre- to post-active NF sessions. Children who did not meet this criterion were considered NF non-learners (NF-NL). Out of the 42 children completing the study, 31 (74%) were able to increase the EI ratio by one-half SD after 20 sessions [$t(45)$ = 5.94, p <0.001. CI(95%): 0.57, 0.28, ES = 1.63].

The baseline parent and teacher ratings of the NF-L versus the NF-NL comparison indicated that the parents rated children more severely symptomatic overall than the teachers; and the NF-L group started with

Table 5.1 Sample characteristics

Males (%)	13 (31%)
Females (%)	29 (69%)
Age M (SD)	
Males	8.93 (1.36)
Females	8.67 (1.44)
Ethnicity	
Caucasian	38
African American	3
Hispanic	1
DSM-IV ADHD diagnoses	
Inattentive type	18 (43%)
Combined type	24 (57%)
Co-occurring diagnoses	
Oppositional defiant	17 (40%)
Dysthymia	7 (17%)
Anxiety spectrum	14 (33%)
Medication status	
Yes: Male/Female	18/6
No: Male/Female	11/7
IQ/Achievement (M, (SD))	
VIQ	107.6 (17.11)
PIQ	107.3 (17.01)
FSIQ	108.4 (16.75)
Reading (Std. Score)	106.1 (14.29)
Math (Std. Score)	101.1 (19.34)
Spelling (Std. Score)	102.3 (14.31)

lower scores than the NF-NL group (see Figure 5.2). Further analyses of the NF-L indicated a significant correlation for the active NF condition between the CTRS-R ADHDtotal and EI change scores ($r^2 = 0.498$, p = 0.01) whereas the placebo condition did not show this effect ($r^2 = 0.02$, n.s.). See Figures 5.3 and 5.4 for correlation results of placebo and active NF conditions.

CTRS-R

Significant treatment effects were noted for ADHDtotal (primary outcome measure) indicating NF-L were superior to placebo $t(50) = -2.97$, p <0.005, CI(95%): −8.6, −1.7, ES = 0.50. Significant treatment effects were also noted on the ADHDin and ADHDhyp sub-scales. See Table 5.2 for change score results.

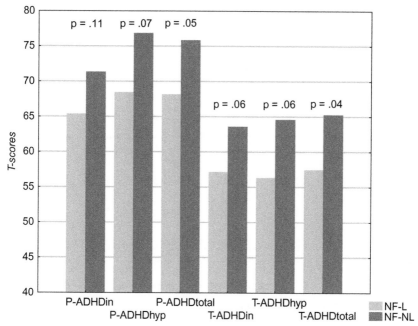

Figure 5.2 Baseline CPRS-R and CTRS-R ADHD scales of neurofeedback learners (NF-L) compared to neurofeedback nonlearners (NF-NL). Note: P is for parent ratings and T for teacher ratings on the Conners' DSM-IV ADHD rating scales (mean = 50, SD = 10): ADHDin = Inattentive, ADHDhyp = Hyperactive/Impulsive, ADHDtotal = Total score.

CPRS-R

For parents' ratings, no treatment effects were found on any of the three CPRS-R scales. Post-hoc analyses indicated all CPRS-R measures showed improvement at the mid-assessment over the post-assessment point regardless of treatment [e.g., ADHD total: $t(62) = -3.71$, p <0.001, CI(95%): -9.4, -2.8, ES = 0.49].

IVA

For the RCQ, there were significant treatment effects favoring NF-L over placebo [$t(59) = 3.09$, p = 0.003, CI(95%): 5.0, 23.2, ES = 0.63). For the AQ there were significant treatment effects for NF-L over placebo ($t(59) = 3.25$, p = 0.002, CI(95%): 5.3, 22.2, ES = 0.60].

DISCUSSION

In the present study we analyzed the effects of neurofeedback (NF) training compared to an identically administered placebo condition. We also

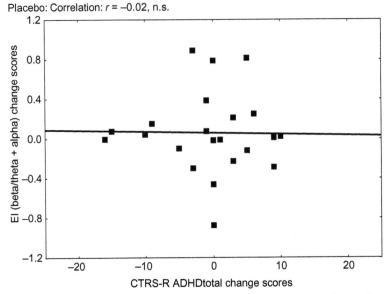

Figure 5.3 Correlations of CTRS-R ADHD Total and EI change scores for NF learners (NF-L) from the placebo condition. Note: EI (Engagement Index) is expressed as a ratio of beta/theta+alpha averaged from first and last three sessions and converted to change scores (post minus pre training). Improvements from baseline to endpoints are noted with positive scores. Teacher's Conners' rating scales (CTRS-R) DSM-IV ADHD Total (ADHDtotal) scale are expressed in T-score changes. Negative numbers indicate improvement from baseline to endpoints.

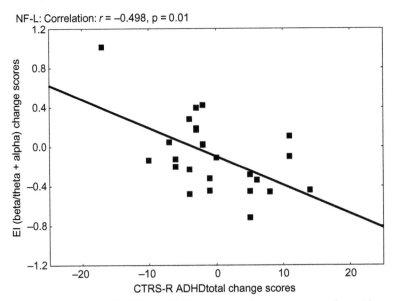

Figure 5.4 Correlations of CTRS-R ADHD Total and EI change scores for NF learners (NF-L) from the active NF condition. See Note to Figure 5.3 for explanations.

Table 5.2 NF learners' (NF-L) comparisons of active NF vs. placebo conditions (N = 31). Teachers and parents behavior T-score changes and IVA quotient changes (mean values and SD)

Measures	NF-L		Placebo		Difference (95%CI)	T-test (p)	ES
	Baseline	Change	Baseline	Change			
CTRS-R Total score	57.9 (10.7)	−3.68 (6.9)	60.0 (9.3)	1.47 (5.5)	−5.15 (−8.6, −1.7)	0.005	0.50
Inattentive	57.7 (9.9)	−2.82 (5.1)	59.3 (9.0)	1.53 (6.6)	−4.35 (−7.7, −0.9)	0.01	0.41
Hyperactive−Impulsive	56.7 (12.7)	−3.96 (9.0)	59.4 (12.3)	0.60 (5.0)	−4.6 (−8.5, −0.6)	0.02	0.37
CTRS-R Total score	68.3 (10.7)	−3.93 (7.7)	70.9 (13.0)	−2.36 (6.5)	−1.56 (−5.1, 1.9)	0.37	
Inattentive	65.7 (11.0)	−2.24 (8.3)	67.8 (12.9)	−1.97 (7.2)	−0.27 (−4.1, 3.6)	0.89	
Hyperactive−Impulsive	68.4 (14.5)	−5.28 (9.0)	71.1 (13.5)	−2.64 (7.0)	−2.6 (−6.6, 1.3)	0.19	
Response control	86.2 (21.7)	12.81 (20.4)	91.6 (19.8)	−1.29 (15.2)	14.10 (5.0, 23.2)	0.003	0.63
Attention	85.3 (25.2)	10.12 (17.4)	86.8 (20.9)	−3.60 (15.4)	13.72 (5.3, 22.1)	0.002	0.60

Note: Change scores are post-training minus baseline. Improvements are indicated with negative changes for teacher and parent ratings and positive changes for IVA quotients. ES = Effect size. ES was only reported for significant findings.

identified NF learners (NF-L) from session EEG data and compared the active and placebo conditions. The primary hypothesis proposed significant positive treatment effects for teacher and parent rating scales and IVA quotients for successful NF-L. The results provided support for the teacher ratings and IVA quotients, but not for the parent ratings.

Neurofeedback Learners vs. Nonlearners

Because there were distinct differences in results between those who responded to NF training and those who did not, only those whose showed response were included in our analysis. That is, participants had to increase their EI (Engagement Index: beta/theta + alpha [12−20 Hz/ 4−12 Hz]) by one-half standard deviation after 20 training sessions to be included in our analysis. This is considered a modest requirement given that participants received 10 hours of operant conditioning that rewarded this exact measure (EI ratio). Participants whose EI did not change in response to EEG operant conditioning were judged non-compliant or "non-learners" (NF-NL) and excluded from analysis. One would not expect symptom change in individuals who could (or would) not make brain-behavior change in spite of many hours of training. Of 42 participants who completed the study, 31 (74%) changed their brainwave activity sufficiently to meet our criteria for NF-L. NF-L success was further supported by an identifiable mechanism of change correlating the primary outcome (CTRS-R, ADHDtotal) with EI changes.

Other researchers have reported using various EEG outcome measures to identify NF learners with successful treatment outcomes. For example, Kropotov and colleagues (2005) reported 72.5% good performers identified as those having increased beta 25% from baseline within session in 60% of 15−22 sessions. Monastra, Monastra, and George (2002) reported 100% participant improvement where the criterion for learner was normalization (within one SD of normal) of the theta/beta ratio in three consecutive sessions (average sessions = 43, range = 34−50). In studies of slow cortical potential (SCP) NF, transfer of learning of negativation (increasing cortical activation) without feedback has been used to separate good from bad performers. Doehnert et al. (2008) reported 50% good performers while Dreschler et al. (2007) reported 47% with both groups completing 30 sessions.

That a quarter of participants were unable to improve their EI significantly may indicate either that there are one or more ADHD subtypes intrinsically resistant to EEG rhythm changes, or require different operant conditioning techniques or tools to achieve such brain function changes. Although we used "broad" reward/inhibit NF training, we did not customize training based on baseline EEG parameters as done by Monastra et al. (2002). Rather, our study consisted of a broad range of EEG subtypes, some of which may be amenable to more specific training protocols and/or more sessions. Future research should address identification of EEG signature(s) specific to those resistant to EI training and/or other protocols. A comparison of our NF-L and NF-NL groups indicated that successful learners presented with lower (more normal) rating scale scores by both parents and teachers, significantly for the ADHD Total scores. Although we would expect the more severe cases to have more room for improvement, our results suggest and we hypothesize that the more severe cases would benefit from more sessions while the moderate cases improved with less sessions. Our operant conditioning involved using Sony PlayStation games which on the surface seem likely to be very engaging for children. However, some of our participants appeared to be more worried about "winning the game" itself leading them to ignore the feedback versus using the feedback to win the game (i.e., the more focused they were, the faster the race car would go, resulting in a win). This type of situation is where a therapist or technician could intervene and redirect the child with metacognitive strategies (Thompson & Thompson, 1998). Although we kept redirections to a minimum in an effort to reduce confounding variables, appropriate engagement or motivation levels of participants is an important factor in the success of NF especially with ADHD children.

Parent, Teacher, and Children Outcomes

As expected, individuals' ability to change their brainwave activity ("learners") improved significantly in behavioral ratings by teachers and in their own attention test scores compared to placebo. However, there was little or no change in parental ratings. This unexpected finding of parents' ratings is inconsistent with most ADHD NF studies that did not use a placebo design.

Parental ratings improved regardless of whether a child was a learner or a placebo participant, suggesting an expectancy bias that teachers did not have. This may have been due in part to the energy put forth in helping their children complete three major assessments and 40 sessions, regardless

of the type of session (to which they were blind). Such perceived improvement is not unusual in non-NF studies. For example, parental placebo
response has also been documented in ADHD crossover studies using
methylphenidate when completing Conners' scales (Grizenko et al., 2004).
Expectancy bias posits that the key factor involved in the placebo effect is
cognitive; that is, what the patient (parent in this case) thinks or expects to
happen as a result of treatment (Kirsch, 1985, 1997). Unfortunately, our
study was not designed to measure the various aspects of the placebo
response or expectancy bias noted in parents' ratings.

Some NF researchers have found no effects of parents' attitudes towards
treatment, motivation of children, and identifying treatment assignment
when comparing NF (SCP and theta/beta) to computerized attention skills
groups (Gevensleben et al., 2009a). Leins et al. (2007) found a difference
with parents' attitudes favoring SCP over a theta/beta group, possibly due
to SCP treatment providers being more qualified than the theta/beta providers. However, since teachers reported similar behavioral improvements in
both treatment groups and were not biased, Leins et al. stated "the efficacy
of treatment protocols is equivalent and that expectancies of parents have
no significant impact on the effects of neurofeedback" (p. 87). Dreschler
et al. (2007) examined parental support (compliance with study homework
assignments) and found no mediating factors related to good versus bad
performance groups. However, Monastra et al. (2002) reported that a systematic parenting style was a mediating factor with behavioral improvements at home on or off medication.

Compared to previous studies we seem to have captured a different
type of parental expectancy which can be attributed to a placebo condition that impacted the results in multiple ways. First, when the placebo-
first group later completed the active NF sessions as their second phase of
the study, there was little room for parent ratings to show improvement.
Second, when the NF-first group completed the placebo condition as
their second phase of the study, scores had a tendency to return to near
baseline levels. This pattern was also noted in the teachers' ratings and
IVA quotients. These findings suggests that treatment lengths may need to
be longer than the 20 sessions used in the study in order for treatment
effects to maintain stability. Finally, because parents' expectancies may
overestimate the actual response to NF, we suggest future studies use
ancillary teacher behavior rating scales to supplement outcomes, and/or
use objective measures such as EEG changes and continuous performance
tests to confirm outcomes.

Teacher behavioral ratings more strongly reflected changes in behavior dependent on participation type — placebo or active NF. Our results of teachers' behavioral ratings indicated placebo-controlled small-to-medium range effect sizes (ES) of 0.37 for Hyperactive-Impulsive (ADHDhyp), 0.41 for Inattention (ADHDin), and 0.50 for the ADHD Total (ADHDtotal) scores. These findings were similar in rank order, but slightly smaller in magnitude, compared to Gevensleben et al. (2009) who used German language ADHD rating scales: 0.40 for Hyperactivity-Impulsivity, 0.50 for Inattention, and 0.64 for Total ADHD symptoms. Our smaller ES may be due to fewer sessions in the current study compared to Gevensleben et al. (2009a).

The children's performance on the Integrated Visual and Auditory continuous performance test (IVA CPT) indicated medium ESs of 0.60 on the Attention (omission) quotient and 0.63 for the Response Control (commission) quotient. These findings are slightly larger than those found by Lévesque, Beauregard, & Mensour (2006): 0.37 for Attention and 0.42 for Response Control after 40 sessions. Monastra et al. (2002) showed larger ESs using the Tests of Variables of Attention (TOVA) with 1.45 on Inattention and 1.27 on Impulsivity scales after an average of 43 NF treatment sessions. The larger ES by Monastra's group may have been due to the EEG theta/beta ratio inclusion criteria, training the ratio, and then using it as completion criteria. This may be one of the best models for obtaining successful outcomes with NF. Identification of EEG criteria and successful NF learning versus NF non-learning as potential mediating variables with CPT outcomes is recommended for future research in this area.

Limitations of the Study

There were several limitations to our study, including using a crossover design, allowing children to be medicated during NF training, not using EEG profiling to guide NF protocol choices, and not enough NF sessions. The crossover design was chosen to use participants as their own controls, and to help with recruitment, i.e., parents probably would be more willing to have their children participate knowing they would eventually receive treatment. Allowing children to be medicated during training was a confounding factor, but it was a compromise in order to protect their rights as participants to still have an option for the "standard of care" stimulant medication. Having participants non-medicated would have been preferable, but we felt allowing children to stay medicated would also be more amenable to parents. Our initial intent was to use EEG profiling using quantitative EEG database comparisons to guide treatment protocols. However, due to equipment restrictions and start up delays this was not implemented. We can only speculate that this may have helped improve outcomes. Finally, we felt that children would have benefited from more sessions, especially the more severe cases, to help optimize the learning potential and improve stability of outcomes.

CONCLUSIONS

Our findings are consistent with many prior studies and expand scientific understanding of the unique effects of NF treatment. Using a placebo-controlled design we have shown that many children diagnosed with ADHD who learn to modulate cortical activity can profit from NF, effectively improving behavioral symptoms as noted by teachers, and performing better on a continuous performance test. Children who present with higher levels of ADHD symptoms may require more sessions in order to benefit from NF. An unexpected finding was a parent expectancy bias exhibited in the placebo condition which made it appear there were no significant changes in behavioral improvements from the NF. We hope these findings will help in planning future studies of NF, especially in regard to the need to consider the variables of success (or lack thereof) in learning of control of brain electrical activity, parental expectations, and use of multiple outcome measure of success.

ACKNOWLEDGMENTS

This research was supported by grants from the Virginia Commonwealth Health Research Board in Richmond, Virginia, and Riverside Healthcare Foundation in Newport News, Virginia. The authors would like to thank Edwin Joseph and Alan Pope for their endless encouragement and support, and all the technicians who worked long hours delivering sessions and assessments. Finally, a special thanks for the schools and teachers who worked with us, and for the parents and children who participated in the study.

REFERENCES

Arnold, L. E. (2004). *Contemporary diagnosis and management of ADHD* (3rd ed.). Newtown, PA: Handbooks in Health Care Co.

Arns, M., de Ridder, S., Strehl, U., Breteler, M., & Coenen, A. (2009). Efficacy of neuro-feedback treatment in ADHD: The effects on inattention, impulsivity and hyperactivity: A meta-analysis. *Clinical Electroencephalography and Neuroscience, 40*(3), 180−189.

Bakhshayesh, A. R. (2007). Die wirksamkeit von neurofeedback im vergleich zum EMG biofeedback bei der behandlung von ADHS-Kindern. PhD thesis, Universität Potsdam, Germany.

Barry, R. J., Clarke, A. R., Johnstone, S. J., McCarthy, R., & Selikowitz, M. (2009). Electroencephalogram theta/beta ratio and arousal in attention-deficit/hyperactivity disorder: Evidence of independent processes. *Biological Psychiatry, 66*, 398−401.

Carmody, D. P., Radvanski, D. C., Wadhwani, S., Sabo, M. J., & Vergara, L. (2001). EEG biofeedback training and attention-deficit/hyperactivity disorder in an elementary school setting. *Journal of Neurotherapy, 43*(3), 5−27.

Chabot, R. J., & Serfontein, G. (1996). Quantitative electroencephalographic profiles of children with attention deficit disorder. *Biological Psychiatry, 40*, 951−963.

Cherkasova, M. V., & Hechtman, L. (2009). Neuroimaging in attention-deficit hyper-activity disorder: Beyond the frontostriatal circuitry. *Canadian Journal of Psychiatry, 54*, 651−664.

Clarke, A. R., Barry, R. J., McCarthy, R., & Selikowitz, M. (2001). EEG-defined sub-types of children with attention-deficit/hyperactivity disorder. *Clinical Neurophysiology, 112*(11), 2098−2105.

Conners, C. K. (2002a). *Conners' Parent Rating Scale-Revised (CPRS-R)* Toronto, ON: Multi-Health Systems Inc.

Conners, C. K. (2002b). *Conners' Teacher Rating Scale-Revised (CTRS-R)* Toronto, ON: Multi-Health Systems Inc.

Doehnert, M., Brandeis, D., Straub, M., Steinhausen, H., & Drechsler, R. (2008). Slow cortical potential neurofeedback in attention deficit hyperactivity disorder: Is there neurophysiological evidence for specific effects? *Journal of Neural Transmission, 115*(10), 1445−1456.

Drechsler, R., Straub, M., Doehnert, M., Heinrich, H., Steinhausen, H., & Brandeis, D. (2007). Controlled evaluation of a neurofeedback training of slow cortical potentials in children with ADHD. *Behavioral and Brain Functions, 3*, 35.

DuPaul, G. J., & Stoner, G. (2003). *ADHD in schools: Assessment and intervention strategies* (2nd ed.). New York: Guilford Press.

Faraone, S. V., Biederman, J., Morley, C. P., & Spencer, T. J. (2008). Effect of stimulants on height and weight: A review of the literature. *Journal of the American Academy of Children and Adolescent Psychiatry, 47*, 994−1009.

Fuchs, T., Birbaumer, N., Lutzenberger, W., Gruzelier, J. H., & Kaiser, J. (2003). Neurofeedback treatment for attention-deficit/hyperactivity disorder in children: A comparison with methylphenidate. *Applied Psychophysiology and Biofeedback, 28*(1), 1−12.

Galland, B. C., Tripp, E. G., & Taylor, B. J. (2009). The sleep of children with attention deficit hyperactivity disorder on and off methylphenidate: A matched case-control study. *Journal of Sleep Research*, doi: 10.1111/j.1365-2869.2009.00795.x.

Gani, C., Birbaumer, N., & Strehl, U. (2008). Long term effects after feedback of slow cortical potentials and of theta-beta-amplitudes in children with attention-deficit/hyperactivity disorder (ADHD). *International Journal of Bioelectromagnetism, 10*(4), 209−232.

Gevensleben, H., Holl, B., Albrecht, B., Schlamp, D., Kratz, O., Studer, P., et al. (2009a). Distinct EEG effects related to neurofeedback training in children with ADHD: A randomized controlled trial. *International Journal of Psychophysiology, 74*, 149−157.

Gevensleben, H., Holl, B., Albrecht, B., Vogel, C., Schlamp, D., Kratz, O., et al. (2009b). Is neurofeedback an efficacious treatment for ADHD? A randomised controlled clinical trial. *Journal of Child Psychology and Psychiatry*, doi:10.1111/j.1469-7610. 2008.02033.x.

Grizenko, N., Lachance, M., Collard, V., Lageix, P., Baron, C., Amor, L. B., et al. (2004). Sensitivity of tests to assess improvement in ADHD symptomatology. *Canadian Child and Adolescent Psychiatry Review*, 13(2), 36−40.

Heinrich, H., Gevensleben, H., Freisleder, F. J., Moll, G. H., & Rothenberger, A. (2004). Training of slow cortical potentials in attention-deficit/hyperactivity disorder: Evidence for positive behavioral and neurophysiological effects. *Biological Psychiatry*, 55, 772−775.

Heywood, C., & Beale, I. (2003). EEG biofeedback vs. placebo treatment for attention-deficit/hyperactivity disorder: A pilot study. *Journal of Attention Disorders*, 7(1), 43−55.

Holtmann, M., Grassmann, D., Cionek-Szpak, E., Hager, V., Panzer, N., Beyer, A., et al. (2009). Spezifische wirksamkeit von neurofeedback auf die impulsivitat bei ADHS − Literaturuberblick und ergebnisse einer prospective, kontrollierten studie. *Kindheit und Entwicklung*, 18, 95−104.

Holtmann, M., & Stadler, C. (2006). Electroencephalograhic biofeedback for the treatment of attention-deficit hyperactivity disorder in childhood and adolescence. *Expert Review of Neurotherapeutics*, 6(4), 533−540.

Jensen, P. S., Arnold, L. E., Swanson, J. M., Vitiello, B., Abikoff, H. B., Greenhill, L. L., et al. (2007). 3-year follow-up of the NIMH MTA study. *Journal of the American Academy of Child and Adolescent Psychiatry*, 46, 989−1002.

Kaiser, D. A., & Othmer, S. (2000). Effects of neurofeedback on variables of attention in a large multi-center trial. *Journal of Neurotherapy*, 4(1), 5−15.

Kirsch, I. (1985). Response expectancy as a determinant of experience and behavior. *American Psychologist*, 40, 1189−1202.

Kirsch, I. (1997). Specifying nonspecifics: Psychological mechanisms of placebo effects. In A. Harrington (Ed.), *The placebo effect. An interdisciplinary exploration*. Cambridge, MA: Harvard University Press.

Klein-Schwartz, W. (2002). Abuse and toxicity of methylphenidate. *Current Opinion in Pediatrics*, 14, 219−223.

Kropotov, J. D., Grin-Yatsenko, V. A., Pomarev, V. A., Chutko, L. S., Yakovenko, E. A., & Nikishena, I. S. (2005). ERPs correlates of EEG relative beta training in ADHD children. *International Journal of Psychophysiology*, 55, 23−34.

Leins, U., Goth, G., Hinterberger, T., Klinger, C., Rumpf, N., & Strehl, U. (2007). Neurofeedback for children with ADHD: A comparison of SCP and theta/beta protocols. *Applied Psychophysiology and Biofeedback*, 32, 73−88.

Lévesque, J., Beauregard, M., & Mensour, B. (2006). Effect of neurofeedback training on the neural substrates of selective attention in children with attention-deficit/hyperactivity disorder: A functional magnetic resonance imaging study. *Neuroscience Letters*, 394, 216−221.

Linden, M., Habib, T., & Radojevic, V. (1996). A controlled study of the effects of EEG biofeedback on cognition and behavior of children with attention deficit disorder and learning disabilities. *Biofeedback & Self-Regulation*, 21(1), 35−49.

Lubar, J. F. (1991). Discourse on the development of EEG diagnostics and biofeedback for attention-deficit/hyperactivity disorders. *Biofeedback & Self-Regulation*, 16, 201−225.

Lubar, J. F. (1997). Neocortical dynamics: Implications for understanding the role of neurofeedback and related techniques for the enhancement of attention. *Applied Psychophysiology and Biofeedback*, 22, 111−126.

Lubar, J. F., & Bahler, W. W. (1976). Behavioral management of epileptic seizures following EEG biofeedback training of the sensorimotor rhythm. *Biofeedback & Self-Regulation*, 1, 77−104.

Lubar, J. O., & Lubar, J. F. (1984). Electroencephalographic biofeedback of SMR and beta for treatment of attention deficit disorders in a clinical setting. *Biofeedback & Self Regulation, 9*(1), 1−23.

Lubar, J. F., & Shouse, M. N. (1976). EEG and behavioural changes in a hyperkinetic child concurrent with training of the sensorimotor rhythm (SMR): A preliminary report. *Biofeedback & Self-Regulation, 3,* 293−306.

Lubar, J. F., Swartwood, M. O., Swartwood, J. N., & O'Donnell, P. H. (1995). Evaluation of the effectiveness of EEG neurofeedback training for ADHD in a clinical setting as measured by changes in T.O.V.A. scores, behavioural ratings, and WISC-R performance. *Biofeedback and Self Regulation, 20,* 83−99.

Margraf, J., Ehlers, A., Roth, W. T., Clark, D. B., Sheikh, J., Agras, W. S., et al. (1991). How "blind" are double-blind studies? *Journal of Consultant and Clinical Psychology, 59,* 184−187.

McCarthy, S., Cranswick, N., Potts, L., Taylor, E., & Wong, I. C. (2009). Mortality associated with attention-deficit hyperactivity disorder (ADHD) drug treatment: A retrospective cohort study of children, adolescents and young adults using the general practice research database. *Drug Safety, 32,* 1089−1096.

Monastra, V. J. (2005). Electroencephalographic biofeedback (neurotherapy) as a treatment for attention deficit hyperactivity disorder: Rationale and empirical foundation. *Child and Adolescent Psychiatric Clinics of North America, 14,* 55−82.

Monastra, V. J., Monastra, D. M., & George, S. (2002). The effects of stimulant therapy, EEG biofeedback and parenting style on the primary symptoms of attention deficit/hyperactivity disorder. *Applied Psychophysiology and Biofeedback, 27*(4), 231−249.

Nash, J. K. (2000). Treatment of attention deficit hyperactivity disorder with neurotherapy. *Clinical Electroencephalography, 31*(1), 30−37.

Norman, G. R., Sloan, J. A., & Wyrwich, K. W. (2003). Interpretation of changes in health-related quality of life: The remarkable universality of half a standard deviation. *Medical Care, 41,* 582−592.

Palsson, O. S., Pope, A. T., Ball, J. D., Turner, M. J., Nevin, S., & deBeus, R. (2001, March). Neurofeedback videogame ADHD technology: Results of the first concept study. Presented at annual meeting of *Association for Applied Psychophysiology & Biofeedback,* Research Triangle Park, NC.

Pappadopulos, E., Jensen, P. S., Chait, A. R., Arnold, L. E., Swanson, J. M., Greenhill, L. L., et al. (2009). Medication adherence in the MTA: Saliva methylphenidate samples versus parent report and mediating effect of concomitant behavioral treatment. *Journal of the American Academy of Child and Adolescent Psychiatry, 48*(5), 501−510.

Pelham, W. E., Jr., & Fabiano, G. A. (2008). Evidence-based psychosocial treatments for attention-deficit/hyperactivity disorder. *Journal of Clinical Child and Adolescent Psychology, 37,* 184−214.

Reeves, G., & Anthony, B. (2009). Multimodal treatments versus pharmacotherapy alone in children with psychiatric disorders: Implications of access, effectiveness, and contextual treatment. *Paediatric Drugs, 11,* 165−169.

Reich, W., Leacock, N., & Shanfeld, K. (1997). *DICA-IV Diagnostic interview for children and adolescents-IV [Computer software]* Toronto, Ontario: Multi-Health Systems, Inc.

Rossiter, T. R., & LaVaque, T. J. (1995). A comparison of EEG biofeedback and psychostimulants in treating attention deficit/hyperactivity disorders. *Journal of Neurotherapy, 1,* 48−59.

Rossiter, T. R. (2004). The effectiveness of neurofeedback and stimulant drugs in treating AD/HD: Part II. Replication. *Applied Psychophysiology and Biofeedback, 29*(4), 233−243.

Satterfield, J. H., Schell, A. M., Backs, R. W., & Hidaka, K. C. (1984). A cross-sectional and longitudinal study of age effects of electrophysiological measures in hyperactive and normal children. *Biological Psychiatry, 19,* 973−990.

Sgrok, M., Roberts, W., Grossman, S., & Barozzine, T. (2000). School board survey of attention deficit/hyperactivity disorder: Prevalence of diagnosis and stimulant medication therapy. *Pediatric Child Health, 5*, 12–23.

Sterman, M. B. (1996). Physiological origins and functional correlates of EEG rhythmic activities: Implications for self-regulation. *Biofeedback & Self-Regulation, 21*, 3–33.

Strehl, U., Leins, U., Goth, G., Klinger, C., Hinterberger, T., & Birbaumer, N. (2006). Self-regulation of slow cortical potentials: A new treatment for children with attention-deficit/hyperactivity disorder. *Pediatrics, 118*, 1530–1540.

Sonuga-Barke, E. J., Coghill, D., Wigal, T., DeBacker, M., & Swanson, J. (2009). Adverse reactions to methylphenidate treatment for attention-deficit/hyperactivity disorder: Structure and associations with clinical characteristics and symptom control. *Journal of Child and Adolescent Psychopharmacology, 19*, 683–690.

Swanson, J. M., Kraemer, H. C., Hinshaw, S. P., Arnold, L. E., Conners, C. K., Abikoff, H. B., et al. (2001). Clinical relevance of the primary findings of the MTA: Success rates based on severity of ADHD and ODD symptoms at the end of treatment. *Journal of the American Academy of Child & Adolescent Psychiatry, 40*, 168–179.

Thompson, L., & Thompson, M. (1998). Neurofeedback combined with training in metacognitive strategies: Effectiveness in students with ADD. *Applied Psychophysiology and Biofeedback, 23*(4), 243–263.

Turner, A. & Sandford, J. A. (1995). *A normative study of IVA: Integrated visual and auditory continuous performance test.* Presented at the Annual Convention of the American Psychological Association, New York, USA.

Wechsler, D. (1999). *Wechsler Abbreviated Scale of Intelligence* San Antonio, TX: The Psychological Corporation.

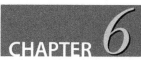

CHAPTER 6

Emerging Empirical Evidence Supporting Connectivity-Guided Neurofeedback for Autistic Disorders

Robert Coben and Lori A. Wagner
Neurorehabilitation and Neuropsychological Services, Massapequa Park, New York, USA

Contents

INTRODUCTION

Autistic spectrum disorders (ASD) are a heterogeneous group of pervasive developmental disorders including Autistic Disorder, Rett Disorder, Childhood Disintegrative Disorder, Pervasive Developmental Disorder–Not Otherwise Specified (PDD-NOS), and Asperger Disorder. Children with ASD demonstrate impairment in social interaction, verbal and nonverbal communication, and behaviors or interests (DSM-IV-TR: APA, 2000).

Neurofeedback and Neuromodulation Techniques and Applications
DOI: 10.1016/B978-0-12-382235-2.00006-8

153

ASD may be comorbid with sensory integration difficulties, mental retardation or seizure disorders. Children with ASD may have severe sensitivity to sounds, textures, tastes, and smells. Cognitive deficits are often associated with impaired communication skills (National Institute of Mental Health; NIMH, 2006). Repetitive stereotyped behaviors, perseveration, and obsessionality, common in ASD, are associated with executive deficits. Executive dysfunction in inhibitory control and set shifting have been attributed to ASD (Schmitz et al., 2006). Seizure disorders may occur in one out of four children with ASD; frequently beginning in early childhood or adolescence (National Institute of Mental Health; NIMH, 2006).

Autistic Disorder includes the following triad of symptoms: (1) impaired social interaction, failure to develop peer relationships, or lack of initiating spontaneous activities; (2) deficits in communication, including delay in or lack of spoken language, inability to initiate or sustain conversation with others, stereotyped repetitive use of language or idiosyncratic language; and (3) restricted repetitive and stereotyped behavior, interests, inflexible adherence to routines or rituals, and repetitive motor patterns (e.g., hand or finger flapping or twisting) (DSM-IV-TR; APA, 2000).

Individuals with Asperger Disorder frequently have high levels of cognitive functioning, engage in literal pedantic speech, experience difficulty comprehending implied meaning, exhibit problems with fluid movement, and manifest inappropriate social interactions. Pervasive Developmental Disorder-Not Otherwise Specified (PDD-NOS) reflects deficits in language and social skills, which do not meet the criteria of other disorders. In contrast, persons with Childhood Disintegrative Disorder and Rett Disorder both have normal periods of early development followed by loss of previously acquired skills. Common features among all these conditions include communication and social skill deficits. There is considerable variability in terms of onset and severity of symptomatology within the Autistic Spectrum of Disorders (Attwood, 1998; Hamilton, 2000; McCandless, 2005; Sicile-Kira, 2004; Siegel, 1996).

Research reviewing the epidemiology of autism (Center for Disease Control and Prevention; CDC, 2009) reported between 1 in 80 to 1 in 240 children in the United States diagnosed with the disorder. In fact, their most recent report (CDC, 2009) suggests a prevalence of 1 in 110, and as high as 1 in 70 boys. According to Blaxill (2004), the rates of ASD were reported to be <3 per 10,000 children in the 1970s and rose to >30 per 10,000 in the 1990s. This rise in the rate of ASD constituted a ten-fold increase over a 20-year interval in the United States. With increased prevalence comes a need to design and empirically validate effective treatments for those impacted by autistic disorders.

Research studies utilizing electroencephalogram (EEG) and single photon emission computed tomography (SPECT) have provided evidence for a neuropathological basis of ASD. A review of numerous EEG studies reported the rate of abnormal EEGs in autism ranged from 10% to 83%, while the mean incidence was 50%. Atypical EEGs often predict poor outcomes for intelligence, speech, and educational achievement (Hughes & John, 1999). In a more recent review of research, Rippon, Brock, Brown, and Boucher (2007) proposed a model of reduced connectivity between specialized local neural networks and overconnectivity within isolated neural assemblies in autism. Disordered connectivity may be associated with an increased ratio of excitation/inhibition in key neural systems. Anomalies in connectivity may be linked to abnormalities in information integration. In SPECT scans of children with autism, abnormal regional cerebral blood flow in the medial prefrontal cortex and anterior cingulate gyrus was related to impaired communication and social interaction, while altered perfusion in the right medial temporal lobe was associated with the obsessive desire for sameness (Ohnishi et al., 2000). Children with autism commonly display executive functioning deficits in planning, cognitive flexibility, and inhibition. These executive deficits are associated with dysfunctional integration of the frontal lobes with other brain regions, and thus also impact upon social, behavioral, and cognitive function (Hill, 2004).

Functional neuroimaging has also linked social cognition dysfunction and language deficits in autism studies to neural substrates (Pelphrey, Adolphs, & Morris, 2004; Welchew et al., 2005). During a sentence comprehension test, individuals with autism showed less functional connectivity between Broca's and Wernicke's areas relative to a control group, suggesting a lower degree of information organization, and neural synchronization during language tasks (Just, Cherkassy, Keller, & Minshew, 2004). A review of neuroimaging studies has found key brain structures including the amygdala, superior temporal sulcus region, and fusiform gyrus to function differently in individuals with autism than in controls (McAlonan et al., 2004).

MAJOR TREATMENTS FOR ASD: AN OVERVIEW

Parents of children with ASD select many different methods of treatment, with an average of seven different therapies being utilized (Green, Pituch,

Itchon, Choi, O'Reilly, & Sigafoos, 2006). Speech therapy (70% of parents) was the most commonly selected treatment, followed by psychopharmacological treatment (52% of parents). Other treatments included visual schedules (43%), sensory integration (38%), and applied behavior analysis (36%). Special diets were implemented by 27% of parents and 43% utilized vitamin supplements. While there may be some benefit to these treatments, many do not lead to long-lasting changes and/or have risks associated with their implementation. The potential benefits and risks of the major treatments for ASD are summarized below.

Applied Behavior Analysis

Applied behavior analysis (ABA), a form of behavior modification, is the method of treatment with the most empirical support for treating ASD. The goal of this therapy is to improve social interaction, behavior, and communication (Bassett, Green, & Kazanjian, 2000). ABA is firmly based on the principles of operant conditioning and measures small units of behavior to build more complex and adaptive behaviors through reinforcement. Typically, imitation, attention, motivation, and compliance are targeted early (Couper, 2004).

The first program that utilized this technique was the Young Autism Project (YAP), which was developed in 1970 by O. Ivar Lovaas (Lovaas, Koegel, Simmons, & Long, 1973). This intensive, highly structured behavioral program was delivered on a one-to-one basis requiring several hours a day. Their findings indicated that therapy delivered with 40 or more hours per week for two or more years showed increased cognitive and academic function (47% of the treatment group versus 2% of controls) (Lovaas, 1987). Follow-up research of these children into late childhood and adolescence reported improved cognitive function and education in regular classrooms (47% of the treatment group versus 0% of controls) (McEachin, Smith, & Lovaas, 1993).

Other studies that measured outcomes of ABA treatment in autism found less promising results than those of Lovaas (1987). Anderson, Avery, DiPietro, Edwards, and Christian (1987) conducted home-based ABA on 14 children for between 15 and 25 hours per week. While modest gains were made in mental ages scores and communication skills, the most impaired children failed to make progress, and none of the children were able to be integrated into regular classrooms following treatment.

Project TEACCH (Treatment and Education of Autistic and Related Communication Handicapped Children), developed by Eric Schopler and colleagues (Schopler & Reichler, 1971) at the University of North Carolina at Chapel Hill, differs from ABA, but utilizes behavioral principles to maximize the skills of children who are autistic (Herbert, Sharp, & Gaudiano, 2002). Ozonoff and Cathcart (1998) investigated the effectiveness of a home-based TEACCH treatment program for children with autism. Children who received the TEACCH treatment from their parents showed significant improvement over the control group on tests of imitation, fine and gross motor, nonverbal conceptual skills, and overall PEP-R scores. Progress was three to four times greater on all outcome tests in the treatment group as compared to the control group.

Ben-Itzchak and Zachor (2007) investigated the effects of intellectual functioning and severity of autistic symptoms on outcome following intensive behavioral intervention. Groups were formed based on IQ scores (high >70 vs. low <70), level of social interaction (high vs. low), and communication deficits (high vs. low) using the Autism Diagnostic Observation Schedule (ADOS; Lord, Rutter, DiLavore, & Risi, 1999), all of which were assessed prior to treatment. After one year of intervention provided one-on-one by a behavioral therapist for at least 35 hours per week, significant improvements were noted in all domains measured by the ADOS, which include imitation, receptive and expressive language, nonverbal communication skills, play skills, and stereotyped behaviors. Children with higher cognitive levels and those with fewer social interaction deficits were more apt to acquire developmental skills post-treatment, particularly in the areas of play skills and receptive and expressive language skills. Play skills progress was more related to the child's cognitive level while progress in expressive language abilities was more related to social abilities.

In their clinical practice guidelines report, the New York State Department of Health Early Intervention Program recommended that ABA and other behavioral interventions be included in the treatment of autism. They specify that intensive behavioral programs should include a minimum of 20 hours of intervention with a therapist per week. Furthermore, the guidelines state that parents should be included in the intervention, and that they be trained in the use of behavioral techniques to provide additional instruction at home with regular therapist consultation. Although promising, intensive behavioral programs are costly and require extensive time on the part of the therapist as well as the family, and debates are ongoing about who should pay for such services (Couper, 2004).

Although behavior therapy improves social, cognitive and language skills, a year or more of intensive training has been used in most research studies that have demonstrated improvement. Furthermore, a strong commitment by parents to complete therapeutic programs is necessary to achieve positive outcomes. While behavioral treatment methods show the most empirical support to date, there remains a need for additional therapies, which may be more easily administered and used in conjunction with the behavioral methods described. It is important to note that, though research has been promising, there has been great variability between studies in their results and outcome measures have often been questionable (e.g., IQ scores, returning to regular classrooms). And, this approach appears to be more effective with those who are higher functioning (i.e., higher IQ), meaning that lower functioning individuals are often left out, even though they are perhaps in greatest need of treatment.

Pharmacological Treatments

Pharmacological and biomedical interventions have also been utilized to treat individuals with ASD. A study conducted at the Yale Child Study Center found that 55% of a group of 109 individuals with a PDD were taking psychotropic medication, with 29.3% taking more than one medication (Martin, Scahill, Klin, & Volkmar, 1999). The most common medications were antidepressants (32.1%), followed by stimulants (20.2%), and neuroleptics (16.5%). The objectives of psychopharmacological treatment for autism include: decreasing the core symptoms of autism; decreasing anxiety and overfocus, improving social skills, reducing aggressive self-injurious behavior; increasing the effects of other interventions, and improving the quality of life for the child and their family. There is no single medication known to be beneficial to all children with ASD, nor that has specifically been developed for individuals with Autistic Spectrum Disorder.

Psychostimulant medications are often used with children who are autistic due to its success in the treatment of ADHD (Jensen et al., 2007). Despite this, stimulant use in children who are autistic remains controversial and largely unproven in terms of efficacy. In the Research Units on Pediatric Psychopharmacology Methylphenidate study (RUPP, 2005b), 49% of the sample were considered positive responders, leaving a significant percentage as non-responders; and there was an 18% side effect rate overall.

Neuroleptics such as haloperidol and thioridazine have been utilized to reduce dysfunctional behaviors associated with ASD. The adverse side effects of sedation, irritability, and extrapyramidal dyskinesias limit the use of these medications, however.

A newer class of neuroleptic, referred to as atypical anti-psychotics, reportedly improves social interaction and decreases aggression, irritability, agitation, and hyperactivity (Barnard, Young, Pearson, Geddes, & Obrien, 2002). They have fewer extrapyramidal adverse side effects than haloperidol and thioridazine. However, most children experience a substantial weight gain within the first months of treatment (Committee on Children with Disabilities, 2001). Risperidone is the only drug that has been approved by the FDA to treat the symptoms (irritability) of autism. A recent meta-analysis of three randomized controlled trials found that the drug was effective in treating the symptoms of irritability and aggression (Jesner, Aref-Adib, & Coren, 2007). The authors concluded that although risperidone may be beneficial, its use must be weighed against its adverse effects, most notably weight gain, and that long-term follow-up is needed prior to determining its efficacy in clinical practice. Risperidone's long-term benefits were studied by the RUPP Autism Network (RUPP, 2005a) in a two-part study. Part one was a 4 month, open-label trial, which was followed by an 8 week randomized, double-blind, placebo substitution study of risperidone withdrawal in those who were considered "responders". Participants whose medication levels were gradually reduced showed a greater return of aggression, temper outbursts, and self-injurious behaviors than those who continued the medication, for whom over 80% maintained their improvements and showed "very good tolerability". Although not a randomized controlled trial, this provided evidence to suggest that risperidone may be effective for time periods of up to one year (Zuddas, Di Martino, Muglia, & Cichetti, 2000). The relapse rate for those maintained on this medication has ranged from 12.5 to 25% (RUPP, 2005a; Troost et al., 2005). Santangelo and Tsatsanis (2005) reported that there are currently no drugs that produce major improvement in the core social or pragmatic language deficits in autism, although several have limited effects on the behavioral features of the disorder.

Repetitive stereotypical and perseverative behaviors have been shown to be characteristic of both obsessive—compulsive disorder (OCD) and autism (McDougle et al., 1995). The overlap between these disorders and the success of selective serotonin reuptake inhibitors (SSRIs) in treating OCD (Geller et al., 2001) has led to the use of SSRIs in treating symptoms of autism. One of the first trials of the SSRI Prozac (fluoxetine) found that doses ranging from 20 to 80 mg per day were effective based on Clinical Global Impressions in 15 of 23 individuals with autism (Cook, Rowlett, & Jaselskis, 1992). However, 6 out of the 23 experienced significant side effects such as restlessness, hyperactivity, agitation, increased appetite, and insomnia. A more rigorous 20 week placebo-controlled crossover study found that fluoxetine significantly reduced repetitive behaviors compared to placebo (Hollander et al., 2005). Although there were no significant side effects, there also were no significant improvements in measures of speech or social interaction. DeLong, Ritch, and Burch (2002) reported a 69% positive response rate for fluoxetine in children, aged 2–8, who were autistic. Treatment parameters were quite variable, with treatment duration ranging from 5 to 76 months and doses ranging from 4 mg/day to 40 mg/day.

A 12 week, double-blind, placebo-controlled study of fluoxetine reported this drug to be efficacious (McDougle et al., 1996). Eight out of 15 adult subjects were rated as "responders", with improvements occurring for repetitive thoughts and behaviors, maladaptive behaviors, and repetitive language use. Side effects were noted to be mild and included sedation and nausea. However, a more recent study by McDougle, Kresch, and Posey (2000) with children and adolescents found only 1 of 18 responded to the drug, with common side effects including insomnia, hyperactivity, agitation, and aggression. Martin, Koenig, Anderson, and Scahill (2003) found similar results in children, reporting only 3 out of 18 subjects to be responsive to fluvoxamine.

At least four other SSRIs have been reported to have at least some beneficial effect, although none have demonstrated efficacy through placebo-controlled studies. Zoloft (sertraline) was found to be effective for aggression and repetitive behavior in 42 adults with PDD, including adults with autism, Asperger's, and PDD-NOS, though 3 of the subjects dropped out of the study due to either agitation or anxiety (McDougle et al., 1998). Social relatedness did not appear to improve. The researchers found sertraline to be more effective for those with autism and PDD-NOS than for those with Asperger's.

Very limited support has been reported for the SSRI Paxil (paroxetine). Two retrospective studies of the SSRI Celexa (citalopram) have reported improvement in some of the symptoms of autism. Couturier and Nicolson (2002) found improvement in 10 out of 17 children in aggression, anxiety, stereotypies, and preoccupations, though not in social interactions and communication. In addition, four children developed adverse side effects such as increased agitation and insomnia causing their treatment to be stopped. Namerow, Thomas, Bostic, Prince, & Monuteaux (2003) found similar improvements in children and adolescents in repetitive behavior, mood, and anxiety. Mild side effects were reported in one-third of their sample, two of whom discontinued treatment due to side effects.

The fourth SSRI that has been studied to treat the symptoms of PDD is Lexapro (escitalopram). In an open-label design of children and adolescents with autism, Asperger's, or PDD-NOS, Owley and colleagues (2005) found significant improvement in 17 of 28 patients based on ratings from the Aberrant Behavior Checklist Irritability subscale (Aman, Singh, & Stewart, 1985). There was wide variability in dose response, which could not be accounted for by weight or age. Due to the limited research on this drug, more rigorously controlled trials are suggested.

Based on the research cited, it appears that the limited benefits of psychopharmacology come at the cost of side effects and rebound of aggressive behavior when medication is discontinued. Furthermore, these drugs appear to be only treating certain symptoms, and typically not the core symptoms of ASD. Many children require multiple medications to improve their symptoms, and often the benefits do not outweigh the side effects. In addition to patients responding to highly variable doses, the majority of studies reviewed indicate that not all children with ASD respond to these various medications, and there is no good explanation for why some are considered responders and some are not. In summary, the research published thus far suggests that some medications may be helpful in managing some of the behavioral disturbances seen in autism.

Diet and Diet-Related Treatments

Research has suggested that individuals with autism may not properly metabolize the proteins in casein (dairy) and gluten (wheat and related grains), resulting in an opioid effect on the brain as they enter the bloodstream (Reichelt, 2001). Autism may be comorbid with metabolic anomalies including: (1) failure of the digestive tract to fully metabolize casein and gluten into amino acids; and (2) "leaky gut" syndrome which allows undigested peptides to pass into the bloodstream (Reichelt, 2001). Cade and colleagues (1999) reported that following a gluten—casein-free diet, children with autism experienced an 81% improvement in symptoms within three months based on parent and physician ratings of severity on a Likert scale. It was also noted, qualitatively, that the mothers of four of the children in this study reported seizure frequency had significantly decreased in three children and had ceased completely in the fourth.

Knivsberg, Reichelt, Hoien, and Nodland (2002) conducted a randomized single-blind controlled study of 10 children with autism on the gluten-free/casein-free (GFCF) diet. At 1 year follow-up, the experimental group had showed significantly greater improvement in autistic behavior, non-verbal cognitive ability, and motor problems. In a 4 year longitudinal single-blind controlled pair-wise study of children with autism, following a GFCF diet resulted in significant improvement on outcome measures of cognitive function, language, and social skills (Reichelt & Knivsberg, 2003). More recently, Elder, Shankar, Shuster, Theriaque, Burns, and Sherrill (2006) conducted a rigorous double-blinded controlled trial of the GFCF diet in autism. Fifteen (12 boys, 3 girls) children with ASD between the ages of 2 and 16 were studied over the course of 12 weeks. The researchers reported no significant differences between groups on their primary measure, the Childhood Autism Rating Scale, while parents reported improvement in their children. The researchers noted that the children were quite heterogeneous (which may have masked any group differences), and noted the relatively small sample size.

An obvious limitation to this type of treatment is the lack of strict control over the diet of these children. When immunoglobulin A anti-gliadin and antiendomysium antibodies were measured to assess compliance, some studies indicated that roughly only half strictly follow dietetic prescriptions (Paolo et al., 1998). It may be difficult for parents to know which foods should be restricted, and some children may respond more slowly than others, requiring greater effects to be noticed. One of the major problems with the GFCF diet is that it may lead to reduced bone cortical thickness (Hediger et al., 2008). Indeed, in this study boys between the ages of 4 and 8 who were autistic showed a 18.9% deviation in metacarpal bone cortical thickness, which was nearly twice that of boys on minimally restricted or non-restricted diets. Furthermore, the GFCF diet may induce nutritional imbalances by limiting the foods that may be eaten. It has also been shown to increase the risk of becoming over-weight/obese (Paolo et al., 1998).

Vitamin Supplements and Enzymes

One supplement that has generated a great deal of interest as a treatment for autism is the gastrointestinal hormone secretin. After receiving intra-venous administration of secretin for upper gastrointestinal (GI) endoscopy, there was improvement in the gastrointestinal symptoms of three children with ASD (Horvath et al., 1998). In addition, within 5 weeks of the secretin administration the children's parents noticed behavioral improvements as evidenced by improved eye contact, alertness, and increased expressive language. The authors suggested that these clinical observations may indicate an association between GI functioning and brain functioning in autism. However, these behavioral observations were incidental and not an expected outcome in the procedure. As a result, there was no control group utilized and the non-experimental nature of the procedure precludes drawing any firm conclusions about its use in treating autistic behaviors. However, in October 1998, Horvath et al.'s (1998) results were reported on national television on NBC's *Dateline*, which likely sparked the demand and sharp increase in price that followed (NIH News Alert, 1999). Anecdotal reports followed, with some parents reporting dramatic improvements in their children, and others reporting no change (NIH News Alert, 1999). The National Institutes of Child Health and Human Development (NICHD) soon funded a study to investigate the use of secretin in the treatment of autism (Sandler et al., 1999). In the double-blind placebo-controlled study the researchers found no difference on any of the standardized behavioral measures utilized between the secretin and placebo groups. Commenting on the results of this study, the director of the NICHD, Duane Alexander stated, "These findings strongly suggest that secretin should not be recommended to treat autism until the results of our other ongoing studies are known" (NIH News Alert, 1999). Similarly, the American Academy of Child and Adolescent Psychiatry released a policy statement on the use of secretin in treating autism: "the available evidence does not suggest that secretin is a useful treatment for children with autism" (American Academy of Child and Adolescent Psychiatry Policy Statement, 1999).

Roberts et al. (2001) investigated the effects of repeated doses of intravenous secretin on 64 children diagnosed with autism in a randomized, placebo-controlled study. Outcome measures included assessment of cognitive, social, language, and gastrointestinal function. Following treatment, receptive and expressive language skill improvement occurred to the same extent in the secretin and placebo groups. However, parents anecdotally reported sleep improvement, toilet training success shortly after the injection, and more connectedness. Untoward side effects of secretin were evident for some of the children; 21% had generalized flushing in the neck, face, or chest following injection; 6.25% experienced irritability and hyperactivity; and 4.68% had an increase in aggression. Although no significant effects were reported for secretin, parent reports of improvement suggest there is a small subgroup of autistic children with GI symptoms who may benefit from treatment with secretin (Roberts et al., 2001). However, it is important to note that repeated use has not been approved by the FDA, and there is the possibility of an allergic reaction with multiple doses (Hirsch, 1999). Thus, extreme caution must be taken when using secretin in this manner.

A comprehensive review of research studies utilizing secretin to treat autism was conducted by Esch and Carr (2004). Seventeen quantitative studies were reviewed, encompassing approximately 600 children aged 2–15, and 12 adults with ASD. Only one of the studies reviewed found a causal relationship between secretin administration and amelioration of autistic symptoms across various treatment variables (type of secretin, dosage potency, frequency), observation times, and participant characteristics (e.g., GI status, severity of ASD, age, history of medication use). Twelve of the 13 placebo-controlled studies reviewed obtained negative results. Despite the lack of empirical support for secretin, parents of autistic children continue to seek out secretin treatment from their physicians (Esch & Carr, 2004). The reviewers attempted to explain this by the media attention that secretin received early on, coupled with the fact that parents of these children are often desperate to find a treatment for this debilitating condition.

In addition to secretin, it has been suggested that the consumption of omega-3 fatty acids may have a positive effect on the symptoms of autism (Amminger et al., 2007). These highly unsaturated fatty acids are essential for normal brain development and functioning (Wainright, 2002), and some studies have found fatty acid deficiencies in children who are autistic (Bell et al., 2004; Bell, Sargent, Tocher, & Dick, 2000; Vancassel et al., 2001). Amminger and colleagues (2007) recently completed a double-blind, randomized controlled trial of omega-3 fatty acid supplementation in children who were autistic. They found that with administration of 1.5 g/day, the treatment group showed no significant change in hyperactive behaviors including disobedience, distractibility, and impulsivity, relative to the control group. Potential limitations to this study include that it was conducted with only 12 subjects, and pre-selection of these subjects was based on high irritability scores based on the Aberrant Behavior Checklist (Aman et al., 1985).

Anecdotal reports that methyl–B12 (methylcobalamin) injections may improve the symptoms of autism have been plentiful; however, there have been very few controlled research studies to support the efficacy of this treatment. In May of 2002, Dr James Neubrander discovered (reportedly accidentally) the effects of this coenzyme. He reported that following injections of methyl-B12 in a child with autism he had been treating, the mother reported dramatic improvements in the child's behavior (Neubrander, 2005). He then began using the treatment on his other patients, again, anecdotally reporting dramatic improvements by the parents. He has reported that in his practice, "94% of children have been found to respond to methyl-B12 therapy". He has reported that executive functioning improved in 90% of children, speech and language improved in 80% of children, and "socialization/emotion" improved in 70% of children (Neubrander, 2005). Richard Deth (2004) reported his results on the administration of 75 μg/kg of methyl-B12, given every three days, in 85 children, between the ages of 3 and 11, who were autistic. A "parental questionnaire" demonstrated improvements in speech and language in 71%, cognitive function in 52%, and socialization/emotional stability in 35% of the children. He also reported that stopping treatment resulted in a worsening of symptoms, which reversed upon reinstatement of the injections.

The only published study found by the authors was an open trial of methyl-B12 conducted in Japan with 13 children with autism, ranging from 2 to 18 years of age (Nakano et al., 2005). Dosages of 25−30 g/kg/day were administered for between 6 and 25 months. The authors found a significant increase in the intelligence and developmental quotients, as well as improvement on the Childhood Autism Rating Scale (Schopler, Reichler, DeVellis, & Daly, 1980). Even after the children were allocated into subgroups based on age and intelligence, these effects did not diminish. This was not a controlled study, however. In contrast, a preliminary report of a double-blind crossover study presented at the American Academy of Child and Adolescent Psychiatry conference revealed no significant benefits in the 14 patients in their study after three months (Deprey et al., 2006). Specifically, there were no differences between the methyl-B12 injections and the placebo on the Clinical Global Impression Scale Improvement, Peabody Picture Vocabulary Test, or Social Communication Questionnaire verbal results.

Chelation

A controversial theory to explain the increase in incidence of ASDs over the past 30 years is that it is related to environmental factors such as exposure to heavy metals (Bradstreet, Geier, Kartzinel, Adams, & Geier, 2003), mercury (Hg) in particular. The medical literature indicates that autism and Hg poisoning have numerous similarities in their symptom profiles, including psychiatric disturbances, speech, language, and hearing difficulties, sensory impairment, and cognitive difficulties (Bernard et al., 2000). In autism, heavy metal toxicity seems to occur from a decreased ability to excrete heavy metals (Adams et al., 2009). Because of this, some health care providers are performing chelation therapy, which utilizes Di-mercaptosuccinic-Acid (DMSA) to clear the body of mercury and other toxic metals.

Results of a study by Holmes (2001) suggest that chelation therapy may be effective only for young children with autism (under age 6), with minimal benefit for older children and adolescents (Kirby, 2005).

Recently, Adams et al. (2009) reported the results of a two-phase study intended to determine the efficacy of DMSA/glutathione in treating children with autism. In phase I, children (N = 65) received nine doses of DMSA over 3 days; levels of metal excretion were measured at baseline and following the first and ninth dose. Those with "high" levels of toxic metal excretion (N = 41) continued to phase II of the study, which involved a 3 month, double-blind, controlled treatment study, in which children were given DMSA for 3 days, followed by 11 days off, repeated six times. The researchers found that DMSA greatly increased excretion of lead, tin, and bismuth, and also increased excretion of mercury, thallium, antimony, and tungsten. In order to assess changes in the severity of autism during the course of the study, five different measures were used: Autism Treatment Evaluation Checklist (ATEC), Severity of Autism Scale (SAS), Pervasive Developmental Disorders Behavior Inventory (PDD-BI), Autism Diagnostic Observation Schedule (ADOS), and Parent Global Impressions (PGI). The ADOS was evaluated by a certified ADOS evaluator while the rest of the measures were assessed by the participants' parents. On these behavioral measures, one round of DMSA provided almost as much benefit as seven rounds. On average across all five measures (ATEC, SAS, PDD-BI, ADOS, and PGI), 77% reported improvement, 12% reported no change, and 11% reported worsening (in both one-round and seven-round groups combined). Stepwise linear regression analyses revealed significant coefficients for the ATECT, SAS, PDD-BI, and ADOS for the seven-round group. According to the authors, these findings suggest that there is a significant relationship between changes in autism severity and urinary excretion of toxic metals for the seven-round group. There have even been reports of death following chelation therapy in autism (Sinha, Silove, & Williams, 2006), making it one of the more risky forms of intervention.

Hyperbaric Oxygen Therapy (HBOT)

Among other brain abnormalities that have been identified, numerous studies using PET and SPECT have shown cerebral hypoperfusion in autism (George, Costa, Kouris, Ring, & Ell, 1992; Mountz, Tolbert, Lill, Katholi, & Liu, 1995; Ohnishi et al., 2000; Starkstein et al., 2000; Zilbovicius et al., 2000), leading to the hypothesis that hyperbaric oxygen therapy (HBOT) may be beneficial in the treatment of autism (Rossignol & Rossignol, 2006). HBOT involves the inhalation of 100% oxygen in a pressurized chamber, usually above one atmosphere absolute (ATA). It has been shown that HBOT can lead to improved functioning in various neurological populations that show cerebral hypoperfusion including stroke (Nighoghossian, Trouillas, Adeleine, & Salord, 1995), cerebral palsy (Montgomery et al., 1999), chronically brain injured (Golden et al., 2002), and even a teenage male with Fetal Alcohol Syndrome (Stoller, 2005). It has been suggested that the increased oxygen delivered by HBOT could counteract the hypoxia caused by hypoperfusion, and lead to a reduction in symptoms of autism.

In a retrospective case study of six children with autism who had undergone low-pressure HBOT at 1.3 ATA and 28–30% oxygen over the course of 3 months, Rossignol and Rossignol (2006) found an average improvement of 22.1% based on ratings from the ATEC. An average improvement of 12.1% was reported based on the CARS, and a 22.1% improvement on the SRS. All children in this study, however, continued all other therapies they were previously receiving, and were also able to initiate new therapies during the study. Furthermore, the study was retrospective, parents were not blinded to the treatment, and there was no control group.

Rossignol, Rossignol, James, Melnyk, and Mumper (2007) treated 18 children with autism with 40 sessions of HBOT at either 1.5 atm at 100% oxygen, or at 1.3 atm and 24% oxygen. They reported a trend toward improvement in C-reactive protein measurements (a marker of inflammation) and no significant increase in oxidative stress. Parental reports revealed statistically significant improvements in irritability, social withdrawal, hyperactivity, motivation, speech, and sensory/cognitive awareness. However, parents were not blinded as to the type of therapy their children were receiving and there was no placebo or control group. These results remain preliminary and further studies are needed with more rigorous experimental designs (blinded, placebo-controlled, randomized). This study does suggest, however, that it is a relatively safe treatment, as no adverse events were reported and all children were able to complete the 40 treatment sessions.

In summary, this review of the autism treatment literature reveals there are no treatments, except possibly behavior therapy, that have been well validated or that have exhibited favorable long term results. In addition, many forms of intervention include the possibility of adverse effects, require long-term use, or were not developed specifically for Autistic Spectrum Disorders. Neurofeedback represents an alternative that may have the potential to decrease symptomatology on a long-term basis with little risk of harm.

NEUROFEEDBACK FOR ASD

Neurofeedback is designed to use sophisticated computer technology to train individuals to improve poorly regulated brainwave patterns. In EEG Biofeedback, information regarding brainwave activity is fed to a computer that converts this information into game-like displays that can be auditory, visual, or both. During a typical session, EEG electrodes (which measure brainwaves) are placed on the scalp and ear lobe(s). Individuals instantly receive feedback about the amplitude and/or synchronization of their brainwaves and learn to improve their brainwave functioning. An example of a typical set-up is displayed in Figure 6.1.

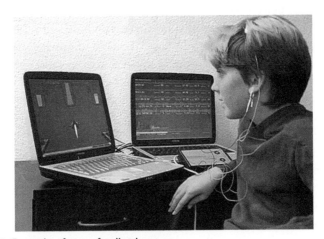

Figure 6.1 Example of neurofeedback set-up.

The only way to succeed at the games involved is for children to control and improve their brainwave patterns (following an operant conditioning paradigm). In research and clinical treatment for children with ADHD, this conditioning process has resulted in improvements that have persisted for up to 5−10 years or more (e.g., Lubar, 1995).

Individuals who participate in EEG biofeedback learn to inhibit brainwave frequencies that may produce negative symptoms and enhance specific frequencies that produce positive results. Table 6.1 displays the typical EEG brainwave frequency bands and lists their normal occurrences and respective significance [information adapted from resources contained in Demos (2005) and Thompson and Thompson (2003a,b)]. Within these general frequency bands there may also be more detailed breakdowns of EEG activity. For example, mu rhythm abnormalities are associated with excesses in the alpha frequency band and have a characteristic morphologic and topographic distribution (Coben & Hudspeth, 2006). Subdivisions of beta power have also been presented and related to clinical characteristics (Rangaswamy et al., 2002).

Table 6.1 EEG frequency bands

Name	Frequency	Normal occurrence	Significance
Delta	0.5−3.5 Hz	Deep sleep and infants	Sign of significant brain dysfunction, lethargy/drowsiness or cognitive impairment
Theta	4−7.5 Hz	Young children, drowsiness, some aspects of learning	Slowing often related to attention/cognitive impairments, internal focus
Alpha	8−13 Hz	Eyes closed, relaxation, self awareness	Excessive alpha during demand states can be a sign of difficulties with learning, emotional stability, relating to the environment or others
Beta	13−30 Hz	Fast activity associated with alertness and activity	Excessive beta is often associated with anxiety, irritability and poor integration
Gamma	Greater than 30 Hz	May be associated with problem-solving and memory consolidation	Unknown

Adapted from Demos (2005) and Thompson and Thompson (2003b).

Individuals with poorly regulated cortical activity can learn to develop a fluid shift in brainwaves to meet task demands utilizing neurofeedback. Through the process of operant conditioning, this treatment modality can result in improvement of brainwave patterns as well as behavior. These changes in EEG patterns have been shown to be associated with regulation of cerebral blood flow, metabolism, and neurotransmitter function (Lubar, 1997).

Neurofeedback is a non-invasive treatment with no known significant or lasting negative side effects that has been shown to enhance neuroregulation and metabolic function in ASD (Coben & Padolsky, 2007). Positive neurofeedback treatment outcomes are often achieved over the course of several months, in contrast to behavior therapy, which often takes a year or more of intensive training. Furthermore, the therapeutic treatment outcomes of neurofeedback training with individuals with ADHD (increased attention, reduced impulsivity and hyperactivity) have been reported to be maintained over time and not reverse after treatment is withdrawn, as in drug therapy and diet therapy (Linden, Habib, & Radojevic, 1996; Lubar, Swartwood, Swartwood, & O'Donnell, 1995; Monastra et al., 2005; Tansey, 1993).

Over 30 years of research on using neurofeedback to treat ADHD has consistently shown that it leads to improvements in attention, impulsivity, hyperactivity, and IQ (see Monastra et al., 2005, for a review and analysis). This success was the foundation for the emergence of using neurofeedback with ASD.

qEEG EVALUATION AND ASD

Quantitative electroencephalographic (qEEG) evaluation or mapping is an assessment procedure designed to pinpoint anomalies in brain function (Hammond, 2005). qEEG analyses measure abnormalities, instabilities, or lack of proper communications pathways (connectivity) necessary for optimal brain functioning. qEEG Maps, collected using 19 electrodes based on the International 10–20 system (Jasper, 1958), reflect quantitative analyses of EEG characteristics of frequency, amplitude and coherence during various conditions or tasks. These data can be statistically compared to an age-matched normative database to reveal a profile of abnormalities. Such regions and aspects of dysfunctional neurophysiology may then be targeted specifically through individualized neurofeedback protocols.

qEEG analyses are conducted to assess underlying neurophysiological patterns related to the symptoms and challenges of children with ASD. In addition, assessment of the raw EEG can be used to evaluate neurological abnormalities such as seizure disorders, which are common in children with autism. qEEG data are important for developing the most individualized, specific, and successful neurofeedback protocols for patients with ASD (Coben & Padolsky, 2007; Linden, 2004).

Linden (2004) identified four qEEG patterns of autism and two of Asperger's based on 19-channel EEG recordings and analysis of raw EEG, absolute power, relative power, and multivariate connectivity. The four autism qEEG subtype patterns are: (1) High Beta activity, which corresponds to obsessing, overfocusing, and anxiety; (2) High Delta/Theta activity, which corresponds to cortical slowing and inattention, impulsivity, and hyperactivity; (3) Abnormal EEG/Seizure activity; and (4) Metabolic/Toxic pattern of lower overall EEG activity (voltage). The High Beta subtype was the most common subtype, occurring in approximately 50—60% of the subjects with ASD. The Delta/Theta subtype occurred in 30—40%, the Abnormal EEG subtype in 33% and the Metabolic/Toxic subtype in 10%. In addition, coherence abnormalities were usually present in the qEEG profiles.

The qEEG patterns of subjects with Asperger's primarily occurred in the right temporal and parietal regions, sites involved in social and emotional recognition mechanisms. The qEEG patterns of those with Asperger's were: (1) high theta/alpha slowing in the right temporal/parietal areas and (2) low coherence between right temporal/parietal brain regions and other regions. More than one qEEG subtype pattern was frequently present in the students with ASD.

Coben, Hirshberg, and Chabot (2010) identified five relative power subtypes in individuals with autism. However, they noted that many types of dysfunction overlap in people with autism and most reveal a combination of findings. In over 83% of the individuals with autism, connectivity anomalies could be identified when compared to the normative group. Coben and Myers (2008) used qEEG multivariate connectivity data to develop a typology of autism connectivity patterns including: (1) patterns of hyperconnectivity across bilateral frontotemporal regions and between left hemisphere locations, and (2) hypoconnectivity involving orbitofrontal, frontal to posterior, right posterior or left hemisphere sites. A pattern of hypoconnectivity that underlies a mu rhythm complex was identified as well.

Neurofeedback: Case Studies, Case Series, Group Pilot Studies

There have been numerous case and group pilot studies conducted with clients diagnosed with autistic spectrum disorders. In general, these studies have shown that neurofeedback improved symptomatology and these improvements were maintained at follow-up. For a more thorough review of these, see Coben, Linden, and Myers (2009).

Controlled Group Studies of Neurofeedback for ASD

In 2007, Coben and Padolsky published a study investigating the effects of neurofeedback treatment for autistic disorders. The study included 49 children on the autistic spectrum, with 37 participants receiving qEEG connectivity-guided neurofeedback and 12 participants in a wait-list control group. Treatment included 20 sessions performed twice per week. The control group was matched for age, gender, race, handedness, other treatments, and severity of ASD. According to the parents, there was an 89% success rate for neurofeedback and an average of 40% reduction in core ASD symptomatology. There were significant improvements on neuropsychological measures of attention, visual-perceptual skills, language functions, and executive functioning. Importantly, reduced cerebral hyperconnectivity was associated with positive clinical outcomes and in all cases of reported improvement, positive outcomes were supported by neurophysiological and neuropsychological assessment.

Mu rhythm abnormalities are a sign of mirror neuron dysfunction, which is thought to be impaired in many children with autism (Oberman et al., 2005). In two studies focused on reducing abnormal mu rhythms in children with autism, Pineda et al. (2008) found that, according to parents, participants showed a small but significant reduction in symptoms but increased ratings of sensory-cognitive awareness. In another study related to mu rhythms, Coben and Hudspeth (2006) studied 14 children with ASD who were identified as having significantly high levels of mu activity and a failure to suppress mu during observational activity. They all received assessment guided neurofeedback, with a strong focus on aspects of mu power and connectivity. The participants were non-randomly assigned to an interhemispheric bipolar training (N = 7) or a coherence training (N = 7) group designed to increase connectivity between central regions and the peripheral frontal cortex. All patients were given neurobehavioral, neuropsychological testing, and qEEG assessment. Both groups of patients improved significantly on neurobehavioral and neuropsychological measures. However, only in the coherence training treatment group was mu activity significantly reduced. Increased coherence was associated with diminished mu and improved levels of social functioning.

Lastly, Coben (2007) conducted a controlled neurofeedback study focused on intervention for prominent social skill deficits based on a facial/emotional processing model. Fifty individuals with autism were included in these analyses and all had previously had some neurofeedback training. All patients underwent pre- and post-neuropsychological, qEEG, and parent rating scale assessments. Twenty-five individuals were assigned to either an active neurofeedback or a wait list control group, in a randomized fashion. The two groups were matched for age, gender, race, handedness, medication usage, autistic symptom severity, social skill ratings, and visual-perceptual impairment levels. Neurofeedback training was qEEG connectivity-guided and included coherence training (along with amplitude inhibits) between maximal sights of hypocoherence over the right posterior hemisphere. The group that received the coherence training showed significant changes in symptoms of autism, social skills, and visual-perceptual abilities such that all improved. Regression analyses showed that changes in visual-perceptual abilities significantly predicted improvements in social skills. EEG analyses were also significant, showing improvements in connectivity and source localization of theta power related to brain regions (fusiform gyrus, superior temporal sulcus) associated with enhanced visual/facial/emotional processing.

In the five controlled group studies that have been completed, a total of 180 individuals with autism have been studied and positive results reported in each study. These findings have included positive changes as evidenced by parental report, neuropsychological findings, and changes in the EEG (Coben, 2007). Both Coben and Padolsky (2007) and Yucha and Montgomery (2008) have viewed these data as demonstrating a level of efficacy of "possibly efficacious" based on the standards put forth by the Association for Applied Psychophysiology and Biofeedback (AAPB, 2006). Added to these initial findings of efficacy is preliminary evidence that the effects of neurofeedback on the symptoms of autism are long-lasting (1−2 years) (Coben, 2009; Kouijzer, DeMoor, Gerrits, Buitelaar, & van Schie, 2009). While these findings are initially encouraging, there are many limitations that prevent firm conclusions to be drawn from the data collected thus far.

First, these studies have largely included non-randomized samples. It is possible that an unknown selection bias exists which could have impacted the findings. Second, none of these studies have included participants or therapists/experimenters who were blind to the condition. Knowledge of group placement could have impacted the findings such that those in treatment (and their parents) would be prone to report significant changes. Third, there has been no attempt to control for placebo effects, attention from a caring professional or expectations of treatment benefit. A randomized, double-blinded, placebo-controlled study is clearly needed to further demonstrate efficacy.

In terms of generalization of these findings to the larger population of individuals who are autistic, very young children and adults have not been well represented in these group studies. Lastly, there is the question of whether neurofeedback may be applicable to persons who are lower functioning or who have more severe symptoms associated with autism. These populations also should be the focus of future investigations.

Efficacy of Connectivity-Guided Neurofeedback for ASD

Coben (2009) has presented a study of the effects of an entire course of connectivity-guided neurofeedback treatment on autistic children. This included 110 subjects on the autistic spectrum, with 85 in the experimental and 25 in the control (wait list) group. The mean age of these subjects was 9.7 years (range = 4–20). Seventy-seven percent of these subjects were not on medication at the time, while 14% were on one medication, 7% on two medications, and 1% on three medications. The mean IQ of this group was 93 (range = 50–130). The mean ATEC score was 50 (range = 40–170). There were no significant differences between the experimental and control groups for age, gender, handedness, race, medications, IQ, or ATEC scores.

The experimental group underwent an average of 74 neurofeedback sessions. They were assessed using qEEG, neuropsychological testing, and parent rating scales before treatment and then again after treatment. In order to evaluate the efficacy of neurofeedback treatment for reducing ASD symptomatology, the subjects' scores on the ATEC and neuropsychological testing were compared before and after treatment. A univariate analysis of variance (ANOVA) revealed that ATEC scores changed significantly after treatment ($F = 117.213$; $p = 7.3570e{-}018$; see Figure 6.2). Furthermore, 98.8% of parents reported a reduction in ASD symptoms on the ATEC after treatment

On objective neuropsychological testing, 100% of subjects demonstrated some degree of improvement. An ANOVA revealed improvements on tests of visual-perceptual skills ($F = 53.6$, $p = 1.6074e{-}010$), language abilities ($F = 31.24$, $p = 1.2653e{-}006$), attentional skills ($F = 54.04$, $p = 7.1610e{-}011$), and executive functioning ($F = 15.65$, $p = 0.00015$). In fact, visual-perceptual

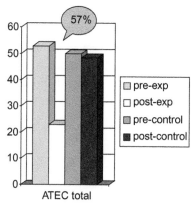

Figure 6.2 Pre-and post-treatment ATEC scores.

skills improved 43%, language abilities improved 47%, attentional skills improved 56%, and executive functioning improved 48%.

Once it was determined that the therapy was efficacious, the next question investigated was whether it had greater efficacy depending on level of functioning or severity of autistic symptoms. We investigated the effects of pre-treatment ATEC and IQ scores on treatment outcome by dividing the groups into quartiles based on ATEC and IQ scores and re-analyzing the data. There were no significant differences for any of these analyses. This revealed that: (1) ASD symptomatology improved with treatment regardless of IQ and (2) severity of ASD symptoms did not affect treatment outcomes. These results suggest that neurofeedback is an effective treatment regardless of the child's intellectual ability or severity of symptoms, at least within the parameters of the subjects that were included in this study.

DISCUSSION

There are few interventions with proven efficacy for children with autism. Behavioral modification interventions currently have the most empirical support, while pharmacologic interventions, hyperbaric oxygen, and vitamin supplementation have shown some potential. It is our opinion that neurofeedback is in a similar position with respect to efficacy for ASD, but more research is needed.

Neurofeedback is an intervention that may prove to be efficacious in the treatment of symptoms of autism. At present, it should be viewed as possibly efficacious with potential, as is the case with most interventions used with this population. Measuring brain-related changes that may occur as a result of neurofeedback is one way of demonstrating its efficacy and mechanism of action. Additional well-designed, more rigorous studies, and longer follow-up periods should be included in the future to measure the efficacy of neurofeedback in treating children on the autistic spectrum.

REFERENCES

AAPB (Association for Applied Psychophysiology & Biofeedback). (2006). Efficacy: How we rate the efficacy of our treatments or how to know if our treatments actually work. Retrieved February 22, 2006 from <www.aapb.org/i4a/pages/index.cfm?pageid=3336>.

Adams, J. B., Baral, M., Geis, E., Mitchell, J., Ingram, J., Hensley, A., et al. (2009). Safety and efficacy of oral DMSA therapy for children with autism spectrum disorders: Part A — Medical results. *BMC Clinical Pharmacology, 9*, 16.

Aman, M. G., Singh, N. N., & Stewart, A. W. (1985). The Aberrant Behavior Checklist: A behavior rating scale for the assessment of treatment effects. *American Journal of Mental Deficiency, 5*, 485—491.

American Academy of Child & Adolescent Psychiatry. (1999, March 3). Secretin in the treatment of autism. [Policy statement]. Retrieved March 19, 2010 from: www.aacap.org/cs/root/policy_statements/secretin_in_the_treatment_of_autism.

American Psychiatric Association. (2000). *Diagnostic and statistical manual of mental disorders, fourth edition-text revision (DSR-IV-TR)* Washington, DC: Author.

Amminger, G. P., Berger, G. E., Schafer, M. R., Klier, C., Friedrich, M. H., & Feucht, M. (2007). Omega-3 fatty acids supplementation in children with autism: A double-blind randomized, placebo-controlled study. *Biological Psychiatry, 61*, 551—553.

Anderson, S. R., Avery, D. L., DiPietro, E. K., Edwards, G. L., & Christian, W. P. (1987). Intensive home-based early intervention with autistic children. *Education and Treatment of Children, 10*, 352—366.

Attwood, T. (1998). *Asperger's syndrome: A guide for parents and professionals.* London: Jessica Kingsley.

Barnard, A. L., Young, A. H., Pearson, A. D. J., Geddes, J., & Obrien, G. (2002). A systematic review of the use of atypical antipsychotics in autism. *Journal of Psychopharmacology, 16*, 93—102.

Bassett, K., Green, C. J., & Kazanjian, A. (2000). *Autism and Lovaas treatment: A systematic review of effectiveness evidence.* British Columbia Office of Health Technology Assessment, The University of British Columbia, Vancouver, BC.

Bell, J. G., MacKinlay, E. E., Dick, J. R., MacDonald, D. J., Boyle, R. M., & Glen, A. C. (2004). Essential fatty acids and phospholipase A2 in autistic spectrum disorders. *Prostoglandins, Leukotrienes, and Essential Fatty Acids, 71*, 201—204.

Bell, J. G., Sargent, J. R., Tocher, D. R., & Dick, J. R. (2000). Red blood cell fatty acid compositions in a patient with autistic spectrum disorder: A characteristic abnormality in neurodevelopmental disorders? *Prostaglandins, Leukorienes, and Essential Fatty Acids, 63*(1-2), 21—25.

Ben-Itzchak, E., & Zachor, D. A. (2007). The effects of intellectual functioning and autism severity on outcome of early intervention for children with autism. *Research in Developmental Disabilities, 28*, 287—303.

Bernard, S., Enayati, A., Binstock, T., Roger, H., Redwood, L., & McGinnis, W. (2000). *Autism: A unique type of mercury poisoning* ARC Research. Available from the Autism Research Institute.

Blaxill, M. F. (2004). What's going on? The question of time trends in autism. *Public Health Reports, 119,* 536—551.

Bradstreet, J., Geier, B. A., Kartzinel, J. J., Adams, J. B., & Geier, M. R. (2003). A case-control study of mercury burden in children with autistic spectrum disorders. *Journal of American Physicians and Surgeons, 8*(3), 76—79.

Cade, R., Privette, M., Fregley, M., Rowland, N., Sun, Z., Zele, V., et al. (1999). Autism and schizophrenia: Intestinal disorders. *Nutritional Neuroscience, 3,* 57—72.

Center for Disease Control and Prevention (2009). Prevalence of the Autism Spectrum Disorders — Autism and Developmental Disabilities Monitoring Network, United States, 2006. *Morbidity and Mortality Weekly Report,* 58 (SS10; 1-20).

Coben, R. (2007, September). Autistic spectrum disorder: A controlled study of EEG coherence training targeting social skill deficits. Presented at the 15th annual conference of the International Society for Neurofeedback and Research, San Diego, CA.

Coben, R. (2009). Efficacy of connectivity-guided neurofeedback for Autistic Spectrum Disorder: Controlled analysis of 75 cases with a 1 to 2 year follow-up. *Journal of Neurotherapy, 13*(1), 81.

Coben, R., Hirshberg, L.M., & Chabot, R. (2010). EEG discriminant power and subtypes in Autistic Spectrum Disorder. (submitted for publication).

Coben, R., & Hudspeth, W. (2006, September). Mu-like rhythms in Autistic Spectrum Disorder: EEG analyses and neurofeedback. Presented at the 14th annual conference of the International Society for Neuronal Regulation, Atlanta, GA.

Coben, R., Linden, M., & Myers, T. E. (2009). Neurofeedback for Autistic Spectrum Disorder: A review of the literature. *Applied Psychophysiology and Biofeedback, 35*(1), 83—105.

Coben, R., & Myers, T. E. (2008). Connectivity theory of Autism: Use of connectivity measures in assessing and treating Autistic Disorders. *Journal of Neurotherapy, 12*(2-3), 161—179.

Coben, R., & Padolsky, I. (2007). Assessment guided neurofeedback for autistic spectrum disorder. *Journal of Neurotherapy, 11*(3), 5—18.

Committee on Children with Disabilities. (2001). Technical report: The pediatrician's role in the diagnosis and management of autistic spectrum disorder in children. *Pediatrics, 107*(5), 1—35.

Cook, E. H., Rowlett, R., & Jaselskis, C. (1992). Fluoxetine treatment of children and adults with autistic disorder and mental retardation. *Journal of the American Academy of Child and Adolescent Psychiatry, 31,* 739—745.

Couper, J. (2004). Who should pay for intensive behavioural intervention in autism? A parent's view. *Journal of Paediatrics and Child Health, 40*(9-10), 559—561.

Couturier, J. L., & Nicolson, R. (2002). A retrospective assessment of citalopram in children and adolescents with pervasive developmental disorders. *Journal of Child and Adolescent Psychopharmacology, 12,* 243—248.

DeLong, G. R., Ritch, C. R., & Burch, S. (2002). Fluoxetine response in children with autistic spectrum disorders: Correlation with familial major affective disorder and intellectual achievement. *Developmental Medicine and Child Neurology, 44,* 652—659.

Demos, J. N. (2005). *Getting started with neurofeedback.* New York: W. W. Norton & Company.

Deth, R.C. (2004, October) Methylcobalamin for Autistic Children. Presented at the 34th annual meeting of the Society for Neuroscience, San Diego, CA.

Deprey, L.J., Brule, N., Widjaja, F., Sepheri, S., Blank, J., Neubrander, J., et al. (2006, October). Double-blind placebo-controlled, cross-over trial of subcutaneous methylcobalamin in children with Autism: Preliminary results. Poster presented at the annual meeting of the American Academy of Child and Adolescent Psychiatry, San Diego, CA.

Elder, J. H, Shankar, M., Shuster, J., Theriaque, D., Burns, S., & Sherrill, L. (2006). The gluten-free, casein-free diet in autism: Results of a preliminary double blind clinical trial. *Journal of Autism and Developmental Disorders, 36,* 413–420.

Esch, B. E., & Carr, J. E. (2004). Secretin as a treatment for Autism: A review of the evidence. *Journal of Autism and Developmental Disorders, 34,* 543–556.

Geller, D. A., Hoog, S. L., Heiligenstein, J. H., Ricardi, R. K., Tamura, R., Kluszynski, S., et al. (2001). Fluoxetine treatment for obsessive compulsive disorder in children and adolescents: A placebo controlled clinical trial. *Journal of the American Academy of Child and Adolescent Psychiatry, 40,* 739–773.

George, M. S., Costa, D. C., Kouris, K., Ring, H. A., & Ell, P. J. (1992). Cerebral blood flow abnormalities in adults with infantile autism. *Journal of Nervous and Mental Disease, 180,* 413–417.

Golden, Z. L., Neubauer, R., Golden, C. J., Greene, L., Marsh, J., & Mleko, A. (2002). Improvement in cerebral metabolism in chronic brain injury after hyperbaric oxygen therapy. *International Journal of Neuroscience, 112,* 119–131.

Green, V. A., Pituch, K. A., Itchon, J., Choi, A., O'Reilly, M., & Sigafoos, J. (2006). Internet survey of treatments used by parents of children with autism. *Research in Developmental Disabilities, 27,* 70–84.

Hamilton, L. (2000). *Facing autism: Giving parents reasons for hope and guidance for help* Colorado Springs, CO: WaterBrook Press.

Hammond, D. C. (2005). *What is neurofeedback?* Retrieved July 25, 2006 from <www.isnr.org/pubarea/whatisnfb.pdf>.

Hediger, M. L., England, L. J., Molloy, C. A., Yu, K. F., Manning-Courtney, P., & Mills, J. L. (2008). Reduced bone cortical thickness in boys with autism or autism spectrum disorder. *Journal of Autism and Developmental Disorders, 38,* 848–856.

Herbert, J. D., Sharp, I. R., & Gaudiano, B. A. (2002). Separating fact from fiction in the etiology and treatment of autism. A scientific review of the evidence. *The Scientific Review of Mental Health Practice, 1*(1). Accessed online at: http://www.srmhp.org/0101/autism.html

Hill, E. L. (2004). Executive dysfunction in autism. *Trends in Cognitive Sciences, 8*(1), 26–32.

Hollander, E., Phillips, A., Chaplin, W., Zagursky, K., Novotny, S., Wasserman, S., et al. (2005). A placebo controlled crossover trial of liquid fluoxetine on repetitive behaviors in childhood and adolescent autism. *Neuropsychopharmacology, 30,* 582–589.

Holmes, A. (2001). *Autism treatments: Chelation of mercury.* Retrieved March 30, 2010, from http://www.healing-arts.org/children/holmes.htm.

Horvath, K., Stefanatos, G., Sokolski, K. N., Wachtel, R., Nabors, L., & Tildon, J. T. (1998). Improved social and language skills after secretin administration in patients with autistic spectrum disorders. *Journal of the Association for Academic Minority Physicians, 9,* 9–15.

Hughes, J. R., & John, E. R. (1999). Conventional and quantitative electroencephalography in psychiatry. *Journal of Neuropsychiatry and Clinical Neurosciences, 11,* 190–208.

Hirsch, D. (1999). Secretin in the treatment of autism. *The Exceptional Parent, 29,* 94.

Jasper, H. (1958). The ten-twenty electrode system of the International Federation. *Electroencephalography and Clinical Neurophysiology, 10,* 371–375.

Jensen, P. S., Arnold, L. E., Swarson, J. M., Vitiello, B., Abikoff, H. B., Greenhill, L. L., et al. (2007). 3-Year follow-up of the NIMH MTA study. *Journal of the American Academy of Child and Adolescent Psychiatry, 46*(8), 989–1002.

Jesner, O.S., Aref-Adib, M., & Coren, E. (2007). Risperidone for autism spectrum disorder. Cochrane Database of Systematic Reviews, 1(CD005040). Retrieved July 18, 2008, from Cochrane Database of Systematic Reviews database.

Just, M. A., Cherkassy, V. L., Keller, T. A., & Minshew, N. J. (2004). Cortical activation and synchronization during sentence comprehension in high-functioning autism: Evidence of underconnectivity. *Brain, 127,* 1811–1821.

Kirby, D. (2005). *Evidence of harm: Mercury in vaccines and the autism epidemic: A medical controversy* New York: St Martin's Press.

Knivsberg, A. M., Reichelt, K. L., Hoien, T., & Nodland, M. (2002). A randomized, controlled study of dietary intervention in autistic syndromes. *Nutritional Neuroscience, 5,* 251–261.

Kouijzer, M. E. J., de Moor, J. M. H., Gerrits, B. J. L., Buitelaar, J. K., & van Schie, H. T. (2009). Long-term effects of neurofeedback treatment in autism. *Research in Autism Spectrum Disorders, 3*(2), 496–501.

Linden, M. (2004, August). *Case studies of qEEG mapping and neurofeedback with autism.* Presented at the 12th annual conference of the International Society for Neuronal Regulation, Fort Lauderdale, FL.

Linden, M., Habib, T., & Radojevic, V. (1996). A controlled study of the effects of EEG biofeedback on cognition and behavior of children with attention deficit disorder and learning disabilities. *Biofeedback and Self-Regulation, 21,* 35–50.

Lord, C., Rutter, M., DiLavore, P. C., & Risi, S. (1999). *Autism diagnostic observation schedule-WPS (ADOS-WPS).* Los Angeles, CA: Western Psychological Services.

Lovaas, O. I. (1987). Behavioral treatment and normal educational and intellectual functioning in young autistic children. *Journal of Consulting and Clinical Psychology, 55,* 3–9.

Lovaas, O. I., Koegel, R., Simmons, J. Q., & Long, J. S. (1973). Some generalization and follow-up measures on autistic children in behavior therapy. *Journal of Applied Behavior Analysis, 6*(1), 131–165.

Lubar, J. F. (1995). Neurofeedback for the management of attention-deficit/hyperactivity disorders. In M. S. Schwartz (Ed.), *Biofeedback: A practitioner's guide* (3rd ed., pp. 493–522). New York: Guilford.

Lubar, J. F. (1997). Neurobiological foundation for neurofeedback treatment of attention deficit hyperactivity disorder (ADD/HD). *Biofeedback, 25*(10), 4–23.

Lubar, J. F., Swartwood, M. O., Swartwood, J. N., & O'Donnell, P. H. (1995). Evaluation of the effectiveness of EEG training for ADHD in a clinical setting as measured by TOVA scores, behavioral ratings, and WISC-R performance. *Biofeedback and Self-Regulation, 20,* 83–99.

Martin, A., Koenig, K., Anderson, G., & Scahill, L. (2003). Low dose fluvoxamine treatment of children and adolescents with pervasive developmental disorders: A prospective, open-label study. *Journal of Autism and Developmental Disorders, 33*(1), 77–85.

Martin, A., Scahill, L., Klin, A., & Volkmar, F. R. (1999). Higher functioning pervasive developmental disorders: Rates and patterns of psychotropic drug use. *Journal of the American Academy of Child and Adolescent Psychiatry, 38,* 923–931.

McAlonan, G. M., Cheung, V., Cheung, C., Suckling, J., Lam, G. Y., Tai, K. S., et al. (2004). Mapping the brain in autism: A voxel-based MRI study of volumetric differences and intercorrelations in autism. *Brain, 128*(Pt 2), 268–276.

McCandless, J. (2005). *Children with starving brains: A medical treatment guide for autism spectrum disorder.* Putney, VT: Bramble Books.

McDougle, C. J., Brodkin, E. S., Naylor, S. T., Carlson, D. C., Cohen, D. J., & Price, L. H. (1998). Sertraline in adults with pervasive developmental disorders: A prospective, open-label investigation. *Journal of Clinical Psychopharmacology, 18,* 62–66.

McDougle, C. J., Kresch, L. E., Goodman, W. K., Naylor, S. T., Volkmar, F. R., Cohen, D. J., et al. (1995). A case-controlled study of repetitive thoughts and behavior in adults with autistic disorder and obsessive—compulsive disorder. *American Journal of Psychiatry, 152*, 772—777.

McDougle, C. J., Kresch, L. E., & Posey, D. J. (2000). Repetitive thoughts and behavior in pervasive developmental disorders: Treatment with serotonin reuptake inhibitors. *Journal of Autism and Developmental Disorders, 30*, 427—435.

McDougle, C. J., Naylor, S. T., Cohen, D. J., Volkmar, F. R., Heninger, G. R., & Price, L. H. (1996). A double-blind, placebo controlled study of fluvoxamine in adults with autistic disorder. *Archives of General Psychiatry, 53*, 1001—1008.

McEachin, J. J., Smith, T., & Lovaas, O. I. (1993). Long-term outcome for children with autism who received early intensive behavioral treatment. *American Journal of Mental Retardation, 97*, 359—372.

Monastra, V. J., Lynn, S., Linden, M., Lubar, J. F., Gruzelier, J., & LaVaque, T. J. (2005). Electroencephalographic biofeedback in the treatment of attention-deficit/hyperactivity disorder. *Applied Psychophysiology and Biofeedback, 30*, 95—114.

Montgomery, D., Goldberg, J., Amar, M., Lacroix, V., Lecomte, J., Venasse, M., et al. (1999). Effects of hyperbaric oxygen therapy on children with spastic diplegic cerebral palsy: A pilot project. *Undersea and Hyperbaric Medicine, 26*, 235—242.

Mountz, J. M., Tolbert, L. C., Lill, D. W., Katholi, C. R., & Liu, H. G. (1995). Functional deficits in autistic disorder: Characterization by technetium-99m-HMPAO and SPECT. *Journal of Nuclear Medicine, 36*, 1156—1162.

Nakano, K., Noda, N., Tachikawa, E., Urano, M., Takazawa, M., Nakayama, T., et al. (2005). A preliminary study of methylcobalamin therapy in autism. *Journal of Tokyo Women's Medical University, 75*(3/4), 64—69.

Namerow, L. B., Thomas, P., Bostic, J. Q., Prince, J., & Monuteaux, M. C. (2003). Use of citalopram in pervasive developmental disorders. *Journal of Developmental and Behavioral Pediatrics, 24*(2), 104—108.

National Institute of Child Health and Human Development. (1999, December 8). [National Institutes of Health News Alert]. Study shows secretin fails to benefit children with autism. Retrieved March 8, 2010, from www.nichd.nih.gov/news/releases/secretin.cfm.

National Institute of Mental Health (2006). *Autism Spectrum Disorders (Pervasive Developmental Disorders).* Retrieved February 12, 2010, from www.nimh.nih.gov/health/publications/autism/complete-index.shtml.

Neubrander, J.A. (2005, May). Methyl-B12: Making it work for you! Presented at the Autism One Conference, Chicago, IL.

Nighoghossian, N., Trouillas, P., Adeleine, P., & Salord, F. (1995). Hyperbaric oxygen in the treatment of acute ischemic stroke. *Stroke, 26*, 1369—1372.

Oberman, L. M., Hubbard, E. M., McCleery, J. P., Altschuler, E. L., Ramachandran, V. S., & Pineda, J. A. (2005). EEG evidence for mirror neuron dysfunction in autism spectrum disorders. *Cognitive Brain Research, 24*, 190—198.

Ohnishi, T., Matsuda, H., Hashimoto, T., Kunihiro, T., Nishikawa, M., Uema, T., & Sasaki, M. (2000). Abnormal regional cerebral blood flow in childhood autism. *Brain, 123*, 1838—1844.

Ozonoff, S., & Cathcart, K. (1998). Effectiveness of a home program intervention for young children with autism. *Journal of Autism & Developmental Disorders, 28*, 25—32.

Owley, T., Walton, L., Salt, J., Guter, S. J., Winnega, M., Leventhal, B. L., et al. (2005). An open-label trial of escitalopram in pervasive developmental disorders. *Journal of the American Academy of Child and Adolescent Psychiatry, 44*, 343—348.

Paolo, M., Viti, M. G., Montouri, M., LaVecchia, A., Cipolletta, E., Calvani, L., et al. (1998). The gluten-free diet: A nutritional risk factor for adolescents with celiac disease? *Journal of Pediatric Gastroenterology and Nutrition, 27*, 519—523.

Pelphrey, K., Adolphs, R., & Morris, J. P. (2004). Neuroanatomical substrates of social cognition dysfunction in autism. *Mental Retardation and Developmental Disabilities Research Reviews, 10*, 259–271.

Pineda, J. A., Brang, D., Hecht, E., Edwards, L., Carey, S., Bacon, M., et al. (2008). Positive behavioral and electrophysiological changes following neurofeedback training in children with autism. *Research in Autism Spectrum Disorders, 2*(3), 557–581.

Ramachandran, V. S., & Pineda, J. A. (2005). EEG evidence for mirror neuron dysfunction in autism spectrum disorders. *Cognitive Brain Research, 24*, 190–198.

Rangaswamy, M., Porjesz, B., Chorlian, D. B., Wang, K., Jones, K. A., Bauer, L. O., et al. (2002). Beta power in the EEG of alcoholics. *Biological Psychiatry, 52*, 831–842.

Reichelt, K. (2001, October). Opioid peptides. Paper presented at the Defeat Autism Now Conference, San Diego, CA.

Reichelt, K., & Knivsberg, A.M. (2003, October). Why use the gluten-free and casein-free diet in autism and what the results have shown so far: Peptides and autism. Paper presented at the Defeat Autism Now Conference, Portland, OR.

Rippon, G., Brock, J., Brown, C., & Boucher, J. (2007). Disordered connectivity in the Autistic brain: Challenges for the "new psychophysiology". *International Journal of Psychophysiology, 63*(2), 164–172.

Roberts, W., Weaver, L., Brian, J., Bryson, S., Emelianova, S., Griffiths, A. M., et al. (2001). Repeated doses of porcine secretin in the treatment of autism: A randomized, placebo-controlled trial. *Pediatrics, 107*(5), 71–80.

Rossignol, D. A., & Rossignol, L. W. (2006). Hyperbaric oxygen therapy may improve symptoms in autistic children. *Medical Hypotheses, 67*, 216–228.

Rossignol, D. A., Rossignol, L. W., James, S. J., Melnyk, S., & Mumper, E. (2007). The effects of hyperbaric oxygen therapy on oxidative stress, inflammation, and symptoms in children with autism: An open-label pilot study. *BMC Pediatrics, 7*, 36–49.

RUPP (Research Units on Pediatric Psychopharmacology Autism Network). (2005a). Risperidone treatment of autistic disorder: Longer-term benefits and blinded discontinuation after 6 months. *American Journal of Psychiatry, 162*, 1361–1369.

RUPP (Research Units on Pediatric Psychopharmacology Autism Network). (2005b). Randomized, controlled, crossover trial of methylphenidate in pervasive developmental disorders with hyperactivity. *Archives of General Psychiatry, 62*(11), 1266–1274.

Sandler, A. D., Sutton, K. A., DeWeese, J., Girardi, M. A., Sheppard, V., & Bodfish, J. W. (1999). Lack of benefit of a single dose of synthetic human secretin in the treatment of autism and pervasive developmental disorder. *New England Journal of Medicine, 341*, 1801–1806.

Santangelo, S. L., & Tsatsanis, K. (2005). What is known about autism: Genes, brain, and behavior. *American Journal of Pharmacogenomics, 5*(2), 71–92.

Schopler, E., & Reichler, R. J. (1971). Parents as cotherapists in the treatment of psychotic children. *Journal of Autism and Childhood Schizophrenia, 1*, 87–102.

Schopler, E., Reichler, R. J., DeVellis, R. F., & Daly, K. (1980). Toward objective classification of childhood autism: Childhood Autism Rating Scale (CARS). *Journal of Autism and Developmental Disorders, 10*(1), 91–103.

Schmitz, N., Rubia, K., Daly, E., Smith, A., Williams, S., & Murphy, D. G. (2006). Neural correlates of executive function in autistic spectrum disorders. *Biological Psychiatry, 59*(1), 7–16.

Sicile-Kira, C. (2004). *Autism spectrum disorders: The complete guide to understanding autism, Asperger's syndrome, pervasive developmental disorder, and ASDs.* New York: The Berkley Publishing Group.

Siegel, B. (1996). *The world of the autistic child: Understanding and treating autistic spectrum disorders.* New York: Oxford University Press.

Sinha, Y., Silove, N., & Williams, K. (2006). Chelation therapy and autism. *British Medical Journal, 333*(7571), 756.

Starkstein, S. E., Vazquez, S., Vrancic, D., Nanclares, V., Manes, F., Piven, J., et al. (2000). SPECT findings in mentally retarded autistic individuals. *Journal of Neuropsychiatry and Clinical Neurosciences, 12,* 370–375.

Stoller, K. P. (2005). Quantification of neurocognitive changes before, during, and after hyperbaric oxygen therapy in a case of fetal alcohol syndrome. *Pediatrics, 116*(4), e586–591.

Tansey, M. A. (1993). Ten-year stability study of EEG biofeedback results for a hyperactive boy who failed a fourth grade perceptually impaired class. *Biofeedback and Self-Regulation, 18*(1), 33–44.

Thompson, L., & Thompson, M. (2003a, March). Neurofeedback treatment for Autistic Spectrum Disorders: Review of 60 cases – principles and outcome. Citation paper presented at the 34th Annual Meeting of the Association for Applied Psychophysiology and Biofeedback, Jacksonville, FL.

Thompson, M., & Thompson, L. (2003b). *The neurofeedback book: An introduction to basic concepts in applied psychophysiology.* Wheat Ridge, CO: Association for Applied Psychophysiology and Biofeedback.

Troost, P. W., Lahuis, B. E., Steenhuis, M. P., Ketelaars, C. E., Buitelaar, J. K., van Engeland, H., et al. (2005). Long-term effects of risperidone in children with autism spectrum disorders: A placebo discontinuation study. *Journal of the American Academy of Child & Adolescent Psychiatry, 44*(11), 1137–1144.

Vancassel, S., Durand, G., Barthelemy, C., Lejeune, B., Martineau, J., Guilloteau, D., et al. (2001). Plasma fatty acid levels in autistic children. *Prostaglandins, Leukotrienes, and Essential Fatty Acids, 65*(1), 1–7.

Wainright, P. E. (2002). Dietary essential fatty acids and brain function: A developmental perspective on mechanisms. *Proceedings of the Nutrition Society, 61,* 61–69.

Welchew, D. E., Ashwin, C., Berkouk, K., Salvador, R., Suckling, J., Baron-Cohen, S., et al. (2005). Functional disconnectivity of the medial temporal lobe in asperger's syndrome. *Biological Psychiatry, 57,* 991–998.

Yucha, C., & Montgomery, D. (2008). *Evidence-based practice in biofeedback and neurofeedback.* Wheat Ridge, CO: Association for Applied Psychophysiology and Biofeedback.

Zilbovicius, M., Boddaert, N., Belin, P., Poline, J. B., Remy, P., Mangin, J. F., et al. (2000). Temporal lobe dysfunction in childhood autism: A PET study. *American Journal of Psychiatry, 157,* 1988–1993.

Zuddas, A., Di Martino, A., Muglia, P., & Cichetti, C. (2000). Long-term risperidone for pervasive developmental disorder: Efficacy, tolerability, and discontinuation. *Journal of Child and Adolescent Psychopharmacology, 10,* 79–90.

CHAPTER 7

Neurofeedback and Epilepsy

Gabriel Tan[1,2], D. Corydon Hammond[3], Jonathan Walker[4], Ellen Broelz[5], and Ute Strehl[5]

[1]Michael E. DeBakey Veterans Affairs Medical Center, Houston, Texas, USA
[2]Baylor College of Medicine, Houston, Texas, USA
[3]University of Utah School of Medicine, Salt Lake City, Utah, USA
[4]Neurotherapy Center of Dallas, Texas, USA
[5]Institute of Medical Psychology and Behavioral Neurobiology, University of Tübingen, Tübingen, Germany

Contents

INTRODUCTION

Nearly 50 million people currently suffer from epilepsy; 0.8% of the general population, according to the World Health Organization (2009). Medication successfully controls seizures in two-thirds of cases, but potential side effects and health risks associated with long-term usage of antiepileptics remain a concern. When medications fail, neurosurgery is another treatment option, but it has limited success (Witte, Iasemidis, & Litt, 2003). All told, about one in three epilepsy patients will continue to experience the disability of uncontrollable seizures throughout their lifetime (Iasemidis, 2003).

The use of neurofeedback to reduce intractable seizures has been under serious investigation for 40 years, beginning with cats (Sterman, Wyrwicka, &

Neurofeedback and Neuromodulation Techniques and Applications
DOI: 10.1016/B978-0-12-382235-2.00007-X

Roth, 1969; Wyrwicka & Sterman, 1968), monkeys (Sterman, Goodman, & Kovalesky, 1978), and humans (Sterman & Friar, 1972). Although EEG rhythm training has been associated with clinical improvement as well as electroencephalographic (EEG) normalization of seizure patients (see Sterman, 2000, for a review), few neurologists and epileptologists have adopted this approach to help treat seizure disorder.

This chapter will briefly summarize the published research on neuro-feedback and epilepsy, followed by a description of the clinical protocols typically used and illustrated with case examples when appropriate. Then, the use of qEEG to improve outcome will be described. The chapter will conclude with some observations and implications for future directions.

RESEARCH SYNOPSIS

Research in the United States has emphasized sensorimotor rhythm (SMR) up-training (i.e., increasing 12—15 Hz activity at motor strip) (Lubar et al., 1981; Sterman, 2000; Sterman, Macdonald, & Stone, 1974) with or without simultaneous downtraining of slow rhythms (e.g., decreasing 4—7 Hz activity) (Cott, Pavloski, & Black, 1979; Hansen, Trudeau, & Grace, 1996; Lantz & Sterman, 1988; Tozzo, Elfner, & May, 1988). Research in Europe, on the other hand, has focused principally on slow cortical potentials (SCP), which last several hundred milliseconds and reflect the level of excitability of underlying cortex. Negative SCP-shifts are observed before and during seizures and positive shifts appear after their abatement (Ikeda et al., 1996). To prevent seizure onset, patients learn to suppress negativity (excitation) by producing positive shifts (inhibition).

The research on neurofeedback and epilepsy has historically been lim-ited (of necessity) to small sample sizes and only a single group for which pre- and post-treatment effects are determined. One exception was a study using SCP which was a controlled study with between-group com-parisons (Kotchoubey et al., 2001). Despite these limitations, results have been consistent across studies, generally suggesting that neurofeedback leads to reduction in seizures. For example, one study found that over 80% of 83 patients achieved control over seizures when a combination of interventions was used, including identifying precursors and triggers for seizures, diaphragmatic breathing, and SMR biofeedback (Andrews & Schonfeld, 1992).

Finally, learned alterations in EEG patterns with neurofeedback are neither necessarily conscious nor voluntary, as indicated by associated changes and related clinical shifts during the unconscious state of sleep. As SMR increases, nocturnal epileptiform activity decreases (Sterman, 1982; Sterman & Shouse, 1980; Whitsett, Lubar, Holder, Pamplin, & Shabsin, 1982).

Sterman (2000) summarized peer-reviewed neurofeedback epilepsy research from 1972 to 1996 and determined that four out of every five patients enrolled in these various studies improved clinically (142 of 174 patients, or 82%), and most (66% of reported cases) exhibited "contingency-related EEG changes and a shift towards EEG normalization" (Sterman, 2000, p. 52).

Studies utilizing SCP training, though not as numerous, also show positive outcomes. Kotchoubey et al. (2001) found decreased seizure incidence following SCP training, which was correlated to SCP amplitude. Rockstroh et al. (1993) reported significant seizure reductions, with six participants having longer seizure-free periods. Finally, Holzapfel, Strehl, Kotchoubey, and Birbaumer (1998) also found reductions in seizure rate following SCP training in an individual experiencing generalized clonic—tonic seizure despite taking anticonvulsant medications and after an anterior callosotomy.

While results reported in these and other studies are promising, any study alone is insufficient to determine whether neurofeedback is efficacious for treating epilepsy. Consequently, a meta-analysis was recently published (Tan et al., 2009). In this study, every EEG biofeedback study indexed in MedLine, PsychInfo, and PsychLit databases between 1970 and 2005 on epilepsy which provided seizure frequency change in response to feedback was included. Sixty-three published studies were identified, 10 of which provided enough outcome information to be included in a meta-analysis. All studies consisted of patients whose seizures were not controlled by medical therapies, which is a very important factor to keep in mind when interpreting results. Nine of 10 studies reinforced SMR while one study trained SCP. All studies reported an overall mean decreased seizure incidence following treatment and 64 out of 87 patients (74%) reported fewer weekly seizures in response to EEG biofeedback. Treatment effect was mean log (post/pre) where *pre* and *post* represent number of seizures per week prior to treatment and at final evaluation, respectively. Due to prevalence of small groups, Hedges's g was computed for effect size. As sample heterogeneity was possible (Q test, $p = 0.18$), random effects were assumed and the effect of intervention was -0.233,

SE = 0.057, z = −4.11, p <0.001. The meta-analysis concluded that: "EEG operant conditioning was found to produce a significant reduction on seizure frequency. This finding is especially noteworthy given that the patients treated with neurotherapy often consisted of individuals who had been unable to control their seizures with medical treatment" (Tan et al., 2009, p. 173).

CLINICAL PROTOCOLS

There are several different approaches utilizing neurofeedback that have reported successful outcomes with uncontrolled epilepsy: (1) reinforcing SMR, inhibiting theta; (2) inhibiting theta, reinforcing 15−18 Hz; (3) SCP self-regulation training; (4) the Low Energy Neurofeedback System (LENS); and (5) QEEG-guided neurofeedback. Each of these will be reviewed briefly.

Reinforcing SMR, Inhibiting Theta

In the recent meta-analytic review, Tan et al. (2009) found that the largest volume of controlled research with documented positive effects for treatment of uncontrolled epilepsy involved reinforcing SMR (most commonly defined as 12−15 Hz over the sensorimotor strip), while inhibiting theta activity (3 or 4−7 Hz). Most of the studies identified used a bipolar (sequential) montage; however, today some clinicians use this protocol with monopolar training (one active electrode site on the head, referenced to an earlobe, usually in the same hemisphere).

Inhibiting Theta, Reinforcing 15−18 Hz

Ayers (1988, 1995) reported successfully treating cases of uncontrolled epilepsy using bipolar (sequential) montage training at T3−C3 (or T7−C1) for 15 minutes, followed by 15 minutes of training at T4−C4 (or T8−C2), which inhibited 4−7 Hz while mildly reinforcing 15−18 Hz (e.g., with the reward threshold at only 0.4 μV). Following improvement and greater normalization of the EEG at these sites, Ayers would then perform the same training at T3−F7 and T4−F8 if head trauma was involved, or at T4−F4 and T3−F3 when migraine was involved (Ayers, 2000). Ayers asserted that inhibiting theta activity was most important in neurofeedback treatment, and that significantly reinforcing beta activity may risk adverse effects. Based on clinical experience, Ayers also asserted that if the practitioner only provides treatment in the hemisphere with a seizure focus (e.g., at T4—C4), in some cases the seizure focus would shift to the other hemisphere — something that Hughes, Taber, and Fino (1991) describe as the mirror phenomenon. Thus, the Ayers approach is to provide treatment at homologous sites in both hemispheres (Ayers, 2000).

SCP Self-Regulation Training

Training of SCP is usually accomplished with one electrode at Cz referenced against the mastoids. Kotchoubey et al. (2001) conducted the largest study utilizing this method involving 41 patients. All their recommendations on how to conduct a SCP session are based on the experience gained in this study. During about 35 sessions of SCP-feedback patients learn to produce electrically negative as well as electrically positive shifts. Within each session 120—140 trials comprising both types of tasks are presented with and without feedback. Trials without feedback are believed to help to transfer self-regulation skills from the clinical setting to everyday life. In addition to SCP, training patients receive behavior therapy in a behavior medicine framework. Here, patients learn to identify stimuli or situations that elicit seizures. In addition they were instructed to apply SCP self-regulation in these situations as well as in moments when seizures are developing. Finally, contingency management helps to reduce seizure frequency. See patient history examples in Examples 7.1 and 7.2.

INDIVIDUALIZING NEUROFEEDBACK BASED ON qEEG FINDINGS

Early studies using neurofeedback for epilepsy were done without the benefit of qEEG (reviewed by Sterman, 2000). In the 1970s and 1980s, normative databases were collected and analyzed and became commercially available (John, Prichep, & Easton, 1987). The goal of qEEG-guided training for epilepsy is to normalize the EEG activity.

Nuwer (1988) was the first to look at qEEG power abnormalities in epileptic patients, but he did not look for coherence abnormalities. Walker (2008) described the power and coherence abnormalities in patients with intractable epilepsy (Tables 7.1 and 7.2).

Walker and Kozlowski (2005) were the first to use power and coherence training to normalize the qEEGs of patients with intractable epilepsy. An excess power in any given frequency band was trained down and a

●●●──

Example 7.1 Patient AB

General History

Patient AB is 35 years old and lives with his wife and his two children. He is currently retraining in an academic education. He experienced his first epileptic seizure at the age of 20, and according to the doctor's diagnosis he suffers from epilepsy with simple focal, complex focal, and rare generalized seizures. The attacks occur during the day as well as during the night, and their frequency varies between three and eight attacks per month. Currently he is taking two types of epilepsy medication: carbamazepine and lamotrigine. Up to the start of treatment he did not keep track of his attacks and due to blood-level checks by the doctor, it is assumed that he does not regularly take his medication. The EEG was evaluated by a neurologist as rather normal with some slowing under hyperventilation.

Patient AB had meningitis during his childhood and spent one year in the hospital. In his childhood, he was always over-protected and thus severely limited. He complained that he never had the opportunity to live out his potential and develop his talents further.

Behavioral Analysis

At the start of an attack, AB feels a queasy sweetish sensation crawling up from his stomach.

Antecedents

His wife observes an increasing irritability in the days preceding an attack. He is restless and talks more than usual. He discusses abstruse topics and immediately before the attack his breathing changes, he holds his breath and during the attack switches to panting and flat breathing. Further antecedents and triggers are alcohol consumption, fatigue, imperative urinary urgency, time pressure, fear of failure and other fear-occupied thoughts, anger, listening to specific classical music, dealing with tricky situations.

Consequences

AB feels exhausted, dizzy, experiences headaches, unpleasant taste but also relief. Light attacks make him feel "activated", while after heavy attacks he sleeps. Functionally he procrastinates making decisions; he avoids strenuous activities and uses the epilepsy as a justification for not being able to exploit his full potential.

Diagnostics

Above average intelligence and logical thinking, but reduced attention and below average visual memory. Very good frontal lobe performance (Wisconsin Card Sorting Test; Nelson, 1976). Results of the BDI (Beck-Depression Inventory; Hautzinger, Bailer, Worall, & Keller, 1994) and MMPI (Minnesota Multiphasic Personality Inventory; Gehring & Blaser, 1993) are noteworthy; i.e., the scores for depression, hypochondria and hysteria are elevated. The FLL (Questionnaire about life goals and life satisfaction; Kraak & Nord-Rüdiger, 1989) revealed low life satisfaction. The patient also has low self-esteem and an external locus of control, according to the FKK scores (questionnaire regarding attributions and locus of control; Krampen, 1991). Further, AB is tentatively diagnosed as a narcissistic personality. Crucial for the therapeutic success is the patient's presumption that the epilepsy prevents him from living out his great potential. He also believes that he will finish his education despite bad grades and will not find a job because of his epilepsy.

Course of Therapy Notes

During the first biofeedback training sessions AB learns to differentiate the two tasks but he produces positive shifts (deactivates) when he is supposed to produce negative shifts (activate) and vice versa. Attempts to switch the strategies show only small effects. Later in the course of treatment AB is more successful and in the last training session the hit-score and differentiation between both tasks are nearly perfect. The first therapy sessions accompanying the biofeedback training are mostly concerned with the analysis and reduction of cognitive misperceptions and dysfunctional affects, in order to counteract the positive avoidance function of the seizure attacks. Later, the main focus is on how to transfer the self-regulation strategies into daily life. Emphasized are the antecedents. In moments of great fatigue (after exhausting tasks at work, during work breaks, when AB is driven home, when he is sitting down at the table for meals) AB is supposed to counteract cortical activation or lower it by applying self-regulation.

The biofeedback itself is done while the classical music, which is listed as an antecedent above, is played. The wife is asked to remind him to use his strategies for less conscious events preceding an attack, like urinary urgency, increased talking, and shallow breathing.

Results

Biofeedback

AB learns to differentiate between the cortically activated and deactivated states; this splitting becomes statistically significant in phase 2 of the treatment.

Attacks

The frequency of attacks continuously declines from four per month during baseline, to two attacks during the first follow-up and one in the second follow-up period. From the diary data we know that some of these attacks occur on days on which AB does not take the complete daily dose of his anti-epileptic medicine.

Test Data and Life Events

Almost all tests show improved scores (memory, MMPI, depression, satisfaction with life, locus of control) at the end of therapy and follow up. The emotional stress reaction (UBV, testing the ability to deal with stress; Reicherts & Perez, 1993) also normalizes.

After finishing his education, AB achieves a temporary contract in his desired profession, which is first extended and later changed to an unlimited contract. The family situation is further stabilizing and the family is moving from a flat into their own house.

(Continued)

●●●
———

Example 7.1 (Continued)

Commentary

Many patients suffer from psychological problems as a result of epilepsy. These issues (depressive moods, lack of social competence, fears, etc.) should also be treated during the epilepsy therapy, although the focus remains on acquiring (cortical) self-control. In this case with a probability of a personality disorder, whose onset may date back to a time when AB had no epilepsy, a differential diagnosis in order to exclude psychogenic epilepsy is crucial. Although a personality disorder cannot be sufficiently treated in the given setting, it must at the same time be taken into account, in order to establish an adequate therapeutic relationship.

In the case of patient AB, despite the positive development, it cannot be assumed that along with the reduction in attack frequency, a complete remission of the personality disorder was achieved. However, this case demonstrates that despite other disorders, the neurofeedback treatment of epilepsy can successfully be conducted. In order to do so, a detailed clinical diagnosis and the consideration of additional diagnoses during the therapeutic process are mandatory.

Outcomes (Follow-Up 8 Years After)

Immediately after the end of NFT, patient AB reported the successful use of strategies learned during training in his daily life. He also described a reduction in seizure frequency to one per month. At the 8 year follow-up, AB experienced on average two simple focal seizures monthly. He also claimed still to use the strategies for activation and deactivation and occasionally managed to suppress an attack. He is still taking carbamazepine and lamotrigine.

Biofeedback

AB achieved varying results in the three refresher training sessions at follow-up and reached a hit-score of 88% for activation. Overall the patient showed better performance for activating than deactivating.

Test Results

The IQ was 112, attention test score was slightly below average performance, while memory was above average. Scores for depression (BDI) were subclinical; MMPI scores were within the normal range, except hypochondriasis and hysteria, which were elevated.

EEG

AB showed normal alpha rhythms, with a slight dysrhythmia but no epileptic focus, and no changes under hyperventilation.

MRI

Tests showed discrete signs of cortical atrophy, especially in the occipital lobe and in temporo-basal areas. Also, the patient showed a slight hemispheric difference in hippocampus size (distinctly more narrow on the right side). This difference extends to the amygdala.

●●●

Example 7.2 Patient EB

General History

Patient EB, a 28-year-old university student in a long-term relationship, suffered her first epileptic seizure at the age of 13. According to the diagnosis, the seizures were predominantly simple focal, rarely complex focal, and only a few were generalized attacks. The epileptic seizure occurrence varied between one and four per week. During the baseline phase (12 weeks before treatment) EB experienced on average three to four seizures weekly. This frequency dropped to about one or two weekly in the following 12 weeks of treatment. At the beginning of NFT, patient EB was taking three different anti-seizure medications: carbamazepin, lamotrigine, and gabapentin. Her EEG showed a slight overall alteration. A tendency toward paroxysmal dysrhythmia as well as a discrete non-specific epilepsy focus on the right parieto-occipital junction was seen by the neurologist.

Social Aspects

The patient generally perceived her studies as "going well". During the week she had a regular study and sleep rhythm. EB had a large social network and applied herself in a supervised study group for students. Despite this, EB felt rather "uncomfortable" in town and often longed for the nature surrounding her parents' residence.

Her father seemed calm and had a relaxing influence on the situation; while her mother often blamed herself for her daughter's epilepsy and pushed EB to increase her medication dosage every time she had a more severe seizure. The mother also worried that studying was harmful to EB. EB was planning to get married to her long-term boyfriend after the end of exams. Her boyfriend viewed the epilepsy as unproblematic but, like her mother, was worried that her condition might worsen. Conflicts and fights between the two often ended unfinished because EB sometimes experienced seizures in these situations.

Behavioral Analysis

Clinical Course

EB described her early seizures as a "wave", a somersault under water, a fast elevator or driving over a bump in the road. However, with the outset of larger attacks, EB reported no longer perceiving them as "fun" but became afraid of future episodes. Complex seizures were accompanied by drooling and cramping of the left arm. Falls were rare.

Antecedents

Fights with EB's mother or boyfriend were sometimes followed by attacks. Half a day before seizure onset, EB often felt irritable, unsatisfied, and restless.

Triggers

Lack of sleep, stress (high workload or aiming to understand theoretical concepts), social conflicts (not feeling accepted, doubting herself, fights with her boyfriend), higher temperatures or elevated ozone levels, and hormonal fluctuations.

(Continued)

●●●————————————————————————————————————

Example 7.2 (Continued)

Diagnosis

EB showed average to above-average scores on neuropsychological (WMS 82—98% rank) and intelligence (IQ ∼120) measures. Over the course of the biofeedback training her IQ improved by one standard deviation. The UBV (testing the ability to deal with the stress of treatment) showed normal scores. The MMPI scores were also normal, although EB was reserved, even defensive toward the test.

Course of Therapy

Biofeedback

EB was very successful in the biofeedback training and learned to differentiate between strategies for activation (negative shifts) and deactivation (positive shifts). In order to avoid seizures the patient practiced both strategies learned during the training several times a day. By using these strategies she even sometimes managed to suppress complex focal seizures. However, she showed an increasing number of simple focal seizures.

Other Therapeutic Approaches

EB also practiced relaxation training, taking the instructions home to practice the technique and sharing this therapeutic approach with her friends. EB also learned to deal with stressful situations both in theory and in practice (e.g., for exam situations, times when she felt unjustifiably criticized, or when she felt neglected). She also learned to cope with anger. In order to prepare for exams, EB was taught how to positively present herself and how to handle difficult situations. EB needed to find support actively, not only in her escape to her parents' house on the weekends but also during the week.

Outcomes (Follow-Up 8 Years After)

Biofeedback

EB was still able to differentiate the strategies for activation and deactivation and even reached a hit-ratio of 100%. Overall the patient showed better performance in activation than deactivation. An example of a transfer trial (self-regulation without feedback) is given in Figure 7.1.

Seizure Frequency and EEG

At the beginning of the study, EB reported 15 simple focal/complex focal seizures per month on average. After completing the biofeedback training, the seizure frequency dropped to 11 per month. At the 8 year follow-up, the authors found that EB experienced only eight seizures (simple and complex focal) on average every month. A slight overall alteration in the EEG was found by her neurologist and there was no certain indication of an epileptic focus.

Social Aspects

After the patient took her exams and graduated from university, she married her boyfriend and gave birth to two children. EB still uses the strategies she learned during the biofeedback training and succeeds in suppressing seizures.

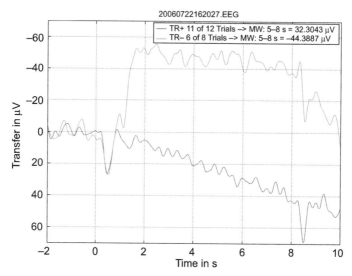

Figure 7.1 Averaged slow cortical potentials shift (negativity: darker line; positivity: lighter line) at 8 year follow-up evaluation.

Table 7.1 Power spectral frequency abnormalities in 25 patients with intractable seizures

Power abnormality (1 or more foci)	Incidence (% of patients)
Excess absolute theta	75
Excess relative theta	33
Deficient relative beta	33
Deficient absolute delta	25
Excessive absolute alpha	18
Deficient absolute alpha	18
Excess absolute beta	18
Excess relative beta	18
Deficient absolute beta	18

deficient power in a given frequency band was trained up. Decreased coherences were trained up and excessive coherences were trained down. Usually one or two sites or combination of sites in coherence were trained, one at a time. Subsequently, a total of 110 patients have been trained with this approach and followed for 1 to 5 years. Ninety-two patients (84%) of them became seizure-free and have remained so. The remainder experienced a sustained reduction in seizure frequency. Eighty-five patients (77%) were off all drugs and remain seizure-free.

Table 7.2 Coherence abnormalities in 25 patients with intractable seizures

Coherence abnormality (1 or more)	Incidence (percent of patients)
Decreased theta coherence	75
Decreased beta coherence	50
Increased beta coherence	50
Increased theta coherence	50
Decreased alpha coherence	42
Increased alpha coherence	33
Decreased delta coherence	25
Increased delta coherence	0
No coherence abnormalities	16

Table 7.3 Comorbid conditions remediated by neurofeedback in 90 intractable epilepsy patients

Condition	Number with condition	Number remediated
Clinical depression	7	7
ADD/ADHD	6	6
Chronic anxiety	5	5
Oppositional defiant disorder	4	4
Migraine	4	4
Dyslexia	4	4
Dysgraphia	4	4
Dyscalculia	4	4
PTSD	4	4

No significant side effects were observed, and there have been no complications.

An added advantage of neurofeedback is the remediation of comorbid conditions in many patients (Table 7.3). These include ADD/ADHD, chronic anxiety, oppositional defiant disorder, migraine, dyslexia, dysgraphia, dyscalculia, and post-traumatic stress disorder.

Neurofeedback training offers many advantages over traditional treatments for patients with drug-resistant epilepsy. It usually eliminates or reduces seizure frequency in these most complex seizure patients, where drugs have failed to do so. It is holistic, promoting normalization of brain activity. It is non-invasive. It is much less expensive than epilepsy surgery, and may succeed where surgery has failed. There is a greater success rate (>90% in the author J.W.'s experience). It can remediate comorbid conditions. It is successful in patients who are not candidates for surgery (no foci or multiple foci).

The disadvantages of qEEG-guided neurofeedback are that different equipment may need to be purchased, and the epileptologist must be trained in qEEG analysis and neurofeedback technique. It requires training and experience for best results.

Recent developments in qEEG and neurofeedback strategies bode well for even better results in the future. In particular, Thatcher, Biver, and North (2007) and Collura (2010) (see also Collura, Guan, Tarrant, Bailey, & Starr, 2010) have developed "live Z-score training", whereby four sites may be simultaneously trained to normalize power, coherence, phase, asymmetry, and/or ratios. Early experience indicates that fewer neurofeedback sessions are usually required, with comparable or better results than with one- or two-site training of power and/or coherence only. See patient history examples in Examples 7.3, 7.4, 7.5, and 7.6.

●●●————————————————————————————————

Example 7.3 Patient History: Example of qEEG-Guided Individualized Training Inhibiting Beta

A new patient provided the following history. He began having petit mal seizures at age 10, was put on an anti-epileptic medication and his seizures remained completely controlled until age 45. At that time he began having liver toxicity from his many years on the medication and his physicians discontinued it and began trying other medications and combinations of medications. During the following two years they were unable to control his seizures and he had remained unemployable. Although he was on three epilepsy medications, he was still having an estimated 100 absence seizures daily, and two or more grand mal seizures a week. In fact, he appeared for our intake appointment with one of his legs in a complete leg cast from having broken his leg in two places during a grand mal seizure the previous week. The neurologist was now recommending neurosurgery and the implantation of a vagal nerve stimulator. When the patient and his wife inquired about the possibility of neurofeedback as another treatment option, the author (D.C.H.) suggested they ask the neurosurgeon what the success rate was of the implant in significantly reducing seizures. They were told 40%, after which they decided to try a less invasive treatment approach before further considering surgery.

Previous clinical EEGs had not revealed a seizure focus. The author did a qEEG and during data-gathering the patient experienced a seizure with classic spike and wave activity, which, when separately analyzed, showed a focus of 3 Hz activity at Fz–Cz (and spreading into F3 and F4) in both absolute and relative power, as well as in the delta/theta ratio. LORETA localized this 3 Hz activity as originating in Brodmann area 10 of the medial frontal gyrus. In eyes-closed and eyes-open conditions, however, when he was not experiencing a seizure, the most prominent activity was excess beta on the frontal

————————————————————————————————

(Continued)

●●●
───

Example 7.3 (Continued)

midline (Fz—Cz) and there was a deficit in absolute power activity from 1—4 Hz, particularly along the midline. This beta excess would generally be considered a sign of cortical irritability.

Although the author (D.C.H.) was tempted to follow the traditional protocol of reinforcing SMR while inhibiting theta (and extending it down to 3 Hz), it was troubling that 13—15 Hz activity was also excessive in the qEEG in central and midline areas. Therefore, it was decided to base training on the qEEG findings and we began training him to inhibit 20—34 Hz, eyes closed, at Fz (with no reinforcement band). Feedback consisted of hearing the sound of the ocean when he reduced the beta below a threshold. The day prior to the first neurofeedback session, he experienced two grand mal seizures. Interestingly, at the time of the second neurofeedback session, he reported that in the previous four days he "felt a lot better" and that there had been fewer absence seizures. Seven days later, as he came for his third neurofeedback session, he reported a 90% reduction in seizure rate. Due to limited finances, the patient only received 12 neurofeedback sessions over a 4 month period of time. During this time when we would have anticipated from his pre-treatment base rate that he may have had 32—48 grand mal seizures, he had only three such seizures and he and his wife labeled his progress as "phenomenal." His absence seizures had been reduced to only 1—4/day, which had been maintained at his 2 month follow-up, at which time he was starting job training through state vocational rehabilitation. He moved soon after the 2 month post-treatment contact and was lost to further follow-up. This case illustrates the potential added value of basing treatment on a qEEG assessment to facilitate the individualization of treatment.

───

●●●
───

Example 7.4 Patient History: Example 1 of Seizure Remediation

A 3-year-old male patient had a correction of situs inversus and an appendectomy at 10 days of age. He had the onset of partial complex seizures at 11 months of age. He was initially treated with carbamazepine which decreased the frequency of the seizures, but made him drowsy. The carbamazepine dosage was decreased and levetiracetam was added. Avoidance of gluten and sugar decreased the frequency of the seizures. Levetiractam made him irritable and aggressive. When he presented to our clinic at age 3 he was having two seizures per month. An MRI of the brain was normal at one year of age. He was considered to be a candidate for epilepsy surgery. He was not particularly hyperactive, but he was impulsive. He was learning his letters and numbers and could repeat words correctly. Walking and running were normal. A typical seizure began with staring into space and blinking repeatedly and being unresponsive, lasting about 2 minutes. He would rarely have jerking movements of the arms and fall to the ground. He would usually sleep for about 2 hours afterwards. He was diagnosed as having partial complex seizures with occasional secondary generalized seizures.

His EEG revealed diffuse 4—5 Hz activity with frequent sharp-and-slow complexes at O1. His qEEG revealed multiple areas of excess focal slow activity (1—10 Hz range) including O1, O2, T5, P3, Pz, T4, C4, P4, T6, F7, T3, FP2, Fp1, C3, Cz, and Fz. There was an excess of 30 Hz activity at P4. There was a decrease in delta coherence in five pairs on the left, an increase in delta coherence in three pairs on the left, a decrease in theta coherence in two pairs on the left, and a decrease in alpha coherence in one pair on the left.

The patient had five sessions to downtrain 1−10 Hz and uptrain 15−18 Hz at each of the following sites (dual training):

> O1 + O2
> T5 + P3
> T4 + PZ
> C4 + P4
> F7 + T6
> F1 + F2
> C3 + CZ
> T3 + FZ

The patient experienced a decline in his seizures as the neurofeedback training progressed. His last seizure occurred after the 30th session. He has had no further seizures (18 months at this point). After neurofeedback training he was paying attention normally and was no longer impulsive, irritable, or aggressive. He no longer requires medication for seizures.

●●●
Example 7.5 Patient History: Example 2 of Seizure Remediation

This young man began having seizures at age 15. He had hit his head several times in motor vehicle accidents (sprint cars) and one bicycle accident at age 7. At age 15 he fell hard on his tailbone, and developed a severe headache. The next morning he had his first grand mal seizure, with a second seizure that afternoon. An EEG was normal, as was an MRI of the brain. He was started on Depakote®, which prevented further seizures, but his headache persisted and he became angry and gained weight. He was switched to Tegretol®, which prevented daytime seizures, but he continued to have one to two nocturnal seizures per month. His pre-existing attention difficulty worsened on Tegretol®. A sleep-deprived EEG revealed a sharp wave abnormality in the right posterior temporal area. He was experiencing initial and terminal insomnia. A continuous performance test was consistent with ADD. He complained of poor memory. His raw EEG on admission to our clinic revealed sharp wave discharges at T5, Cz, T6, and Oz. His QEEG revealed excess slow activity (in the 1−10 Hz range) in the following areas: O1, O2, F8, Pz, P4, T6, FP1, and FPZ. There was a decrease in alpha coherence in two pairs on the left, a decrease in beta coherence in two pairs on the left and one pair on the right. He had neurofeedback training, five sessions to reduce 1−10 Hz and increase 17 Hz for each of the following locations (dual training):

> O1 + O2
> F8 + Pz
> P4 + T6

(Continued)

●●●
──

Example 7.5 (Continued)

F1 + F2
T5 + C3
F3 + F4
P3 + Pz

His last seizure occurred after the 30th session of neurofeedback. After the 35th session he tapered and stopped the Tegretol®, with no recurrence of seizures (for 20 months so far). He began to do very well in school — improving from a GPA of 2.5 in high school to a 4.0 in his first year in college.

──

●●●
──

Example 7.6 Patient History: Example of qEEG Assistance in Recognition of a Tumor

Several years ago one of the authors (D.C.H.) was asked by a physician to use neurofeedback to treat his son's uncontrolled epilepsy. A qEEG (Figure 7.2) revealed some focal delta at electrode site F8. It was recommended to the 21-year-old patient and his father that this could potentially be associated with a lesion which an MRI could rule out. The father indicated that his son had an MRI two years prior, as well as another clinical EEG in recent months, and that he wanted us to simply proceed with treatment. As neurofeedback was performed the seizure frequency mildly decreased and then reached a plateau. After a dozen sessions it was suggested to the father that an MRI might still be a good idea, and particularly since the university had just obtained a new MRI unit that had two and a half times the resolution of the old one. The MRI revealed a tumor beneath this electrode site, and on closer examination of the older MRI they could perceive the fainter image of the tumor, which did not appear to have increased in size. A month later the patient underwent neurosurgery and on 6 year contact had never experienced another seizure. This case illustrates the importance of thorough medical evaluation and in having qualified individuals interpret EEG and qEEG findings.

──

LOW ENERGY NEUROFEEDBACK SYSTEM (LENS)

The Low Energy Neurofeedback System (LENS; Hammond, 2007; Larsen, 2006; Ochs, 2007) is a passive form of neurofeedback which produces its effects through feedback that involves a very tiny electromagnetic field which has field strength of 10^{-18} watts/cm^2 (less than the output of a watch battery). The feedback is delivered in one second intervals down electrode wires while the patient remains motionless, with the feedback being adjusted 16 times per second to remain a certain number of cycles per second faster than the dominant EEG frequency at the electrode site being trained. LENS treatment is traditionally done by providing feedback at all 19 standards

Montage: Laplacian   EEG ID:

Z transformed relative power FFT color maps

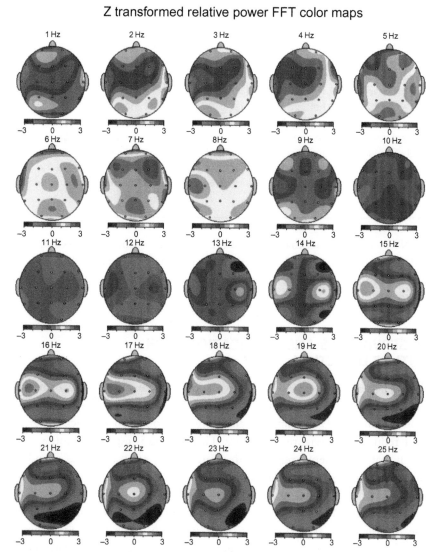

Figure 7.2 (*See Color Plate Section*) qEEG — Example 7.6.

electrode sites proceeding systematically from where the amplitude of the EEG and variability are the least toward electrode sites where the amplitude and variability are greatest. Many anecdotal reports have been made of successful treatment of uncontrolled epilepsy using LENS, including several treated by one of the authors (D.C.H.). Advantages often cited for the use of

●●●
Example 7.7 Patient History: Example of Successful LENS Treatment

A 6-year-old male was brought for treatment of uncontrolled epilepsy and harsh daily headaches. He was on very significant doses of two anti-seizure medications and yet he was still having an average of 10 absence seizures daily and a grand mal seizure once every 6–12 weeks. His eyes-closed qEEG showed excess 8–9 Hz activity that was most prominent in the left hemisphere, particularly in fronto-temporal areas. He also demonstrated excess 18–30 Hz activity in frontal (F3–Fz–F4) and central areas. After two LENS sessions he reported "I hardly had any headaches" in the previous five days and he had not experienced any seizures. A total of 22 LENS sessions was done during which his level of seizure medication was reduced, and after the second session there were no further absence seizures observed and he was having only about one mild headache (that did not require medication) every 3–4 weeks. Improvements were stable at 3 month follow-up.

LENS include the fact that it can be used with very young patients and individuals without the impulse control or stamina to do traditional neurofeedback and that treatment length often appears to be shortened by 35–40%. See patient history example in Example 7.7.

OBSERVATIONS AND IMPLICATIONS FOR FUTURE DIRECTION

This chapter has reviewed and provided an update on the state of the art on neurotherapy and epilepsy. The meta-analysis published in 2009 concluded that: "EEG operant conditioning was found to produce a significant reduction in seizure frequency. This finding is especially noteworthy given that the patients treated with neurotherapy often consisted of individuals who had been unable to control their seizures with medical treatment" (Tan et al., 2009, p. 173).

Since then, there have been exciting new developments, including the use of coherence training, the use of qEEG to guide the neurotherapy, and the use of the Low-Energy Neurofeedback System. Particularly noteworthy is the observation that neurotherapy has been able to help individuals who have been resistant to traditional pharmacotherapy. Furthermore, the value of neurotherapy for epilepsy should be considered from the perspective that this treatment has had minimal side effects as compared to standard pharmacotherapy.

Despite its value, neurotherapy has not been widely accepted and incorporated into the practice of mainstream medicine for the treatment of epilepsy. More well-designed and large scale studies involving control groups are clearly indicated. Comparative efficacy and cost—benefit analysis research could help to further assess its value *vis-à-vis* traditional pharmacotherapy. In this scenario, neurofeedback would be provided to individuals as an alternative to pharmacotherapy rather than as a second line treatment after pharmacotherapy has failed.

Future research should use qEEG to individualize and guide the selection of neurofeedback protocol, much as how it is being done in the treatment of other medical conditions such as closed head injury. In the latter case, a normative database has been developed to guide future treatment.

REFERENCES

Andrews, D. J., & Schonfeld, W. H. (1992). Predictive factors for controlling seizures using a behavioural approach. *Seizure, 1*(2), 111—116. doi:10.1016/1059-1311(92)90008-O.

Ayers, M. E. (1988). Long-term clinical treatment follow-up of EEG neurofeedback for epilepsy. *Epilepsy Support Program Newsletter, 3*(2), 8—9.

Ayers, M. E. (1995). Long-term follow-up of EEG neurofeedback with absence seizures. *Biofeedback & Self-Regulation, 20*(3), 309—310.

Ayers, M.E. (2000). Personal communication.

Collura, T. F. (2010). *Advanced Brainmaster EEG Neurofeedback Practicum* [DVD]. USA: Future Health. Retrieved from www.futurehealth.org/populum/pageproduct.php?f=Advanced-BrainMaster-EEG-N-by-Futurehealth-081113-616.html#cartchoices.

Collura, T. F., Guan, J., Tarrant, J., Bailey, J., & Starr, F. (2010). EEG biofeedback case studies using live Z-scores and a normative database. *Journal of Neurotherapy, 14*(1), 22—46.

Cott, A., Pavloski, R. P., & Black, A. H. (1979). Reducing epileptic seizures through operant conditioning of central nervous system activity: Procedural variables. *Science, 203*(4375), 73—75. doi:10.1126/science.758682.

Gehring, A., & Blaser, A. (1993). *MMPI — Minnesota Multiphasic Personality Inventory. Deutsche Kurzform für Handauswertung. 2. Aufl.* Berne, Göttingen, Toronto, Seattle: Hans Huber.

Hammond, D. C. (2007). *LENS: The low energy neurofeedback system.* New York: Haworth Press.

Hansen, L. M., Trudeau, D. L., & Grace, D. L. (1996). Neurotherapy and drug therapy in combination for adult ADHD, personality disorder, and seizure disorder: A case report. *Journal of Neurotherapy, 2*(1), 6—14. doi:10.1300/J184v02n01.

Hautzinger, M., Bailer, M., Worall, H., & Keller, F. (1994). *Beck-Depressions-Inventar (Bearbeitung der deutschen Ausgabe).* Berne: Hans Huber.

Holzapfel, S., Strehl, U., Kotchoubey, B., & Birbaumer, N. (1998). Behavioral psychophysiological intervention in a mentally retarded epileptic patient with brain lesion. *Applied Psychophysiology and Biofeedback, 23*(3), 189—202. Retrieved from www.aapb.org/aapb_journal.html.

Hughes, J., Taber, J., & Fino, J. (1991). The effect of spikes and spike-free epochs on topographic brain maps. *Clinical EEG (Electroencephalography), 22*(3), 150—160.

Iasemidis, I. D. (2003). Epileptic seizure prediction and control. *IEEE Transactions on Biomedical Engineering, 50*, 549—558. Retrieved from www.ieee.org/portal/site/iportals?WT.mc_id=tu_hp.

Ikeda, A., Terada, K., Mikuni, N., Burgess, R. C., Comair, Y., Taki, W., et al. (1996). Subdural recording of ictal DC shifts in neocortical seizures in humans. *Epilepsia, 37*(7), 662–674. Retrieved from http://www.epilepsia.com/.

John, E. R., Prichep, L. S., & Easton, P. (1987). Normative databanks and neurometrics: Basic concepts, methods and results of norm construction. In A. Remond (Ed.), *Handbook of electroencephalography and clinical neurophysiology* (pp. 449–495). Amsterdam: Elsevier.

Kotchoubey, B., Strehl, U., Uhlmann, C., Holzapfel, S., König, M., Fröscher, W., et al. (2001). Modification of slow cortical potentials in patients with refractory epilepsy: A controlled outcome study. *Epilepsia (Series 4), 42*(3), 406–416. Retrieved from www.epilepsia.com/.

Kraak, B., & Nord-Rüdiger, D. (1989). *Fragebogen zu Lebenszielen und zur Lebenszufriedenheit* Göttingen, Toronto, Zürich: Hogrefe.

Krampen, G. (1991). *Fragebogen zu Kompetenz- und Kontrollüberzeugungen.* Göttingen, Toronto, Zürich: Hogrefe.

Lantz, D., & Sterman, M. B. (1988). Neuropsychological assessment of subjects with uncontrolled epilepsy: Effects of EEG feedback training. *Epilepsia, 29*(2), 163–171. Retrieved from www.epilepsia.com/.

Larsen, S. (2006). *The healing power of neurofeedback: The revolutionary LENS technique for restoring optimal brain function.* Rochester, VT: Healing Arts Press.

Lubar, J. F., Shabsin, H. S., Natelson, S. E., Holder, G. S., Whitsett, S. F., Pamplin, W. E., et al. (1981). EEG operant conditioning in intractable epileptics. *Archives of Neurology, 38*(11), 700–704. Retrieved from http://archneur.ama-assn.org/.

Nelson, H. E. (1976). A modified card sorting test sensitive to frontal lobe defects. *Cortex, 12,* 313–324.

Nuwer, M. R. (1988). Frequency analysis and topographic mapping of EEG and evoked potentials in epilepsy. *Electroencephalography & Clinical Neurophysiology, 69*(2), 118–126.

Ochs, L. (2007). The low energy neurofeedback system (LENS): Theory, background, and introduction. *Journal of Neurotherapy, 10*(2-3), 5–39. doi:10.1300/J184v10n02.

Reicherts, M., & Perez, M. (1993). *Fragebogen zum Umgang mit Belastung im Verlauf-UBV.* Berne, Göttingen, Toronto, Seattle: Hans Huber.

Rockstroh, B., Elbert, T., Birbaumer, N., Wolf, P., Düchting-Röth, A., Reker, M., et al. (1993). Cortical self-regulation in patients with epilepsies. *Epilepsy Research, 14*(1), 63–72.

Sterman, M. B. (1982). EEG biofeedback in the treatment of epilepsy: An overview circa 1980. In L. White, & B. Tursky (Eds.), *Clinical biofeedback: Efficacy and mechanisms* (pp. 311–330). New York: Guilford Press.

Sterman, M. B. (2000). Basic concepts and clinical findings in the treatment of seizure disorders with EEG operant conditioning. *Clinical Electroencephalography, 31*(1), 45–55. Retrieved from www.ecnsweb.com/images/articles2000.htm#JANUARY%202000,% 20Volume%2031.

Sterman, M. B., & Friar, L. (1972). Suppression of seizures in an epileptic following sensorimotor EEG feedback training. *Electroencephalography & Clinical Neurophysiology, 33*(1), 89–95. doi:10.1016/0013-4694(72)90028-4.

Sterman, M. B., Goodman, S. J., & Kovalesky, R. A. (1978). Effects of sensorimotor EEG feedback training on seizure susceptibility in the rhesus monkey. *Experimental Neurology, 62*(3), 735–747. doi:10.1016/0014-4886(78)90281-9.

Sterman, M. B., Macdonald, L. R., & Stone, R. K. (1974). Biofeedback training of the sensorimotor electroencephalogram rhythm in man: Effects on epilepsy. *Epilepsia, 15*(3), 395–416. Retrieved from www.epilepsia.com/.

Sterman, M. B., & Shouse, M. N. (1980). Quantitative analysis of training, sleep EEG and clinical response to EEG operant conditioning in epileptics. *Electroencephalography and Clinical Neurophysiology, 49*(5-6), 558–576. doi:10.1016/0013-4694(80)90397-1.

Sterman, M. B., Wyrwicka, W., & Roth, S. R. (1969). Electrophysiological correlates and neural substrates of alimentary behavior in the cat. *Annals of the New York Academy of Sciences, 157*(2), 723–739. doi:10.1111/j.1749-6632.1969.tb12916.x.

Tan, G., Thornby, J., Hammond, D. C., Strehl, U., Canady, B., Arnemann, K., et al. (2009). Meta-analysis of EEG biofeedback in treating epilepsy. *Clinical EEG and Neuroscience: Official Journal of the EEG and Clinical Neuroscience Society (ENCS), 40*(3), 173–179.

Thatcher, R. W., Biver, C. J., & North, D. M. (2007). Z-score EEG biofeedback: Technical foundations. *Applied Neuroscience*, Retrieved from http://www.appliedneuroscience.com/Z%20Score%20Biofeedback.pdf.

Tozzo, C. A., Elfner, L. F., & May, J. G. (1988). EEG biofeedback and relaxation training in the control of epileptic seizures. *International Journal of Psychophysiology, 6*(3), 185–194. doi:10.1016/0167-8760(88)90004-9.

Walker, J. E. (2008). Power spectral frequency and coherence abnormalities in patients with intractable epilepsy and their usefulness in long-term remediation of seizures using neurofeedback. *Clinical EEG & Neuroscience, 39*(4), 203–205.

Walker, J. E., & Kozlowski, G. P. (2005). Neurofeedback treatment of epilepsy. *Child & Adolescent Psychiatric Clinics of North America, 14*(1), 163–176. doi:10.1016/j.chc.2004.07.009.

Witte, H., Iasemidis, L. D., & Litt, B. (2003). Special issue on epileptic seizure prediction. *IEEE Transactions on Biomedical Engineering, 50*, 537–539. doi:10.1109/TBME.2003.810708.

World Health Organization. (2009). Epilepsy: *Etiology, epidemiology and prognosis*. Retrieved from www.who.int/mediacentre/factsheets/fs999/en/index.html.

Wyrwicka, W., & Sterman, M. B. (1968). Instrumental conditioning of sensorimotor cortex EEG spindles in the walking cat. *Physiology & Behavior, 3*(5), 703–707. doi:10.1016/0031-9384(68)90139-X.

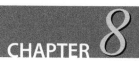

CHAPTER 8

Feedback of Slow Cortical Potentials: Basics, Application, and Evidence

Sarah Wyckoff and Ute Strehl
Institute of Medical Psychology and Behavioral Neurobiology, University of Tübingen, Tübingen, Germany

Contents

Although it has been studied over the last 50 years, the investigation and application of slow cortical potentials (SCP) as a method of brainwave feedback has largely been restricted to the European neurofeedback community. The development of reliable and valid equipment and publication of several meta-analyses demonstrating the clinical efficacy of SCP feedback has spurred new interest in this training modality. This chapter will briefly discuss the origins of SCP activity, followed by a description of the technical requirements. Then feedback, diagnosis, and evaluation requirements will be addressed. Finally, the chapter will conclude with a review

Neurofeedback and Neuromodulation Techniques and Applications
DOI: 10.1016/B978-0-12-382235-2.00008-1

of the published research of SCP feedback and epilepsy, attention deficit/ hyperactivity disorder (ADHD), migraines, and beyond.

BASICS

The electrical activity of the brain has been under investigation for more than a century. Canton (1875) first reported observing electrical currents from the exposed brain surface of live animals with a galvanometer. Fifty years later, Berger (1929) published his discovery of rhythmic alpha brain-wave activity during the first known electroencephalographic recording of a human subject. In their early experiments, both researchers reported distinct changes in electrical current during eyes-open, eyes-closed, and sleep conditions. Electroencephalography (EEG), or monitoring and recording of electrical brain activity with an electronic monitoring device, is currently used as a neurological diagnostic procedure and assessment tool in cognitive behavioral and psychophysiological research. EEG activity reflects the summation of excitatory and inhibitory postsynaptic potentials in the pyramidal cells of the upper layers of the cerebral cortex, with some contribution of granular and glial activity (for reviews, see Lopes da Silva, 1991; Speckmann & Elger, 1999). Large field potentials, which can be recorded on the scalp, are generated from the synchronous extracellular current flow of neurons that have similar spatial orientation, radial to the scalp, as well as by glial sources (Fellin et al., 2009).

EEG wave patterns are classified as synchronized or desynchronized and are linked to specific recording tasks and distinct behavioral states. According to Steriade, Gloor, Llinás, Lopes da Silva, and Mesulam (1990) synchronized EEG activity reflects the occurrence of high-amplitude oscillations of slow frequencies measured during a relaxed, eyes-closed condition. According to their physiological model of rhythmic activity, the intrinsic electrophysiological properties of thalamocortical neurons allows them to oscillate within different frequency spectra; however, they are subject to the controlling influence of the reticular thalamic nucleus that unites individual discharges into simultaneous volleys within the 1–20 Hz frequency range. Desynchronized EEG activity signals the replacement of synchronized rhythms with lower-amplitude oscillations of faster frequencies measured during visual attention, eyes-open conditions. The braking action of the reticular thalamic nucleus is mediated by cholinergic projections from the brain stem to the thalamus and basal forebrain. During desynchronization, acetylcholine is responsible for the direct excitation of thalamic relay neurons and the synaptic decoupling in the thalamic generation of spindle activity, allowing neuronal ensembles to fire freely (acceleration) in response to specific processing demands.

Spontaneous EEG rhythms are traditionally defined within conventional frequency bands called delta (0.5−4 Hz), theta (4−7 Hz), alpha (8−12 Hz), sensorimotor rhythm or SMR (12−15 Hz), beta (13−30 Hz), and gamma (30−100 Hz). Direct current (DC) shifts of less than 1 Hz are referred to as SCPs. Although embedded in oscillatory EEG activity, SCPs do not occur spontaneously and belong to the family of event-related potentials. DC potentials were observed by Canton (1875), but until recently, the assessment of SCP was limited to only a few research labs in Europe. Historically, most DC and low frequency activity have been selectively omitted from EEG recordings, as they existed below the low frequency cut-off of a majority of amplifiers. However, technological advance has led to accessibility of DC-amplifiers capable of monitoring frequencies as low as 0.01 Hz, renewing interest in SCP acquisition and feedback.

As stated previously, SCPs belong to the family of event-related potentials (ERPs). The common feature of brain potentials subsumed under this category is that they are time-locked to a specific event. These events may be external or internal and include physical stimuli, behavioral responses, and cognitive and emotional processes. In order to detect these deflections within the raw EEG, averaging techniques are required. The timing of these responses reflects diverse aspects of brain communication and information processing. ERPs can be observed from ∼50 to 1000 msec after the onset of a stimulus, and sub-divided into early and late components on the basis of their latency and direction of deviance (positive or negative). Early components occur at or before 100 msec, are less sensitive to cognitive variables, and are determined by the physical qualities of the stimulus including intensity and duration. The late components, including the P300, occur after 200 msec and are influenced by endogenous factors such as information processing.

SCPs are negative and positive polarizations in the EEG that last from ∼300 ms to several seconds and the amplitudes may vary from several microvolts (μV) to more than 100 μV (e.g., during seizures). The negative polarizations of SCPs have received many labels depending upon the experimental context in which they are observed. Walter and colleagues developed a paradigm to elicit contingent negative variation (CNV; Walter, 1964; Walter, Cooper, Aldridge, McCallum, & Winter, 1964). The CNV is a wide and prolonged negative deflection, evoked by a GO/NO-GO paradigm, contingent on an individual's conscious perception of a warning stimulus (S1) preceding another imperative stimulus (S2) that requires a specific response. This activity is hypothesized to play a critical role in the preparatory distribution of sensory, motor, and attentional resources.

In the late 1970s, Birbaumer and colleagues at the University of Tübingen began developing a physiological model in which SCPs of EEG reflected the threshold regulation mechanism of cortical activation and inhibition. In simple terms, negative SCP shifts increase the firing probabilities of a cell assembly, while positive SCP shifts inhibit this activity. The exact mechanisms generating these slow potentials are still a matter of controversy. Negative surface SCPs are hypothesized to result from a sink caused by synchronous slow excitatory postsynaptic potentials in the apical dendrites of layer I in the cortex with a source being located in layers IV and V, while positive fluctuations are understood as an inhibition or abatement of negativities reflecting the activity of large cell assemblies (review, see Birbaumer, Elbert, Canavan, & Rockstroh, 1990). However, current data suggest that the modulation of SCPs relies on the coordinated activity of neuronal and glial cell systems (Fellin et al., 2009). Astrocytes have been found to modulate slow cortical oscillations by regulating, simultaneously inhibiting, NMDA and A_1 synaptic receptor functions. Inhibition of cortical synapses in NMDA receptors produces excitatory activity, or hypofunction of postsynaptic receptors, thereby shortening the up-state duration of cortical neurons (negativity). Conversely, the inhibition of A_1 receptors results in the reduction of extracellular adenosine and loss of tonic suppression of cortical synapses (positivity).

Regardless of the mechanism in charge of producing these slow cortical oscillations, significant diurnal variation has been observed in animal research suggesting that DC potentials fluctuate during the day in relation to changes in arousal (Shinba, 2009). DC potentials recorded in the frontal areas of the cerebral cortex referenced to the cerebellum were found to be more positive during light periods (8am–8pm) than dark periods. Spectral correlation and coherence analysis of resting-stated magnetoencephalography (MEG) recordings revealed that ultraslow (<0.1 Hz) spontaneous power modulations are synchronous over large spatial distances, mimicking the temporal-spatial properties of functional magnetic resonance imaging (fMRI) signals (Liu, Fukunaga, de Zwart, & Duyn, 2010). Dominant low frequency (<0.1 Hz) power fluctuations were observed in both gamma (>30 Hz) and sub-gamma (<30 Hz) rhythms and were noticeably stronger during light sleep eyes-closed periods than during awake eyes-open or eyes-closed conditions. These findings are in line with the data indicating that negative SCP shifts, such as the "Bereitschafts potential" (Kornhuber & Deecke, 1965) or the CNV (Walter et al., 1964), indicate local excitatory mobilization, while positive potentials indicate disfacilitation.

Several studies have found a consistent relationship between cortical negativity and reaction time, signal detection, and short-term memory performance (review, see Birbaumer et al., 1990; Birbaumer, 1999). Therefore, SCPs have been conceptualized as a tuning mechanism in attentional regulation, and the self-regulation of SCPs hypothesized as a plausible treatment for disorders characterized by impaired excitation thresholds. In a series of experiments, the ability to self-regulation SCP shifts was investigated. Findings indicated that both healthy and clinical patient populations were able to learn self-regulation of negative and positive SCP shifts over central electrode sites (Birbaumer, Roberts, Lutzenberger, Rockstroh, & Elbert, 1992; Holzapfel, Strehl, Kotchoubey, & Birbaumer, 1998; Schneider, Heimann, Mattes, Lutzenberger, & Birbaumer, 1992; Schneider, Rockstroh et al., 1992; Siniatchkin, Kropp, & Gerber, 2000) as well as demonstrate simultaneous control over right–left-hemispheric differences (Birbaumer et al., 1988; Gruzelier, Hardman, Wild, & Zaman, 1999).

TECHNICAL AND TRAINING REQUIREMENTS

As stated earlier, accessibility of devices capable of recording, analyzing, and providing feedback of SCPs signals has been limited to a handful of research labs for the past few decades. However, recent advancements in DC amplifiers, electrodes, signal processing, and artifact controls have improved the recording quality of very slow EEG signals. The next section presents the common technical standards and training procedures necessary for SCP feedback.

Amplifiers

Historically, frequencies in the range of zero to $1-2$ Hz have been omitted from EEG recordings as the result of high-pass low frequency filtration in an effort to minimize the impact of physiological, mechanical, electrical, and chemical artifacts. However, the recording of SCPs requires a high-pass filter that allows the registration of very low frequencies (<0.01 Hz).

Because SCP shifts are very slow, a time constant of at least 10 seconds and a data sampling rate of 128 Hz (cycles per second) or greater is required. DC amplifiers do not omit any of these ultra-low frequencies and are ideal for capturing SCP data. Nevertheless, it is important to note that, to date, the majority of SCP research conducted has employed low frequency AC amplifiers with a low frequency cutoff of 0.01 Hz.

Artifacts

The inclusion of DC components in EEG recordings results in several challenges, as slow cortical activity is highly susceptible to artifact contamination from a variety of sources. EEG artifacts consist of potential shifts that do not originate from the brain, although some activity can easily be mistaken for legitimate EEG. Therefore artifact control is paramount in the acquisition of "clean" and "noise-free" data. Artifacts can be minimized in a variety of ways.

Eye blinks and horizontal or vertical movements are among the most common and recognizable artifacts occurring in EEG recordings. Because the eye acts as a dipole and produces a significant source of artifact in SCP signals, measurement of electromyography (EOG) components are essential. Eye movements lead to changes in polarity as the result of electrical potentials generated in the neurons of the retina. In fact, eye position alone produces DC signals that influence baseline EEG values; upward gazes shift the baseline upward and downward gazes shift the baseline down (Saab, 2009). During blinks, the eyelid picks up the positive charge of the cornea and generates a positive potential. These artifacts negatively impact the EEG recording, with frontal electrode sites being the most susceptible to contamination. To control these artifacts, reduce signal distortion, and limit inaccurate feedback, several EOG electrodes are placed around the eye. For the detection of horizontal eye-movements electrodes are attached 1.5 cm lateral to the outer canthus of each eye. Two additional electrodes are applied to detect vertical eye-movement and attached 3 mm above the middle of the left eyebrow and 1.5 cm below the middle of the left lower eye-lid. Online correction of ocular potentials can then be subtracted from the EEG signal through the use of several different algorithms (Kübler, Winter, & Birbaumer, 2003; Schlegelmilch, Markert, Berkes, & Schellhorn, 2004).

Body movement is another source of artifact in EEG recordings. Swallowing, tongue movements, and respiration may produce slow

low-frequency artifacts while postural changes, muscle contractions, and tension may produce high-frequency artifacts. In order to reduce artifact, patients are instructed to relax, minimize movements, and breathe at a consistent rate and volume. Despite this, artifacts originating from the frontalis, orbicularis, and temporalis muscles may still be present. To prevent reinforcement of physiological or muscle induced SCP shifts, threshold detection algorithms may be applied to identify "invalid" training trials generating amplitudes of 200 μV or greater.

Finally, DC drifts may be produced by changes in skin resistance caused by perspiration and electrode polarization. Electrode polarization reflects the electro-chemical reaction of the electrode, conductive medium, and the scalp. Once the electrodes are attached to the scalp, ions move across the conductive boundary and accumulate a charge. Electrode voltage stabilizes after a few minutes and should be similar across all electrode sites. Variability in electrode voltage generates an unstable signal, with slow potentials derived from artifacts, which are recorded along with the EEG. These DC drifts can be minimized through thorough cleansing and preparation of the electrode site, use of special electrodes, and development of a light and temperature control assessment environment.

Electrode Application

In neurofeedback paradigms, SCPs are recorded at the vertex (Cz) and referenced to one or both mastoids depending on device requirements. In addition to the active and reference electrodes, a ground sensor and two to four EOG electrodes are used. An impedance of 5—10 kΩ can be obtained by prepping the skin with alcohol, acetone, and/or abrasive creams to remove excess oils, hair, and dead skin. To avoid DC drift, sintered Ag/AgCl (silver/silver chloride) electrodes should be attached firmly with an ample amount of conductive electrode paste containing sodium chloride as the electrolyte.

Training Protocol

During SCP training sessions, patients are seated in a comfortable chair in front of a notebook or desktop computer, with or without the clinician present in the training room. Training of SCP self-regulation requires the monitoring of two different brain states. The patients are cued by a graphic symbol to "activate" or "deactivate" their brain (see Figure 8.1). Each trial period lasts approximately 8 sec and is preceded by a 2 sec passive "resting" phase. The passive phase allows the patient to prepare for

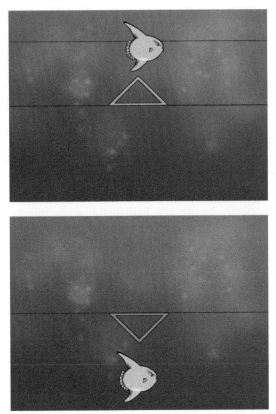

Figure 8.1 *(See Color Plate Section)* Example of SCP feedback training screens for negativity ("Activation", upper panel) and positivity ("Deactivation", lower panel). *(By kind permission of neuroConn GmbH, Germany.)*

the presentation of the next training cue, while serving as the baseline for the following active phase. Baseline data are collected for a period of milliseconds and the mean average is set to zero. A tone marks the beginning of the trial and movement of the feedback symbol reflects the degree of the individual's SCP shifts: feedback moving upward as the result of a negative shift (reduce excitation threshold) and downward as a result of a positive shift (increase excitation threshold). Every 62.5 msec the average SCP amplitude for the preceding 500 msec is calculated and compared to the baseline. If the averaged SCP amplitude increases compared to the baseline, the feedback reflects a negative shift. A decrease in amplitude indicates that the SCP is less negative than during the baseline indicating cortical positivity, or inhibition of negativity.

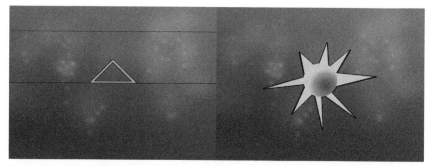

Figure 8.2 *(See Color Plate Section)* Example of SCP transfer training screen for negativity—activation task (left panel). Example of SCP visual feedback reward for successful activation or deactivation (right panel). *(By kind permission of neuroConn GmbH, Germany.)*

Unlike traditional neurofeedback protocols that reward the regulation of specific frequencies or ratios in one direction, SCP training rewards the bi-directional regulation of two tasks, production of negative or positive shifts. The capacity to train shifts in one direction is limited due to the long time constant of SCP shifts and use of a relative baseline. For example, patients may have an easier time producing a negative shift if the relative baseline was already more positive. Therefore, it would be increasingly difficult to shift a potential into the same direction over a series of identical tasks unless the patient was producing a shift in the opposite direction during the baseline phase. For this reason, the distribution of required negative and positive shifts is randomly set. During initial training blocks the task distribution is set to 50/50. In advanced training phases the task distribution is adjusted to 30/70 according to the patient's pathology and treatment goals. Every train (1 to 3–4 trials) of identical tasks is followed by the opposite task in random order. In addition to the immediate feedback successful activation and deactivation is indicated with a visual reward (see Figure 8.2). To generalize newly acquired regulation skills to everyday life situations, 25% of all trials serve as "transfer trials" in which no feedback is presented during the active phase but level of success is indicated with the visual reward system following the trial (see Figure 8.2).

Feedback trials are grouped into three to five training blocks, each followed by a short break. A typical session lasts one hour and consists of 100 to 120 trials. In research settings, the total number of SCP sessions is typically 25 to 35, and training appointments are generally scheduled in several blocks of intensive daily sessions (weekends off), followed by a

4 week break every 10 sessions. During breaks patients practice SCP self-regulation in everyday situations. To facilitate home training and generalization of SCP regulation, patients are instructed to imagine producing the positive and negative shifts and assisted with a visual of the training screen via cue card or DVD. For example, ADHD children are encouraged to focus on producing negative shifts to promote attention and focus while working on homework, whereas individuals with epilepsy are urged to practice self-regulation skills in the wake of seizure activity by trying to shift their brain in an electrically positive direction. Current investigations of SCP training in ADHD populations at the University of Tübingen are examining the efficacy of a biweekly training schedule. Independent clinicians report that such "non-intensive" training schedules also facilitate mastery of SCP self-regulation skills and behavior changes in their clients in a clinical setting.

Introduction to SCP Feedback

As with other neurofeedback and biofeedback modalities, the first session focuses less on training techniques and regulation strategies and typically serves as an information session and introduction to EEG. Patients are provided with basic information on SCP training, the rational for treatment specific to their pathology, and an explanation of the session procedures. The training equipment is explained, and patients are invited to handle the electrodes, touch the prepping gels and conductive pastes, and customize the feedback options. In order to minimize the production of artifacts in subsequent training session, once all the training electrodes and EOG sensors are connected, patients are given the opportunity to view and manipulate their physiological activity. Within a matter of moments, patients begin to discover that their eye and tongue movements, muscle contractions, and teeth clenching impact the EEG signal. During these "experiments" the clinician explains how artifacts may produce the desired SCP shifts but keep the patient from acquiring brain-driven self-regulation skills.

Following the exercise in what "not" to do during the session, patients are encouraged to relax their posture, minimize movement artifact, and attempt to regulate their SCPs. Because the self-regulation of SCPs is more difficult than the self-regulation of EEG frequencies, particularly during early session blocks, the clinician should coach the patient and provide as much positive reinforcement as possible. Patients are prompted to focus on the SCP shift during each trial and search for conscious strategies that produce shifts in the desired direction. The goal is to help the patient connect states of mental activation to positive and negative SCP shift. In many patients, negative shifts are associated with activating images, whereas positive shifts are associated with relaxation, disengagement, and boredom. However, these strategies may not be effective in all patients. Clinician assistance during the process of trial and error can be realized by using a secondary screen and intercom system if the patient is training in an adjacent room. Shaping procedures may be implemented to facilitate the process of learning. Training thresholds can be utilized to increase or decrease the degree of SCP shifts required for a successful trial. Typically training sessions begin with minimal or no threshold. Once a training strategy is identified and a patient builds self-regulation skills it may be useful to increase thresholds during advanced sessions.

DIAGNOSIS AND EVALUATION

As previously stated, the self-regulation of SCPs is theorized as a plausible treatment for disorders characterized by impaired excitation thresholds. Apart from assessment procedures required for confirmatory diagnosis, no specific evaluation of the EEG is necessary to begin SCP training. However, documentation of pre-/post- core symptoms (e.g., behavioral, personality variables, attention, seizure incidence, etc.) and changes in cognitive processing are encouraged. Additionally, a continuous performance test (CPT) can be implemented to assess changes in the latency and amplitude of event-related potentials.

The training method is identical for all patients; only the task distribution is altered according to patient pathology and training goals. Review of the session data following each session facilitates learning and development of self-regulation strategies (see Figure 8.3). Variables of interest include signal amplitudes, hit rates for task-specific trials, and differences between negativities and positivities for both active feedback and transfer conditions. Analysis of hit rate statistics indicates the percentages of time patients are able to produce the required positive or negative shifts. The hit rate distribution is less important than the differentiation between the shifts of both tasks. For example, a patient may demonstrate good task differentiation but be more successful in producing negative shifts rather than positive shifts (see Figure 8.4). Conversely, a patient may demonstrate a hit rate percentage of zero but demonstrate good differentiation. In this

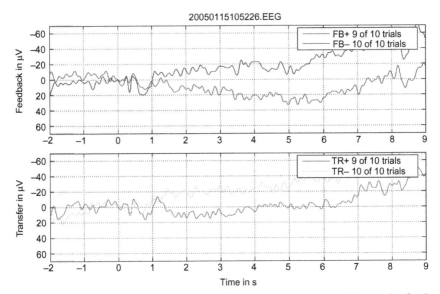

Figure 8.3 Averaged slow cortical potentials in negativity and positivity under feedback (upper panel) and transfer (lower panel) conditions. *(By kind permission of neuroConn GmbH, Germany.)*

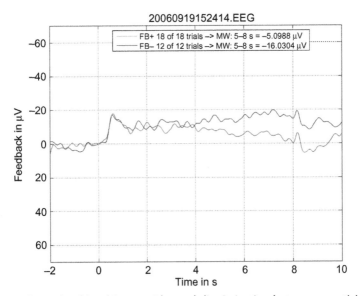

Figure 8.4 Example of low hit rate with good discrimination between negativity and positivity tasks. *(By kind permission by neuroConn GmbH, Germany.)*

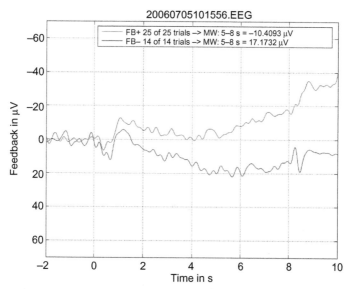

Figure 8.5 Example of low hit rate for both tasks with good differentiation in the opposite training direction. *(By kind permission of neuroConn GmbH, Germany.)*

case, the task differentiation is in the opposite training direction as the result of the patient producing negativities when they are prompted to produce positivities and vice versa (see Figure 8.5). This finding indicates that the patient is capable of producing bi-directional shift changes, but requires additional coaching and training to reverse the activation reactions.

EVIDENCE BASE AND INDICATIONS

Because SCP shifts reflect the threshold regulation mechanism of cortical activation and inhibition, it has been applied as a treatment for disorders characterized by impaired excitation thresholds. A majority of SCP feedback research has focused on treatment of epilepsy, ADHD, and migraine populations. The next section presents the rationale for use of SCP feedback in these populations, as well as the major research findings to date.

Epilepsy

In patients with epilepsy, negative SCP shifts have been observed preceding and during ictal discharges and positive SCP shifts following seizure termination (Ikeda et al., 1997). These and other findings from animal research led researchers to conceptualize epilepsy as a problem in restraining the hyperactivation of neurons in which increased cortical negativity decreases an individual's threshold for paroxysmal activity. Therefore, it was hypothesized that training epileptic patients to suppress negative SCPs (i.e., to produce positive shifts) would attenuate epileptic discharges resulting in seizure frequency reduction (Birbaumer et al., 1991). To date, two multicenter studies have shown that patients with epilepsy are able to learn self-regulation of SCPs and as a result have significantly decreased incidence of seizures (Kotchoubey et al., 2001; Rockstroh et al., 1993).

Rockstroh and colleagues (1993) investigated 25 patients with drug-refractory epilepsies that participated in 28 sessions of SCP feedback in which modulation of SCPs in both positive and negative directions was rewarded. Eighteen patients continued to monitor seizure frequency during a 1-year follow-up period, revealing that, compared to baseline levels, seizure incidence was significantly lower during the follow-up period (p <0.01). Six patients reported post-treatment seizure frequency below the 8 week median baseline values, seven showed seizure frequency reductions, and five did not report changes in seizure incidence. Kotchoubey and colleagues (2001) compared the impact of SCP feedback, respiration training, and anticonvulsive medication treatment on seizure frequency. Thirty-four patients participated in 35 sessions of SCP feedback in which modulation of positive and negative shifts were randomly distributed. Cortical positivity was required in 50% of trials for the first 20 sessions and 67% for the last 15 sessions. Overall, significant seizure reduction was reported for the SCP (p<0.05) and medication conditions but not for the respiration training. For the SCP training group the overall seizure frequency rate decreased by one-third, the rate of simple partial seizures decreased by one-half, and some patients became seizure-free. Stability of SCP self-regulation was observed at 6 month follow-up and seizure reduction was maintained at 12 month follow-up (Kotchoubey et al., 2001; Strehl, Kotchoubey, Trevorrow, & Birbaumer, 2005).

In a meta-analysis of EEG biofeedback studies, indexed in online research databases between 1970 and 2005, data on seizure frequency changes related to treatment were assessed. The results indicated that EEG operant conditioning of sensorimotor rhythm (SMR) or SCPs produced a significant (p<0.005) reduction in seizure frequency for patients with treatment-resistant epilepsy (Tan et al., 2009). Following treatment, an overall mean decreased seizure incidence was reported in all studies and 74% of patients reported fewer weekly seizures in response to neurofeedback.

Attention Deficit Hyperactivity Disorder (ADHD)

Rockstroh, Elbert, Lutzenberger, and Birbaumer (1990) observed impaired regulation of SCPs in children with attentional problems. Children with attention issues were only able to self-regulate SCPs during feedback trials and showed reduced negativities in anticipation of a task. In a series of studies, Helps and colleagues investigated the distribution and function of very low frequency networks (VLF; <0.1 Hz) during resting state and rest-task transitions in adolescents with and without ADHD. In DC-EEG recordings, ADHD children exhibited decreased resting state VLF power and attenuated power during rest-task transitions, and this was significantly different from controls (Helps et al., 2010). Attenuation of power was negatively correlated with task performance, whereby participants who attenuated least made more errors, had greater variability, and slower reaction times. ADHD participants with high self-reported inattention showed significantly less power in 0.06—0.2 Hz and 0.5—1.5 Hz frequency bands then participants with low inattention and healthy controls (Helps, James, Debener, Karl, & Sonuga-Barke, 2008). These findings support the conceptualization of ADHD symptoms as the consequences of impaired excitation threshold regulation, characterized by decreased cortical negativity. Therefore, it was hypothesized that training ADHD patients to augment negative SCPs would increase the capacity to produce cortical activation necessary for concentration and cognitive tasks.

Heinrich, Gevensleben, Freidsleder, Moll, and Rothenberger (2004) investigated the neurophysiologic effects of SCP training in 13 children (7—13 years old) with ADHD and 9 ADHD wait-listed controls. Following 25 sessions of SCP training, participants had a 25% reduction in ADHD symptomatology, a decrease of impulsivity errors and increase of CNV during CPT assessment. Strehl, Leins, Goth, Klinger, and Birbaumer (2006) proved that children with ADHD were able to regulate negative shifts during feedback and transfer trials. Following 30 sessions of SCP training the 23 participants (8—13 years old) had significant improvements in behavioral, attention, and IQ scores, which remained stable over a 6 month follow-up. At a 2-year follow-up of these patients, all improvements in behavior and attention remained stable and an additional significant reduction of core ADHD symptoms and attention improvement were observed (Gani, Birbaumer, & Strehl, 2008). SCP self-regulation skills were preserved and half of the children no longer met criteria for ADHD.

In a controlled evaluation of SCP neurofeedback compared to group treatment for ADHD, the 17 participants (M = 10.5 years old) in the SCP training group underwent 30 sessions and showed greater improvement on parent and teacher rating scales in areas of cognition and attention than their group therapy peers (Drechsler et al., 2007). The group therapy program was based on the principles of cognitive behavioral therapy and comprised components of social skill training, self-management, metacognitive skill training, and enhancement of self-awareness. Investigation of specific and non-specific factors influencing the behavioral improvements revealed that effective parental support and the ability to self-regulate SCPs in transfer conditions had moderate effects on positive training outcomes. Gevensleben et al. (2009) compared a combined neurofeedback training protocol to a computerized attention skills training program within an ADHD population (M = 9.1 years old). The 59 participants in the combined neurofeedback condition participated in counter balanced blocks of theta/beta and SCP training sessions (36 sessions total). Comparable effects were observed for both neurofeedback protocols during intermediate and post-training assessment, both indicating improvements in parent and teacher behavior ratings scales compared to the computerized attention skills training group. In a meta-analysis of research focused on neurofeedback treatment of ADHD in child populations, a large effect size was found for training (both frequency and SCP training) on impulsivity and inattention in controlled studies and those using pre- and post-designs (Arns, de Ridder, Strehl, Breteler, & Coenen, 2009).

Migraines

Welch and Ramadan (1995) hypothesized that disordered mitochondrial oxidative phosphorylation and decreased intracellular free magnesium in the brain and body tissue of migraine patients produce instability of neuronal functions due to neuronal hyperexcitability. Migraines patients appear to produce increased CNV amplitudes and reduced habituation compared to healthy controls (review, see Kropp, Siniatchkin, & Gerber, 2002). Stronger negativity of the CNV apparently results in greater general allocation of attentional and mental resources to tasks in a migraine population. Therefore, it was hypothesized that training migraine patients to suppress negative SCPs (i.e., to produce positive shifts) would attenuate cortical excitation resulting in a reduction of migraine frequency and intensity.

Siniatchkin, Hierundar and colleagues (2000) investigated the clinical efficacy of SCP training in children with migraines. Ten children suffering with migraines were compared with 10 healthy controls and 10 wait-listed migraine sufferers. During the initial two sessions, migraine sufferers demonstrated an impaired ability to regulate negative shifts, especially during the transfer trails. However, following 10 sessions of SCP feedback no significant difference in self-regulation mastery was observed compared to healthy controls, and the migraine patients showed a significant reduction in CNV amplitudes and reported significant reductions in the number of days with migraine or other headache activity.

Other Applications

Although there are no treatment studies of SCP feedback in other clinical conditions, there are several studies that indicate other clinical populations are capable of learning to self-regulate SCP activity. Accordingly, clinicians may wish to use the SCP protocol with other conditions that are characterized by impaired regulation of excitation thresholds. Gruzelier et al. (1999) and Schneider, Rockstroh et al. (1992) demonstrated that although schizophrenic patients showed impaired regulation of SCPs during initial feedback sessions, they were able to reduce negative SCP shifts simultaneously over right−left hemispheres and central electrode sites following 10 to 20 treatment sessions. Additional research by Schneider and colleagues indicated that male inpatients with alcohol dependence (1993), bipolar disorder, and major depression (Schneider, Heimann et al., 1992) also were able to regulate required negativity and negativity suppression following 5 to 20 SCP treatment sessions. Independent SCP clinicians also have reported positive treatment outcomes with Gilles de la Tourette's syndrome, autism, and dyslexia. These case reports and findings are encouraging; however, further research is needed.

Patients suffering from diseases leading to severe or total motor paralysis and loss of communication ability may also benefit from SCP training. Patients who are completely paralyzed but maintain sensory and cognitive functions are said to have "locked-in syndrome". The locked-in state may result from stroke, brain lesions and tumors, brain injuries, or degenerative neuromuscular diseases such as amyotrophic lateral sclerosis (ALS) or Lou Gehrig's disease. Self-regulation of positive and negative SCP shifts can be used to control a cursor on a computer screen required to select letters or words, and is often referred to as "brain−computer communication" (Kübler et al., 2001). This area of SCP research focuses on maintenance of communication and enhanced quality of life for patients with total paralysis.

CONCLUSION

In conclusion, there is a growing interest in SCP feedback due to developments in DC-EEG recording equipment and analysis software. SCPs are very slow shifts of brain activity with a time constant of up to several seconds. These shifts are either positive or negative and reflect regulation of cortical excitation thresholds. Management of DC-EEG specific artifacts and strict training requirements are necessary to ensure the acquisition of valid SCP data and to maximize the clinical outcomes. Research findings and clinical application of SCP feedback in epilepsy, ADHD, and migraine populations have been positive and demonstrated efficacy. Reported side effects are similar to those encountered with other neurofeedback and biofeedback modalities and include headache, fatigue, spaciness, and feelings of agitation or irritability (Hammond & Kirk, 2008). These feelings are generally transient and pass shortly following training sessions. Proper training and supervision, adherence to standards of practice, and an open patient—clinician dialogue can help to reduce these negative training effects. Additional clinical trials and controlled studies now are needed to validate SCP feedback as a treatment method for an even broader range of conditions and populations.

REFERENCES

Arns, M., de Ridder, S., Strehl, U., Breteler, M., & Coenen, A. (2009). Efficacy of neurofeedback treatment in ADHD: The effects on inattention, impulsivity and hyperactivity: A meta-analysis. *Clinical EEG and Neuroscience, 40*(3), 180—189.

Berger, H. (1929). Über das Elektrenkephalogramm des Menschen, 1st report. *Archiv fur Psychiatrie und Nervenkrankheiten, 87*, 527—570.

Birbaumer, N. (1999). Slow cortical potentials: Plasticity, operant control, and behavioral effects. *The Neuroscientist, 5*, 74—78.

Birbaumer, N., Elbert, T., Canavan, A., & Rockstroh, B. (1990). Slow potentials of the cerebral cortex and behavior. *Physiological Reviews, 70*, 1—41.

Birbaumer, N., Elbert, T., Rockstroh, B., Daunm, I., Wolf, P., & Canavan, A. (1991). Clinical-psychological treatment of epileptic seizures: A controlled study. In A. Ehlers (Ed.), *Perspectives and promises in clinical psychology* (pp. 81—96). New York: Plenum Press.

Birbaumer, N., Lang, P., Cook, E., Elbert, T., Lutzenberger, W., & Rockstroh, B. (1988). Slow brain potentials, imagery and hemispheric differences. *International Journal of Neuroscience, 39*, 101—116.

Birbaumer, N., Roberts, L., Lutzenberger, W., Rockstroh, B., & Elbert, T. (1992). Area-specific self-regulation of slow cortical potentials on the sagittal midline and its effects on behavior. *Electroencephalography and Clinical Neurophysiology*, *84*, 353—361.

Canton, R. (1875). The electric currents of the brain. *British Medical Journal*, *2*, 278.

Drechsler, R., Straub, M., Doehnert, M., Heinrich, H., Steinhausen, H. C., & Brandeis, D. (2007). 1 Controlled evaluation of a neurofeedback training of slow cortical potentials in children with attention deficit/hyperactivity disorder (ADHD). *Behavioral and Brain Functions*, *3*, 35.

Fellin, T., Halassa, M. M., Terunuma, M., Succol, F., Takano, H., Frank, M., et al. (2009). Endogenous nonneuronal modulators of synaptic transmission control cortical slow oscillations in vivo. *Proceedings of the National Academy of Sciences of the United States of America*, *106*(35), 15037—15042.

Gani, C., Birbaumer, N., & Strehl, U. (2008). Long-term effects after feedback of slow cortical potentials and of theta-beta-amplitudes in children with attention-deficit/hyperactivity disorder (ADHD). *International Journal of Bioelectromagnetism*, *10*(4), 209—232.

Gevensleben, H., Holl, B., Albrecht, B., Vogel, C., Schlamp, D., Kratz, O., et al. (2009). Is neurofeedback an efficacious treatment for ADHD? A randomized controlled clinical trial. *Journal of Child Psychology and Psychiatry*, *50*(7), 780—789.

Gruzelier, J., Hardman, E., Wild, J., & Zaman, R. (1999). Learned control of slow potential interhemispheric asymmetry in schizophrenia. *International Journal of Psychophysiology*, *34*, 341—348.

Hammond, D. C., & Kirk, L. (2008). First, do no harm: Adverse effects and the need for practice standards in neurofeedback. *Journal of Neurotherapy*, *12*(1), 79—88.

Heinrich, H., Gevensleben, H., Freidsleder, F. J., Moll, G. H., & Rothenberger, A. (2004). Training of slow cortical potentials in ADHD: Evidence for positive behavioral and neurophysiological effects. *Biological Psychiatry*, *55*, 772—775.

Helps, S. K., Broyd, S. J., James, C. J., Karl, A., Chen, W., & Sonuga-Barke, E. J. (2010). Altered spontaneous low frequency brain activity in attention deficit/hyperactivity disorder. *Brain Research*, *31*(1322), 134—143.

Helps, S. K., James, C., Debener, S., Karl, A., & Songura-Barke, E. J. S. (2008). Very low frequency EEG oscillations and the resting brain in young adults: A preliminary study of localization, stability and association with symptoms of inattention. *Journal of Neural Transmission*, *115*, 279—285.

Holzapfel, S., Strehl, U., Kotchoubey, B., & Birbaumer, N. (1998). Behavioral psycho-physiological intervention in a mentally retarded epileptic patient with a brain lesion. *Applied Psychophysiology and Biofeedback*, *23*, 189—202.

Ikeda, A., Yazawa, S., Kunieda, T., Araki, K., Aoki, T., Hattori, H., et al. (1997). Scalp-recorded, ictal focal DC shift in a patient with tonic seizure. *Epilepsia*, *38*(12), 1350—1354.

Kornhuber, H., & Deecke, L. (1965). Hirnpotentiländerungen bei Willkürbewegungen und passiven Bewegungen de Menschen. *Bereitschaftspotential und reafferente Potentiale, Pflügers Archiv*, *284*, 1—17.

Kotchoubey, B., Strehl, U., Uhlmann, C., Holzapfel, S., König, M., Fröscher, W., et al. (2001). Modulation of slow cortical potentials in patients with refractory epilepsy: A controlled outcome study. *Epilepsia*, *42*(3), 406—416.

Kropp, P., Siniatchkin, M., & Gerber, W. D. (2002). On the pathophysiology of migraine — links for "empirically based treatment" with neurofeedack. *Applied Psychophysiology and Biofeedback*, *27*(3), 203—213.

Kübler, A., Neumann, N., Kaiser, J., Kotchoubey, B., Hinterberger, T., & Birbaumer, N. P. (2001). Brain-computer communication: Self-regulation of slow cortical potentials for verbal communication. *Archives of Physical and Medical Rehabilitation*, *82*(11), 1533—1539.

Kübler, A., Winter, S., & Birbaumer, N. (2003). The thought translation device: Slow cortical potential biofeedback for verbal communication in paralyzed patients. In M. Schwartz, & F. Andrasik (Eds.), *Biofeedback: A practitioner's guide* (3rd ed., pp. 471–481). New York: Guilford.

Liu, Z., Fukunaga, M., de Zwart, J. A., & Duya, J. H. (2010). Large scale spontaneous fluctuations and correlates in brain electrical activity observed with magnetoencephalography. *Neuroimage, 51*(1), 102–111.

Lopes da Silva, F. (1991). Neural mechanism underlying brain waves: From neural membranes to networks. *Electroencephalography and Clinical Neurophysiology, 79*, 81–93.

Rockstroh, B., Elbert, T., Birbaumer, N., Wolf, P., Düchting-Röth, A., Reker, M., et al. (1993). Cortical self-regulation in patients with epilepsies. *Epilepsy Research, 14*, 63–72.

Rockstroh, B., Elbert, T., Lutzenberger, W., & Birbaumer, N. (1990). Biofeedback: Evaluation and therapy in children with attentional dysfunctions. In A. Rothenberger (Ed.), *Brain and behavior in child psychiatry* (pp. 345–355). Berlin: Springer.

Saab, M. (2009, January). DC-EEG in psychophysiology applications: A technical and clinical overview. *NeuroConnections Newsletter*, 7–18.

Schlegelmilch, F., Markert, S., Berkes, S., & Schellhorn, K. (2004). Online ocular artifact removal for DC-EEG-signals: Estimation of DC-level. *Biomedizinische Technik, Efgänzungsband 2, Band, 49*, 340–341.

Schneider, F., Heimann, H., Mattes, R., Lutzenberger, W., & Birbaumer, N. (1992). Self-regulation of slow cortical potentials in psychiatric patients: Depression. *Biofeedback Self Regulation, 17*(3), 203–214.

Schneider, F., Rockstroh, B., Heimann, H., Lutzenberger, W., Mattes, R., Elbert, T., et al. (1992). Self-regulation of slow cortical potentials in psychiatric patients: Schizophrenia. *Biofeedback Self Regulation, 17*(4), 277–292.

Shinba, T. (2009). 24-h profiles of direct current brain potential fluctuation in rats. *Neuroscience Letters, 465*, 104–107.

Siniatchkin, M., Hierundar, A., Kropp, P., Kuhnert, R., Gerber, W. D., & Stephani, U. (2000). Self-regulation of slow cortical potentials in children with migraine: An exploratory study. *Applied Psychophysiology and Biofeedback, 25*(1), 12–32.

Siniatchkin, M., Kropp, P., & Gerber, W. D. (2000). Neurofeedback — The significance of reinforcement and the search for an appropriate strategy for the success of self-regulation. *Applied Psychophysiology and Biofeedback, 25*(3), 167–175.

Speckmann, E. J., & Elger, C. E. (1999). Introduction to the neurophysiological basis of the EEG and DC potentials. In E. Niedermeyer, & F. Lopes da Silva (Eds.), *Electroencephalography: Basic principles, clinical applications, and related fields* (4th ed., pp. 13–27). Baltimore, MD: Williams & Wilkins.

Steriade, M., Gloor, P., Llinás, R. R., Lopes da Silva, F., & Mesulam, M. M. (1990). Basic mechanisms of cerebral rhythmic activities. *Electroencephalography and Clinical Neurophysiology, 76*, 481–508.

Strehl, U., Kotchoubey, B., Trevorrow, T., & Birbaumer, N. (2005). Predictors of seizure reduction after self-regulation of slow cortical potentials as a treatment of drug-resistant epilepsy. *Epilepsy & Behavior, 6*, 156–166.

Strehl, U., Leins, U., Goth, G., Klinger, C., & Birbaumer, N. (2006). Physiological regulation of slow cortical potentials-a new treatment for children with ADHD. *Pediatrics, 118*(5), 1530–1540.

Tan, G., Thornby, D., Hammond, D. C., Strehl, U., Canady, B., Arnemann, K., et al. (2009). Meta-analysis of EEG biofeedback in treating epilepsy. *Clinical EEG and Neuroscience, 40*(3), 173–179.

Walter, W. G. (1964). The contingent negative variation: An electrical sign of significant association in the human brain. *Science, 146*, 434.

Walter, W. G., Cooper, R., Aldridge, V. J., McCallum, W. C., & Winter, A. L. (1964). Contingent negative variation: An electric sign of sensorimotor association and expectancy in the human brain. *Nature, 203*, 380–384.

Welch, K. M. A., & Ramadan, N. M. (1995). Mitochondria, magnesium and migraine. *Journal of Neurological Sciences, 134*, 9–14.

CHAPTER 9

Real-Time Regulation and Detection of Brain States from fMRI Signals

Ranganatha Sitaram[1], Sangkyun Lee[1,2], Sergio Ruiz[1,2,4], and Niels Birbaumer[1,3]

[1]Institute of Medical Psychology and Behavioral Neurobiology, University of Tübingen, Tübingen, Germany
[2]Graduate School of Neural and Behavioral Sciences, International Max Planck Research School, Tübingen, Germany
[3]Ospedale San Camillo, Istituto di Ricovero e Cura a Carattere Scientifico, Venezia — Lido, Italy
[4]Department of Psychiatry, Faculty of Medicine, Pontificia Universidad Católica de Chile, Santiago, Chile

Contents

INTRODUCTION

Functional magnetic resonance imaging (fMRI) allows non-invasive assessment of brain function with high spatial resolution and whole brain coverage, by measuring changes of the blood oxygenation level-dependent (BOLD) signal. Although the BOLD response is an indirect measure of neural activity, there is accumulating evidence suggesting the close coupling between BOLD and electrical activity of the neurons

(Logothetis, 2008). It is postulated that the combined effect of increases and decreases in deoxygenated hemoglobin content resulting from changes in cerebral blood volume, cerebral blood flow, and oxygen metabolism following neural firing results in the BOLD signal (Buxton, Uludağ, Dubowitz, & Liu, 2004). fMRI data typically consist of time-series of several hundred 3D images across the brain over a period of time, with each image acquired every few seconds. fMRI usability and applications have been somewhat limited by the offline mode of data analysis, due to the large size of the data, very intensive computation involved in preprocessing and analysis of fMRI images. Fortunately, innovations in high-performance magnetic resonance scanners and computers, combined with developments in techniques for faster acquisition, processing, and analysis of MR images, have burgeoned a fresh round of developments in fMRI methodology for scientific research and clinical treatment. Real time fMRI (rtfMRI) permits simultaneous measurement and observation of brain activity during an ongoing task. Online single subject preprocessing and statistical analysis of functional data is now possible within a single repetition time (TR), of 1.5−2 s. Novel applications based on rtfMRI have been developed in the last decade, including fMRI data quality assessment, neurosurgical monitoring, and neurofeedback for self-regulation of brain activity. Adding to the above developments are more recent advances in multivariate pattern classification of fMRI signals based on which brain activations in a whole neural network, rather than just a single brain region, could be potentially decoded and modulated (LaConte et al., 2007; Sitaram et al., 2010). Here, we first review historical developments in rtfMRI, followed by an overview of a fMRI Brain−Computer Interface (fMRI−BCI) system for enabling decoding and self-regulation of brain activity, and finally discuss the results of several studies on healthy individuals and patient populations for clinical treatment of neuropsychological disorders.

HISTORICAL DEVELOPMENT OF REAL-TIME fMRI

Functional imaging experiments typically follow a serial procedure in which fMRI images are first acquired from one or more participants performing the tasks under investigation, followed by an offline procedure of signal preprocessing of the images and statistical mapping that may take several days. This sequential processing approach has initially developed due to the large size of data generated in neuroimaging experiments, whose processing and analyses incurred high computational costs. However, it is to be admitted that lack of online implementation of fMRI preprocessing and analysis could limit its applicability and usability in several ways.

First, experimenters cannot monitor data quality during scanning in the absence of online processing. Considering the high cost of MRI scanning, a system for monitoring of data quality is useful for saving the costs and efforts to obtain good quality data. If an investigator can detect artifacts correlated to the stimulus in real-time, such as head motion or other physiological artifacts, it enables him or her to re-acquire the data immediately. Furthermore, in the absence of online analysis, it is hard to modify an experimental design based on the physiological and behavioral changes of the participant. These limitations were first overcome by the pioneering work of Cox and colleagues.

Cox and colleagues (Cox, Jesmanowicz & Hyde, 1995) first proposed a method to analyze brain activation in real-time by computing correlation between a voxel's BOLD signal and a reference time-series of the experimental design in a recursive manner to reduce the computational demands. Statistical maps of the brain were obtained in real-time by coloring voxels that show higher correlations than a user-specified threshold. However, this method did not yet correct for non-specific noise originating in the scanning instrument. Voyvodic (1999) reported an approach to improve the flexibility of the experimental paradigm with a software program for accurate, real-time paradigm control and online fMRI analysis. The paradigm control included simultaneous presentation of stimuli, automatic synchronization to an fMRI scanner, and monitoring of a variety of physiological and behavioral responses. The online analysis performed MR image reconstruction, head motion correction in the translational motion, and statistical tests for block or event-related design. Since then, many studies have improved the image acquisition process in terms of data quality, speed, and statistical power (Gao and Posse, 2003; Posse et al., 1999, 2001, 2003; Weiskopf et al., 2005; Yoo et al., 1999) and algorithms (Bagarinao et al., 2003; Cox & Savoy, 2003; Cox et al., 1995; Cox & Jesmanowicz, 1999; Gao & Posse 2003; Gembris, Taylor, Schor, Frings, Suter, & Posse, 2000; LaConte et al., 2007; Sitaram et al., 2010; Smyser et al., 2001; Voyvodic, 1999).

Further developments in multiecho echo-planar imaging (mEPI) increased the functional contrast-to-noise ratio (CNR) by sampling multiple echoes in a single shot of radio frequency (RF) pulse (Posse et al.,

1999). This method is suitable for rtfMRI as it allows the detection of small signal changes within each echo (of 30–40 ms in a 3T scanner). Adaptive multi-resolution EPI (Panych & Jolesz, 1994) achieved high spatial and/or temporal resolution in regions of functional activations distributed throughout the brain by selectively detecting those regions with RF encoding in multiple stages. Such a method can zoom into the regions of activations while ignoring quiescent regions. Yoo and his colleagues (Yoo et al., 1999) implemented a real-time adaptive acquisition system with a multi-resolution EPI to extract signals from cortex and allow more efficient data acquisition time.

Another notable improvement in imaging was in removing magnetic susceptibility artifacts. Due to the differences in magnetic susceptibilities of different imaged parts, such as air, bone, different brain tissues, the static magnetic field is not homogenous near borders of two brain regions. Particularly, in air–tissue interfaces such as the regions of the basal brain and frontal sinuses greater geometric distortions occur. When one radio-frequency excitation pulse is applied to a slice in single-shot imaging and a read-out time (T_{RO}) of about 10–40 ms is used to encode the slice, the inhomogeneities cause local shifts near the air–tissue interfaces (the misalignment of the functional images to wrong anatomical structure) in the resonance frequency ($1/T_{RO} = 25-100$ Hz). Several methods (Andersson, Hutton, Ashburner, Turner, & Friston, 2001; Jezzard & Balaban, 1995; Kybic et al., 2000; Studholme, Constable, & Duncan, 2000; Zaitsev, Hennig, & Speck, 2004) have been suggested to reduce the geometric distortion. However, not every one of these methods may be suitable for real-time applications as they require additional reference scans and computational time. Weiskopf and colleagues (Weiskopf et al., 2005) developed a real-time method to allow for simultaneous acquisition and distortion correction of functional images contributing further to the development of real-time fMRI.

Taken together, many different algorithms have been developed for the acquisition and real-time processing of fMRI signals. To improve the sensitivity of functional imaging, correction of head movement artifacts is a challenging problem. According to Cox and Jesmanowicz (1999), if two neighboring voxels differ in intrinsic brightness by 20%, then a motion of 10% of a voxel dimension can result in a 2% signal change – comparable to the BOLD signal change at 1.5T (Bandettini et al., 1992; Cox & Jesmanowicz, 1999). In addition, if movement correlates with a given task/stimuli, it can elicit false activations (Hajnal et al., 1994). If movement is not correlated with the task/stimuli, signal changes due to the movement can change or reduce the actual activation in functional images (Cox & Jesmanowicz 1999). Cox and his colleagues (1999) reported an online method for head-movement correction by an algorithm for three-dimensional (3D) image rotation and shifting (a rigid body model; since the head moves as a whole, it is assumed that motion of the head can be estimated in three directions for translation and three directions for rotation) by generalizing the shears factorization directly to three dimensions. However, this approach is not suitable for real-time applications as the time needed for realignment of 80 images is estimated to be several minutes. Mathiak and Posse (2001) reported a real-time method of head motion correction in which rigid body (from six parameters including three for translation and three for rotation) transformation was applied in the interval between acquisitions of two functional images. Besides improving the performance of realignment of the functional images, an error (indicating potentially noise or artifact) added by the realignment process also would need to be considered. Mathiak and Posse (2001) proposed that at least three slices with an image matrix of 64×64 would be required to reduce the error in the estimated movement parameters to less than 1% of the voxel size.

Further concerning realignment, a variety of real-time pre-processing techniques for the corrections of respiration artifacts, spatial smoothing (Posse et al., 2003) and spatial normalization to stereotactic space (Gao & Posse, 2003) have been developed. To identify significant voxels in online analysis, methods such as correlation (Cox et al., 1995), general linear model (Caria et al., 2007, 2010; Rota et al., 2009; Ruiz et al., 2008; Smyser et al., 2001; Weiskopf, Veit, Wilhelm, & Elena, 2003), and t-tests (Voyvodic, 1999) have been used.

The above technical advances in rtfMRI enabled the development of fMRI-BCI systems (see the following sections) for self-regulation of brain activity with neurofeedback to study plasticity and functional reorganization. Neurofeedback is based on the psychological theory of instrumental learning, i.e., training in the presence of contingent reward (Skinner, 1938; Weiskopf et al., 2004). Studies have reported different methods for the generation of reward. Yoo and Jolesz (2002) used the statistical map of brain activations as visual feedback. Posse et al. (2003) gave participants verbal feedback of the BOLD signal change in the amygdala at intervals of 60 s. Weiskopf et al. (2003) introduced real-time feedback by showing two time courses of the BOLD signal in two circumscribed brain regions, namely, rostral—ventral and dorsal anterior cingulate cortex, which were updated at an interval of 2 s. DeCharms, Christoff, Glover, Pauly, Whitfield, & Gabrieli (2004) built an fMRI-BCI system to guide self-regulation of the somatomotor cortex with visual feedback of three different time courses, in the target ROI, in a background ROI (irrelevant to the task performance), and difference between the two ROIs. Recent studies (Caria et al., 2007, 2010; deCharms et al., 2004, 2005; Rota et al., 2009) have used visual feedback in the interval of 1—2 s.

OVERVIEW OF THE fMRI—BCI SYSTEM

fMRI—BCI could be defined as a closed loop system that extracts brain signals from regions of interest and/or classifies patterns of brain activity from a whole neural network in real-time, so that this information can be provided to the subject as contingent feedback to enable him to volitionally control the brain activity. In general, an fMRI—BCI system is comprised of the following subsystems: (1) the subject, (2) signal acquisition, (3) pre-processing, (4) signal analysis, and (5) feedback generation. Depending on the purpose of the experiment, the subject would be instructed and trained to perform mental tasks guided by the feedback information. Here, we describe the last four subsystems mainly based on the fMRI—BCI system built in the Institute of Medical Psychology and Behavioral Neurobiology, University of Tübingen, Germany. The word real-time in the following sections implies that signal processing is performed within a single TR (for example, 1.5 s).

Signal Acquisition

Experiments are conducted on a 3T whole body scanner using a standard 12 channel head coil (Siemens Magnetom Trio Tim, Siemens, Erlangen, Germany). In principle, scanners from other manufacturers and with other field strengths could be used for fMRI—BCI development. Whole brain images of the subject are acquired using an EPI pulse sequence which is modified to export functional images to the host computer of the scanner. Pulse sequence parameters used for signal acquisition in our experiments were as follows: repetition time $TR = 1.5$ seconds, echo time $TE = 45$ msec, flip angle $= 70$ degree, number of slices $= 16$, bandwidth $= 1.3$ KHz/pixel, $FOV_{PE/RO} = 210$, image matrix $= 64 \times 64$, voxel size $= 3 \times 3 \times 5mm^3$. These parameters could be modified keeping in mind, however, the trade-off between signal-difference to noise ratio, also called the contrast-to-noise ratio (CNR), and the spatio-temporal resolution. Intrinsic parameters that modify the inherent signal produced by a volumetric element (voxel) of the tissue, such as TR, TE, and flip angle affect the CNR. Extrinsic parameters do not affect the measured tissue, but influence the mechanics of the data collection, e.g., spatio-temporal resolution (Brown & Semelka, 1999). In the setup of the parameters for real-time signal acquisition, a suitable compromise must be made between spatial resolution, i.e., FOV, image matrix and slice thickness, number of slices, and temporal resolution, i.e., TR. In our fMRI–BCI experiments, the repetition time was reduced to 1.5 seconds (compared to 2–3 s in a conventional fMRI experiments) to increase the temporal resolution of BOLD signal, while the number of slices was reduced to 16 (from 25–30 slices in conventional fMRI measurement) and slice thickness was increased to 5 mm. With these parameters, adequate spatial and temporal resolutions for functional image acquisition were provided. However, the older MRI operating software provided by manufacturers (e.g., Syngo, version VB13 and before, Siemens Medical Solutions, Erlangen, Germany) did not have a provision for online export of functional images. To retrieve images in real-time for online processing, a generalized image reconstruction module was inserted into the conventional EPI sequence provided by Siemens (Caria et al., 2007, 2010; Rota et al., 2009; Sitaram et al., 2010; Weiskopf et al., 2003). This module receives EPI k-space raw data from the MRI scanner hardware, reconstructs whole brain images before start of the next volume of the brain, and stores them in a pre-specified directory that could be immediately accessed for another program to perform online preprocessing and analysis. Fortunately, recent versions of scanner operating software (e.g., Siemens Syngo version VB15, VB17 and VA30) have provided a standard option to enable real-time export of functional images, simplifying and standardizing the future development of real-time fMRI.

Pre-processing

After the acquisition of each volume of EPI images, various online pre-processing steps could be performed for artifact removal and noise reduction. To prevent artifactual signals caused by head movement, head padding and bite bars could be used. In addition, through a head-motion correction step, we could monitor how much the participants move in 6 directions (3 translations and 3 rotations) in real-time, and instruct them to avoid such movement. Head movement can be inferred by monitoring the time courses of the head movement parameters. Patients could then be reminded to avoid moving if excessive head movement is observed. In addition to this motion correction, pre-processing also includes spatial smoothing to reduce the effect of noise, and de-trending to remove linear trends in the BOLD time-series.

Signal Analysis

After completion of pre-processing steps, whole-brain images are used for statistical analysis and generation of functional maps. For real-time statistical analysis, a variety of algorithms that perform subtraction of two different conditions, correlation analysis, or general linear model could be used. Real-time statistical analysis is usually performed either by analyzing recent time samples of data extracted from a sliding window or by incrementally analyzing all data acquired up to a given time point. The sliding-window method is superior in reflecting the current brain state as it uses the most recent information. However, this method is not statistically powerful because a limited number of samples are used in the statistical test. In contrast, the incremental method provides more robust information by using all the data acquired up to a given time point.

Studies (Caria et al., 2007, 2010; deCharms et al., 2004; Rota et al., 2009) have also used the subtraction method of determining activation maps where signals in the baseline condition are subtracted from the activation condition in a sliding window to provide feedback information in the ROIs. The correlation method (Cox et al., 1995; Gembris et al., 2000; Posse et al., 2001) is applied by computing the correlation coefficient between the time-series of the measured BOLD signal at each voxel and the reference (or design) time-series representing the change in the task conditions, and assessing the coefficients with a specified threshold. The correlation method can be used in either a sliding-window fashion or an incremental fashion.

General Linear Model (GLM) is now a standard method of analysis of functional images to estimate the parameters that fit the measured time-series of BOLD signal at each voxel, with a linear summation of multiple experimental and confounding effects weighted by the corresponding parameters. A GLM for two different conditions and one confounding effect produces three parameters to best fit the measured time-series of BOLD signal at a voxel. These parameters are computed independently for all the voxels of the brain and then used for statistical tests such as the *t*-test and the F-test. As an example, the *t*-test can be applied on the first parameter values over all the brain voxels, where the parameter magnitudes correspond to involvement of each voxel in the first condition. These statistical tests identify the voxels that are significant (i.e., activated solely in the corresponding condition) in the tests. However, since the number of samples (i.e., scanned images) is limited in real-time applications, Bagarinao et al. (2003) developed a method of real-time GLM by updating the parameters in GLM as new data become available. Similarly, the commercially available real-time fMRI analysis software, Turbo Brain Voyager (TBV, Brain Innovations, Maastricht, Netherlands) used in our fMRI–BCI setup (Caria et al., 2007, 2010; Rota et al., 2009; Ruiz et al., 2008; Weiskopf et al. 2003) uses real-time GLM by applying the recursive least squares regression algorithm (Pollock, Green, & Nguyen, 1999) to update GLM estimation incrementally.

All of the above methods are univariate methods as all the statistical tests are separately performed at each voxel. In contrast, multivariate methods can recognize spatial and temporal patterns of activity from multiple distributed voxels in the brain. Multivariate methods accumulate weak information available at multiple locations to jointly decode cognitive states although information at any single location cannot differentiate between the states (Haynes & Rees, 2006). Recent studies (Cox & Savoy, 2003; Haynes & Rees, 2006; Haynes, Sakai, Rees, Gilbert, Frith, & Passingham, 2007; Harrison & Tong 2009; Kamitani & Tong, 2005; Lee et al., 2010; Mitchell et al., 2003) have applied multivariate methods to increase sensitivity of fMRI analysis. Laconte and his colleagues (2007) developed an fMRI–BCI system by employing a multivariate pattern classification method called support vector machines (SVM). While most fMRI–BCI studies to date have investigated self-regulation of brain activity at one or two ROIs using univariate analysis, multivariate methods allow for real-time feedback of a whole network of brain activity pertaining to a task.

We have recently implemented a real-time classification method for automatically recognizing multiple emotional brain states from fMRI signals (Sitaram et al., 2010; see Figure 9.1). In our study, participants were instructed to recall two (happy and disgust) or three (happy, disgust, and sad) salient emotional episodes in a block design paradigm. While participants performed emotional imagery, whole brain images were acquired and pre-processed in real-time to correct for head-motion artifacts and

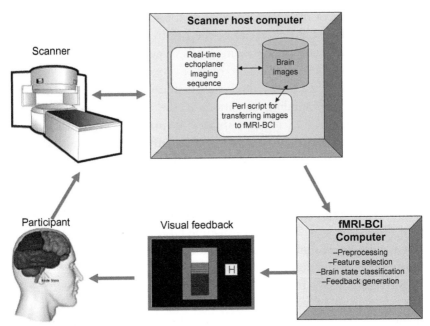

Figure 9.1 The Tübingen real-time fMRI brain state classification system is comprised of the following subsystems: an image acquisition subsystem, which is a modified version of the standard echo-planar imaging (EPI) sequence written in C and executed on the scanner host computer; and an fMRI–BCI subsystem, which performs image preprocessing, brain state classification and visual feedback, implemented in C and Matlab scripts (Mathworks, Natwick, MA) and executed on a 64-bit Windows desktop. A Perl-script on the scanner host transfers the acquired images after every scan (at an interval of 1.5s) to the fMRI-BCI computer. (*Reproduced from Sitaram et al., with permission.*)

spatially smoothed to improve signal-to-noise ratio. As the number of voxels in the brain images is too large (tens of thousands, depending on the scanning parameters) for a pattern classifier to handle efficiently, a computational method called feature selection needs to be carried out to reduce the data size and improve the efficacy of classification. We have developed a novel method of feature selection called effect mapping (Lee et al., 2010). In practice, the emotion classifier is first trained for each participant on a set of initial data taken out of two sessions of the experiment. The trained classifier is then used to recognize online (at intervals of 1.5 s) the states of emotion, namely, happy, disgust or sad, as the participant engages in emotional imagery. In our study, participants were provided real-time visual feedback of the state of their brain based on the classifier output. Our study, performed on 18 healthy individuals, showed that fMRI—BCIs built using a pattern classifiers can robustly decode multiple brain states (average classification accuracy >80%) in real time and provide feedback of the states.

Feedback Generation

As explained earlier, the results of real-time signal analysis in the ROI or in the network determined by the pattern classifier can be transformed to generate contingent feedback to the participant. Recent studies have shown the usefulness of feedback in learning to regulate the BOLD signal in one or more regions of the brain with fMRI—BCI (Caria et al., 2007, 2010; deCharms et al., 2004, 2005; Posse et al., 2003; Rota et al., 2009; Ruiz et al., 2008). In addition, Lee and his colleagues (2008) reported the effects of neurofeedback in self-regulation training by showing that insula-regulation training with feedback leads to cerebral reorganization in the brain regions relevant to emotion processing (Lee, Sitaram, Ruiz, & Birbaumer, 2008). In studies with rtfMRI (Caria et al., 2007, 2010; deCharms et al., 2004, 2005; Posse et al., 2003; Rota et al., 2009; Ruiz et al., 2008), different forms of feedback have been used. Except for one study that used verbal feedback (Posse et al., 2003), most studies to date (Caria et al., 2007; deCharms et al., 2004, 2005; Rota et al., 2009; Ruiz et al., 2008) have used visual feedback. Hinterberger et al. (2004) showed that visual feedback compared to auditory feedback leads to better learning in self-regulation of slow cortical potential (SCP; change of cortical potential below 1 Hz) using an EEG-BCI. As fMRI experiments generally have more acoustic background noise, visual feedback is presumably more effective. Visual feedback has been provided in a variety of forms such as time courses of BOLD activity in target areas updated in real-time, functional maps based on online statistical analysis, and virtual reality based animation. Using the conventional univariate method of analysis, feedback can be based on one or more ROIs by combining them in the form of additive or subtractive contrasts. The subtraction of BOLD signals of the reference area from that of the ROI can result in more robust feedback as the BOLD activity in the reference area reflects the global change of brain due to head movements, swallowing and systemic changes in BOLD. More sophisticated methods of feedback computation could potentially include correlational analysis between time-series of BOLD activations in the ROIs, bivariate or multivariate methods of functional connectivity computation using Granger causality modelling (GCM), and multivariate pattern classification (Laconte et al., 2007; Sitaram et al., 2010). Future developments in the adaptation of existing brain signal analysis methods to real-time requirements will dictate how well these methods could be used in fMRI-BCI applications.

fMRI—BCI IN RESEARCH AND CLINICAL TREATMENT

In the last decades, neurofeedback based on electrical brain signals has been successfully applied to train subjects to self-regulate different components of the electroencephalogram, leading to measurable behavioral changes. EEG neurofeedback has been therapeutically applied to neurological and psychiatric disorders, such us intractable epilepsy, stroke, locked-in syndrome and amyotrophic lateral sclerosis (Birbaumer, 2006; Fuchs, Birbaumer, Lutzenberger, Gruzelier, & Kaiser, 2003; Kotchoubey et al., 2001; Kubler, Kotchoubey, Kaiser, Wolpaw, & Birbaumer, 2001; Murase, Duque, Mazzocchio, & Cohen, 2004; Strehl et al., 2006). For its part, the development of real-time fMRI and fMRI—BCI has been more recent. In the next sections, we will review the studies that have been conducted so far with this new technique on healthy subjects, and the attempts to implement this methodology on clinical populations.

fMRI—BCI Studies in Healthy Populations
Regulation of Brain Regions of Emotion
The modulation of brain areas related to emotional processing has been of particular interest for fMRI—BCI research. Posse and colleagues (Posse et al., 2003) used rtfMRI and feedback of amygdala activation to reinforce mood induction. Amygdala modulation can be of special importance due to its role in emotion processing and learning, and due to its involvement in several neuropsychiatric disorders (Buchanan, 2007; Lawrie, Whalley, Job, & Johnstone, 2003; Pause, Jungbluth, Adolph, Pietrowsky, & Dere, 2010). A group of six healthy subjects performed a paradigm of self-induction of mood to alternate between neutral and sad affective states while in the scanner. After each trial, subjects received verbal feedback of the signal change of BOLD activation in the amygdala. Subjects successfully achieved sad induction, and their self-mood ratings correlated with the level of activity in the amygdala. Therefore, this study showed that real-time fMRI could be used to monitor the activations of a particular brain area, and suggested that feedback may influence perceived mood. However, as both the task of self-induction and BCI feedback were

presented simultaneously, it was not possible to ascertain whether amygdala self-regulation was actually achieved due to the BCI feedback.

Weiskopf and colleagues from our group (Weiskopf et al., 2003) investigated whether fMRI−BCI could be applied to achieve self-regulation of the anterior cingulate cortex (ACC). The ACC is part of the limbic system and is subdivided into a dorsal "cognitive division" (ACcd), and a rostral-ventral "affective division" (Acad) (Bush, Luu, & Posner, 2000). A healthy subject was instructed to upregulate the activations of these areas, presented to him as a continuously updated visual feedback (delay <2 s), introducing the concept of "immediate feedback" of the BOLD signal. Using imagery of landscapes, sports, and social interaction in many training sessions, the subject achieved a significant increase of the BOLD signal between up-regulation and baseline blocks. Additionally, the signal in the affective ACC increased across the sessions of training, suggesting a "learning effect". Although it was not possible to correlate the BOLD signal change with any behavioral measurement, the participant rated the valence and arousal of his affective state as more positive for regulation blocks compared to baseline blocks. Hence, this single subject study was one of the first that convincingly showed that BOLD signal of circumscribed brain regions can be self-regulated using fMRI−BCI, and that self-regulation by fMRI−BCI training might lead to affective modifications. Studies have shown (Caria et al., 2007, 2010) that a robust ability to self-regulate a brain region can be learned with contingent feedback, and not with sham feedback, nor with mental imagery without feedback.

Further to this study, our group investigated whether healthy subjects can voluntarily gain control over anterior insular activity using fMRI−BCI (Caria et al., 2007). The insula cortex is an anatomically complex mesocortical structure, part of the paralimbic system that plays a central role in sensory integration, emotion, and cognition, including such functions as olfaction, gustation, autonomic functions, temperature and pain perception, and self-awareness (for reviews see Augustine, 1996; Craig, 2009; Ture, Yasargil, Al-Mefty, & Yasargil, 1999). Modulation of the insular activity with fMRI−BCI training might be relevant for treatment of different psychiatric diseases as social phobia, antisocial behavior, schizophrenia, and addictive disorders (Nagai, Kishi, & Kato, 2007; Naqvi & Bechara, 2009). In this study, nine healthy subjects were trained to voluntarily control the BOLD signal of the anterior insular cortex, using fMRI−BCI in four feedback sessions. The visual feedback was the normalized and continuously updated average BOLD signal from the right anterior insula, presented to the subjects by means of thermometer bars. All participants were able to successfully regulate the BOLD signal, and training resulted in a significantly increased activation cluster in the anterior portion of the right insula across sessions. However, self-regulation could not be achieved by a control group trained with sham feedback, suggesting that successful self-regulation is achieved by contingent fMRI feedback. This work was the first group study that showed that volitional control of emotionally relevant brain areas can be attained by fMRI–BCI training.

Given this, can learned self-regulation produce a measurable behavioral modification? In a later study, Caria and colleagues (Caria et al., 2010) explored the relationship between brain self-regulation and emotional behavior using fMRI–BCI. Healthy participants underwent four fMRI–BCI scanning sessions to modulate the BOLD response in the left anterior insula guided by visual feedback (as in the previous study). After each modulation block of self-regulation and baseline, participants were presented with either an emotionally negative or a neutral picture taken from the International Affective Picture System (IAPS; Lang, Bradley, & Cuthbert, 1997). Immediately after presentation, participants were required to rate the picture using the Self-Assessment Manikin (Lang, 1980). Participants learned to increase and decrease the BOLD response significantly in the anterior insula guided by contingent feedback, and behavioral data showed a significant difference of valence ratings of the aversive pictures in the last session. These results demonstrate that fMRI–BCI manipulation of paralimbic regions such as insula is possible and can modulate a specific emotional response.

A question that arises from these studies is whether, in addition to behavioral modification, self-regulation of circumscribed brain areas also leads to cerebral reorganization. In a further analysis of our data reported in Caria et al. (2007), we investigated (Lee et al., 2008) changes in brain connections associated with anterior insula self-regulation. We used multivariate support pattern analysis and effective connectivity analysis with Granger causality modeling (Seth, 2009). Our analyses revealed changes in the neural network of emotion regulation represented by an inverted U-curve of connectivity densities across the sessions of self-regulation. Feedback training resulted in an initial increase of the density of the connections among regions such as the left and right insula, ACC, medial prefrontal cortex, dorsolateral prefrontal cortex, and amygdala. Further training seemed to indicate pruning of presumably redundant connections and strengthening of potentially relevant connections. This effect can be of special importance as it shows that BCI might be used to build a more efficient neural pathway, especially for conditions in which abnormal neural connectivity is implied (as in autism and schizophrenia).

In a very recent study, Hamilton and colleagues (Hamilton et al., 2010) tested whether healthy individuals can downregulate the activity of the subgenual anterior cingulate (sACC) cortex with fMRI−BCI. Studies have shown that downregulation of this region produced by deep brain stimulation led to a sustained antidepressive effect in patients with treatment-resistant depression, suggesting that endogenous modulation by BCI might be used as a therapeutic approach (Lozano et al., 2008; Mayberg et al., 2005). Using "positive affect strategies" and visual contingent feedback of the BOLD signal, eight healthy women were able to downregulate the BOLD signal from sACC. The learned downregulation, however, did not persist in a subsequent session where subjects were not provided with feedback. However, the study included a psychophysiological interaction (PPI) analysis of functional connectivity (Friston et al., 1997) which showed that BCI training was associated with a decreased correlation (connectivity) between sACC and posterior cingulate cortex. Similar to the study performed by Lee and colleagues (2008), this finding indicates that fMRI−BCI training leads to changes in the effective connectivity of a network subserving a task.

Prediction of emotional states from brain activity constitutes a major scope of affective neuroscience. It could solve several pressing clinical problems such as the assessment of affect in verbally incompetent people with dementia, minimally conscious state, and locked-in-syndrome, and the detection of deception. Recent advances in multivariate pattern classification of functional magnetic resonance imaging (fMRI) signals are especially important due to the high spatial resolution, whole brain coverage, and non-invasiveness of fMRI. As mentioned earlier, in a recent study (Sitaram et al., 2010) we showed that an online support vector machine (SVM) can be built to recognize two discrete emotional states, such as happiness and disgust, from fMRI signals in healthy individuals instructed to recall emotionally salient episodes from their lives. The classifier also showed robust prediction rates in decoding three discrete emotional states (happiness, disgust, and sadness) in an extended group of participants. Subjective reports collected from participants ascertained that they performed emotion imagery, and that the online classifier decoded emotions and not arbitrary states of the brain. This study also showed a relationship between the participants' affect scores as measured by positive and negative affect scores (PANAS) and the subjective ratings of their performance in the emotion imagery task, indicating that participants who report greater negative affect rate themselves relatively lower in their ability to perform the imagery task. Offline whole-brain classification (see Figure 9.2) as well as region-of-interest classification in 24 brain areas previously implicated in emotion processing revealed that the frontal cortex was critically involved in emotion induction by imagery. Finally, we demonstrated an adaptive pattern classifier-based real-time feedback system with which subjects were trained to enhance the functional network of emotion regulation by repeated training.

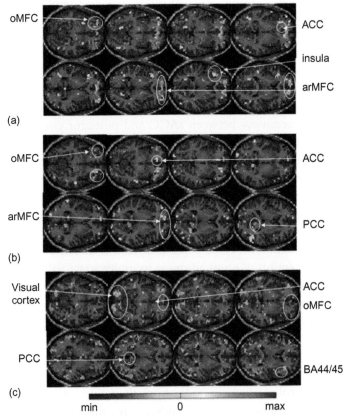

Figure 9.2 *(See Color Plate Section)* Exemplary brain activation maps generated from a single subject whole brain SVM classification showing discriminating voxels for: (a) happy vs. disgust classification, (b) happy vs. sad classification, and (c) disgust vs. sad classification. Brain regions: oMFC, orbital medial frontal cortex; arMFC, anterior rostral MFC (based on Amodio & Frith, 2006); OFC, orbitofrontal cortex; ACC, anterior cingulate cortex; PCC, posterior cingulate cortex.

Motor System

In one of the earliest fMRI–BCI studies, Yoo and Jolesz (2002) tested whether subjects could self-regulate the activity of motor areas by fMRI neurofeedback. Brain activations from sensorimotor regions produced by a simple finger-tapping task were extracted by fMRI, in five healthy participants. Through sessions of regulation, participants were asked to adapt their hand motor strategies in order to expand the functional activations in the motor cortex, guided by the brain activations maps provided as visual feedback, at the end of each block of regulation. After a few trials of training, all participants were able to adapt their motor strategies to successfully expand their brain activations in the ROI.

DeCharms and colleagues (deCharms et al., 2004) used a hand motor imagery task in six participants who were instructed to optimize their strategies in order to increase the activations in the somatomotor cortex, while receiving ongoing real-time fMRI visual feedback of the level of activations in these brain regions. A significant monotonic activation increase in the ROI across training was also found. Furthermore, a control group of subjects who were trained in the scanner in an identical task, but without valid rtfMRI information (sham feedback), did not achieve self-regulation.

Other studies have attempted to use fMRI–BCI technology to translate brain activity into direct control of computers and robots. Yoo and colleagues (Yoo et al., 2004) used fMRI to decode brain activities associated with four distinct covert functional tasks (mental calculation, mental speech generation, and motor imagery of sequential finger position of right and left hand), and subsequently translated these activations into predetermined computer commands for moving four directional cursors. Three healthy participants were able to make a cursor navigate in a 2D maze demonstrating "spatial navigation by thought". The same group (Lee, Ryu, Jolesz, Cho, & Yoo, 2009), later explored the use of fMRI–BCI to control a robotic arm. The BOLD signal extracted from primary motor areas (M1) of right and left hemispheres were used to adjust vertical and horizontal coordinates of this external device. Three healthy subjects attempted to move the robotic arm using motor imagery to activate M1 with the help of visual feedback to adjust the level of cortical activation. With different degrees of success, participants were able to gain voluntary control of two-dimensional movement of the robotic device. These preliminary studies can be of crucial importance for future therapeutic attempts in patients with motor dysfunctions due to stroke, brain or spinal injury, or degenerative disorders.

Auditory System

Yoo and colleagues tested the feasibility of using fMRI neurofeedback for the regulation of cortical activations related to auditory attention (Yoo et al., 2006). Eleven healthy participants passively received auditory stimulation in the scanner to determine the auditory areas as regions of interest. During the regulation sessions, participants were instructed to engage in an attentional task (listening to the auditory stimuli) in order to increase the volume of activation within the ROI. Between scanner sessions, verbal feedback of the activation of auditory areas was given to the subjects. The experimental group successfully increased the BOLD signal in left auditory areas and other extra-temporal areas. A control group that was not given feedback of the activations in the auditory cortex did not achieve consistent increase in activations in the region, indicating the importance of feedback in self-regulation.

Language Processing

In an experiment conducted by our team, fMRI–BCI was used to train subjects to achieve self-control of right inferior frontal gyrus (BA 45), and to measure whether this voluntary increase of the BOLD signal would modulate language processing (Rota et al., 2009). All seven subjects of the experimental group achieved voluntary self-regulation of the activation-level recorded in the target ROI, with a progressive increase of the level of activation in the right BA 45 across training sessions. Short-term behavioral effects of self-regulation with regard to language processing were explored by comparing accuracy levels and reaction times before and after feedback training in prosodic and syntactic tasks. During the self-regulation of BA 45, experimental subjects significantly improved their accuracy for the identification of affective prosodic stimuli (but not for syntactic stimuli), confirming the role of inferior frontal gyrus in the processing of emotional information. These results pointed out that self-regulation of prefrontal cortical areas by fMRI–BCI is possible, and could be explored as a means to normalize dysfunctional cortical networks to enhance cognitive and/or behavioral disturbances associated with clinical disorders.

fMRI–BCI Studies in Clinical Populations

The studies described above showed that fMRI–BCI can enable healthy subjects to achieve voluntary control of circumscribed brain areas. Some of these studies have also shown behavioral changes and cerebral changes due to fMRI–BCI practice. The next paragraphs describe how far we have gone in the applications of fMRI–BCI with neurological and psychiatric disorders.

Pain Perception

Chronic pain is a major health problem causing untold suffering for millions of patients, and economic burden worldwide. DeCharms and colleagues (deCharms et al., 2005) focused on the use of self-regulation of rostral ACC (rACC) to investigate the modulation of pain perception. This area, among others, is involved in mediating the conscious perception of pain (Mackey & Maeda, 2004; Petrovic & Ingvar, 2002; Wager et al., 2004). The results of fMRI–BCI training in a group of healthy subjects showed that is it possible to gain deliberate control of the rACC activation aided by contingent fMRI feedback, and that self-regulation is significantly associated with changes in the perception of pain caused by a noxious thermal stimulus. Going one step further, they demonstrated that similar self-regulation can be achieved by a group of chronic pain patients who reported decrease in the level of ongoing pain after the fMRI–BCI training. It remains to be seen if such behavioral changes persist in the long term.

Stroke Rehabilitation

In recent work by our group, Sitaram and colleagues (2010) assessed the feasibility of fMRI–BCI feedback training for enabling healthy individuals and stroke patients to regulate the ventral premotor cortex (PMv), an area involved in observation, imagery, and execution of movement (Grezes & Decety, 2001). The authors hypothesized that upregulation of the BOLD signal in the PMv would facilitate motor cortical output from primary motor cortex (M1). Each fMRI–BCI feedback session consisted of four runs of self-regulation training. Results showed that training enabled participants to learn to upregulate the BOLD response of PMv. To measure behavioral effects of self-regulation, the authors used paired pulses of transcranial magnetic stimulation (TMS) to induce intracortical inhibition and facilitation, and simultaneously measured motor evoked potential (MEP) on the participant's finger. Results showed evidence for reduction in intracortical inhibition after feedback training compared to the same situation before feedback training, and even further reduction during self-regulation of PMv.

Tinnitus Treatment

Tinnitus, the perception of sound in the absence of an auditory stimulus, is a common chronic disorder with limited treatment options that can adversely impact the quality of life of the patients. Current views of its neural basis include an over-activation of the auditory network (Eggermont, 2005; Kleinjung et al., 2005). Six patients with chronic tinnitus were examined by Haller, Birbaumer, & Veit (2010). After localizing the primary auditory cortex, patients were instructed to downregulate the BOLD activity of this area aided by contingent visual feedback. Most of the patients learned to downregulate their activations in the auditory ROI. Furthermore, a linear decrease in the auditory activations was detected over training sessions. After a single day of BCI training there was a decrease of the subjective report of tinnitus in two of six participants. This preliminary data suggests that fMRI–BCI potentially could produce beneficial effects for the treatment of this disorder.

Mental Disorders

So far, two chronic and irreversible mental disorders have been the focus of interest in our group: psychopathy and schizophrenia. Psychopathy is a severe personality disorder often considered untreatable. Studies by our group have shown that persons diagnosed with psychopathy fail to activate prefrontal cortex and limbic regions (including insula cortex, cingulate cortex, left amygdala, and orbitofrontal cortex) during a fear-conditioning task (Birbaumer et al., 2005; Veit et al., 2002). Therefore, we hypothesized that upregulation of these areas could facilitate the acquisition of aversive conditioning, potentially modifying the behavioral manifestations of the disorder. Using a similar paradigm as Caria et al. (2007), we trained individuals with criminal psychopathy to self-regulate anterior insula cortex with fMRI–BCI. Preliminary results showed for the first time that such persons can learn self-regulation of left anterior insula. Furthermore, self-regulation led to an increase in the effective connectivity of the brain network involved in emotional processing.

In a second study, we made the first attempt to apply fMRI–BCI with schizophrenic patients (Ruiz et al., 2008; full article in press). The first aims of this study were to evaluate whether schizophrenic subjects can achieve volitional regulation of anterior insula cortex activity by fMRI–BCI training, and to explore the relationship between the capability to self-regulate and other aspects of their symptomatology. Insula cortex was chosen as the ROI based on the increasing evidence that insula dysfunction might be critically involved in different aspects of schizophrenic psychopathology. Secondly, we explored whether self-regulation is associated with a behavioral modification of facial emotion recognition. Finally, we studied whether learned self-regulation can modulate the functional connectivity of the emotional brain network (measured by Granger causality modelling). Nine chronic schizophrenic patients, moderately symptomatic and under antipsychotic medication, were recruited. The training consisted of twelve sessions of fMRI-BCI during which patients were trained using online visual feedback of bilateral anterior insula activity. Our results showed that after a few sessions of training, patients learned to self-regulate the BOLD response in the insula cortex (see Figure 9.3). Self-regulation was not achieved, however, in a later session conducted without fMRI-feedback (transfer session).

The capability to self-regulate was negatively correlated with the severity of negative symptoms and the duration of the illness. After learned insula self-regulation, patients detected significantly more disgust faces, in line with the extensive evidence of the role of insula in face disgust recognition. However, for reasons that need more exploration,

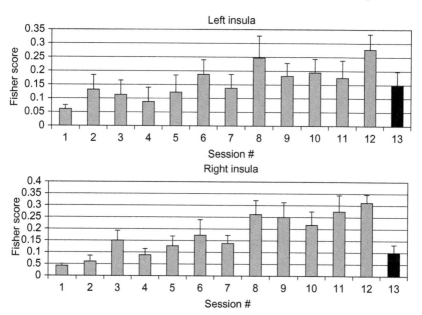

Figure 9.3 Group analysis of self-regulation in the left and right anterior insula. Gray bars represent the Fisher score (as a measure of signal change in the ROI) and standard error across training sessions. The black bars represent the mean and standard error for the transfer session.

patients detected less happy faces during self-regulation. Volitional control of insula was also associated with a modulation of the perception of emotion intensity. Finally, volitional self-regulation led to a significant enhancement of the effective connectivity arising from the insula cortex on both hemispheres, and of the emotional network in general.

These results showed that with adequate training these schizophrenic subjects were able to learn volitional regulation of the insula cortex by fMRI−BCI. Learned self-regulation led to changes in the perception of emotional faces, one of the hallmarks of schizophrenic dysfunction, thus providing evidence that behavioral modulation by this new technique in schizophrenia is possible. The enhancement of the connectivity in brain emotional network suggests that fMRI−BCI may be useful in "re-connecting" abnormal neural connections in schizophrenia.

CONCLUSIONS

New developments in computer and device technology, and signal processing have brought fresh enthusiasm and interest in real-time neuroimaging. Several new applications of this technique, most significantly led by research in brain−computer interfaces, are being developed and tested. rtfMRI has inspired a promising new approach to cognitive neuroscience. There is growing evidence that learned control of the local brain activity through rtfMRI can be used as an independent variable to observe its effects on behavior. fMRI−BCI has enabled anatomically specific control of subcortical and cortical areas (some of them not accessible to electrophysiological methods), such as amygdala, insular regions, cingulate regions, and sensorimotor cortex. Encouraged by the behavioral modifications following self-regulation training, there have been several new attempts to apply this methodology to neuropsychiatric disorders.

The above studies and novel developments of BCI methodology can open up opportunities for studies in psychiatric populations and possible future therapeutic applications. However, before the full clinical application of fMRI−BCI, some important aspects have to be addressed and explored by further studies. fMRI−BCI is an expensive and difficult to implement technology. Furthermore, to date none of the mentioned studies has convincingly shown that self-regulation can be generalized "out of the scanner setting", without the help of on-going contingent feedback. Whether the behavioral changes produced by fMRI−BCI are more than a short-term effect has yet to be explored.

Finally, these findings have opened a fundamental question, that is, "How does learned regulation of the BOLD signal in the brain influence behavior?" A clearer understanding of the neural mechanisms underlying the BOLD response perhaps will lead us to answer this question. Perhaps fMRI—BCI will, itself, be employed to help understand the relationships between neural activity, the BOLD response, and behavior.

REFERENCES

Andersson, J. L., Hutton, C., Ashburner, J., Turner, R., & Friston, K. J. (2001). Modeling geometric deformations in EPI time series. *Neuroimage, 13*(5), 903—919.

Augustine, J. R. (1996). Circuitry and functional aspects of the insular lobe in primates including humans. *Brain Research Brain Research Reviews, 22*, 229—244.

Bagarinao, E., Matsuo, K., Nakai, T., & Sato, S. (2003). Estimation of general linear model coefficients for real-time application. *Neuroimage, 19*(2 Pt 1), 422—429.

Bandettini, P. A., Wong, E. C., Hinks, R. S., et al. (1992). Time course EPI of human brain function during task activation. *Magnetic Resonance in Medicine, 25*(2), 390—397.

Birbaumer, N. (2006). Breaking the silence: Brain—computer interfaces (BCI) for communication and motor control. *Psychophysiology, 43*, 517—532.

Birbaumer, N., Veit, R., Lotze, M., Erb, M., Hermann, C., Grodd, W., et al. (2005). Deficient fear conditioning in psychopathy: A functional magnetic resonance imaging study. *Archives of General Psychiatry, 62*, 799—805.

Brown, M. A., & Semelka, R. C. (1999). *MRI basic principles and applications.* Hoboken, NJ: Wiley—Blackwell.

Buchanan, T. W. (2007). Retrieval of emotional memories. *Psychology Bulletin, 133*, 761—779.

Bush, G., Luu, P., & Posner, M. I. (2000). Cognitive and emotional influences in anterior cingulate cortex. *Trends in Cognitive Sciences, 4*, 215—222.

Buxton, R. B., Uludağ, K., Dubowitz, D. J., & Liu, T. T. (2004). Modeling the hemodynamic response to brain activation. *Neuroimage, 23*(Suppl 1), S220—S233.

Caria, A., Sitaram, R., Veit, R., Begliomini, C., & Birbaumer, N. (2010). Volitional control of anterior insula activity modulates the response to aversive stimuli: A real-time functional magnetic resonance imaging study. *Biological Psychiatry,* June 4. Epub ahead of print.

Caria, A., Veit, R., Sitaram, R., Lotze, M., Weiskopf, N., Grodd, W., et al. (2007). Regulation of anterior insular cortex activity using real-time fMRI. *Neuroimage, 35*, 1238—1246.

Cox, D. D., & Savoy, R. L. (2003). Functional magnetic resonance imaging (fMRI) brain reading: Detecting and classifying distributed patterns of fMRI activity in human visual cortex. *Neuroimage, 19*(2 Pt 1), 261—270.

Cox, R. W., & Jesmanowicz, A. (1999). Real-time 3D image registration for functional MRI. *Magnetic Resonance in Medicine, 42*(6), 1014—1018.

Cox, R. W., Jesmanowicz, A., & Hyde, J. S. (1995). Real-time functional magnetic resonance imaging. *Magnetic Resonance in Medicine, 33*(2), 230—236.

Craig, A. D. (2009). How do you feel — now? The anterior insula and human awareness. *Nature Reviews Neuroscience, 10*, 59—70.

deCharms, R. C., Christoff, K., Glover, G. H., Pauly, J. M., Whitfield, S., & Gabrieli, J. D. (2004). Learned regulation of spatially localized brain activation using real-time fMRI. *Neuroimage, 21*, 436—443.

deCharms, R. C., Maeda, F., Glover, G. H., Ludlow, D., Pauly, J. M., Soneji, D., et al. (2005). Control over brain activation and pain learned by using real-time functional MRI. *Proceedings of the National Academy of Sciences of the U S A*, *102*, 18 626–18 631.

Eggermont, J. J. (2005). Tinnitus: Neurobiological substrates. *Drug Discovery Today*, *10*, 1283–1290.

Friston, K. J., Buechel, C., Fink, G. R., Morris, J., Rolls, E., & Dolan, R. J. (1997). Psychophysiological and modulatory interactions in neuroimaging. *Neuroimage*, *6*, 218–229.

Fuchs, T., Birbaumer, N., Lutzenberger, W., Gruzelier, J. H., & Kaiser, J. (2003). Neurofeedback treatment for attention-deficit/hyperactivity disorder in children: A comparison with methylphenidate. *Applied Psychophysiology and Biofeedback*, *28*, 1–12.

Gao, K., & Posse, S. (2003). TurboFIRE: Real-time fMRI with automated spatial normalization and Talairach Daemon database [Abstract]. 9th Annual Meeting of the OHBM, New York, USA.

Gembris, D., Taylor, J. G., Schor, S., Frings, W., Suter, D., & Posse, S. (2000). Functional magnetic resonance imaging in real-time (FIRE), sliding-window correlation analysis and reference-vector optimization. *Magnetic Resonance in Medicine*, *43* (2), 259–268.

Grezes, J., & Decety, J. (2001). Functional anatomy of execution, mental simulation, observation, and verb generation of actions: A meta-analysis. *Human Brain Mapping*, *12*, 1–19.

Haller, S., Birbaumer, N., & Veit, R. (2010). Real-time fMRI feedback training may improve chronic tinnitus. *European Radiology*, *20*, 696–703.

Hajnal, J. V., Myers, R., Oatridge, A., Schwieso, J. E., Young, I. R., & Bydder, G. M. (1994). Artifacts due to stimulus correlated motion in functional imaging of the brain. *Magnetic Resonance in Medicine*, *31*(3), 283–291.

Hamilton, P., Glover, G. H., Hsu, J., & Johnson, R. (2010). Modulation of subgenual anterior congulate cortex activity with real-time neurofeedback. *Human Brain Mapping*, May 10. Online publication.

Harrison, S. A., & Tong, F. (2009). Decoding reveals the contents of visual working memory in early visual areas. *Nature*, *458*(7238), 632–635.

Haynes, J. D., & Rees, G. (2006). Decoding mental states from brain activity in humans. *Nature Reviews Neuroscience*, *7*(7), 523–534.

Haynes, J. D., Sakai, K., Rees, G., Gilbert, S., Frith, C., & Passingham, R. E. (2007). Reading hidden intentions in the human brain. *Current Biology*, *17*(4), 323–328.

Jezzard, P., & Balaban, R. S. (1995). Correction for geometric distortion in echo planar images from B0 field variations. *Magnetic Resonance in Medicine*, *34*(1), 65–73.

Kamitani, Y., & Tong, F. (2005). Decoding the visual and subjective contents of the human brain. *Nature Neuroscience*, *8*(5), 679–685.

Kleinjung, T., Eichhammer, P., Langguth, B., Jacob, P., Marienhagen, J., Hajak, G., et al. (2005). Long-term effects of repetitive transcranial magnetic stimulation (rTMS) in patients with chronic tinnitus. *Otolaryngology Head and Neck Surgery*, *132*, 566–569.

Kotchoubey, B., Strehl, U., Uhlmann, C., Holzapfel, S., Konig, M., Froscher, W., et al. (2001). Modification of slow cortical potentials in patients with refractory epilepsy: A controlled outcome study. *Epilepsia*, *42*, 406–416.

Kubler, A., Kotchoubey, B., Kaiser, J., Wolpaw, J. R., & Birbaumer, N. (2001). Brain–computer communication: Unlocking the locked in. *Psychology Bulletin*, *127*, 358–375.

Kybic, J., Thevenaz, P., Nirkko, A., & Unser, M. (2000). Unwarping of unidirectionally distorted EPI images. *IEEE Transactions on Medical Imaging*, *19*(2), 80–93.

LaConte, S. M., Peltier, S. J., & Maciuba, A. (2007). Real-time fMRI using brain-state classification. *Human Brain Mapping, 28*(10), 1033–1044.

Lang, P. J. (Ed.), (1980). Behavior treatment and bio-behavioral assessment: Computer applications. *Technology in Mental Health Care Delivery Systems.* Norwood, NJ: Ablex.

Lang, P. J., Bradley, M. M., & Cuthbert, B. N. (Eds.), (1997). *International Affective Picture System (IAPS): Technical manual and effective ratings.* The Center for Research in Psychophysiology. Gainesville, FL: University of Florida.

Lawrie, S. M., Whalley, H. C., Job, D. E., & Johnstone, E. C. (2003). Structural and functional abnormalities of the amygdala in schizophrenia. *Annals of the New York Academy of Sciences, 985*, 445–460.

Lee, S., Halder, S., et al. (2010). Effective functional mapping of fMRI data with support-vector machines. *Human Brain Mapping,* [Epub ahead of print].

Lee, J. H., Ryu, J., Jolesz, F. A., Cho, Z. H., & Yoo, S. S. (2009). Brain-machine interface via real-time fMRI: Preliminary study on thought-controlled robotic arm. *Neuroscience Letters, 450*, 1–6.

Lee, S., Sitaram, R., Ruiz, S., & Birbaumer, N. (2008). Measure of neurofeedback effects in an fMRI Brain–Computer Interface with support vector machine and Granger causality model. Xth International Conference on Cognitive Neuroscience, Bodrum, Turkey.

Logothetis, N. K. (2008). What we can do and what we cannot do with fMRI (Review). *Nature, 453*, 869–878.

Lozano, A. M., Mayberg, H. S., Giacobbe, P., Hamani, C., Craddock, R. C., & Kennedy, S. H. (2008). Subcallosal cingulate gyrus deep brain stimulation for treatment-resistant depression. *Biological Psychiatry, 64*, 461–467.

Mackey, S. C., & Maeda, F. (2004). Functional imaging and the neural systems of chronic pain. *Neurosurgery Clinics of North America, 15*, 269–288.

Mathiak, K., & Posse, S. (2001). Evaluation of motion and realignment for functional magnetic resonance imaging in real time. *Magnetic Resonance Medicine, 45*(1), 167–171.

Mayberg, H. S., Lozano, A. M., Voon, V., McNeely, H. E., Seminowicz, D., Hamani, C., et al. (2005). Deep brain stimulation for treatment-resistant depression. *Neuron, 45*, 651–660.

Mitchell, T. M., Hutchinson, R., et al. (2003). Classifying instantaneous cognitive states from FMRI data. *AMIA Annual Symposium Proceedings*: 465–9.

Murase, N., Duque, J., Mazzocchio, R., & Cohen, L. G. (2004). Influence of interhemispheric interactions on motor function in chronic stroke. *Annals of Neurology, 55*, 400–409.

Nagai, M., Kishi, K., & Kato, S. (2007). Insular cortex and neuropsychiatric disorders: A review of recent literature. *European Psychiatry, 22*, 387–394.

Naqvi, N. H., & Bechara, A. (2009). The hidden island of addiction: The insula. *Trends in Neuroscience, 32*, 56–67.

Panych, L. P., & Jolesz, F. A. (1994). A dynamically adaptive imaging algorithm for wavelet-encoded MRI. *Magnetic Resonance in Medicine, 32*(6), 738–748.

Pause, B. M., Jungbluth, C., Adolph, D., Pietrowsky, R., & Dere, E. (2010). Induction and measurement of episodic memories in healthy adults. *Journal of Neuroscientific Methods, 189*(1), 88–96.

Petrovic, P., & Ingvar, M. (2002). Imaging cognitive modulation of pain processing. *Pain, 95*, 1–5.

Pollock, D. S. G., Green, R. C., & Nguyen, T. (1999). *Handbook of Time Series Analysis, Signal Processing, and Dynamics.* San Diego, CA: Academic Press.

Posse, S., Binkofski, F., Schneider, F., Gembris, D., Frings, W., et al. (2001). A new approach to measure single-event related brain activity using real-time fMRI:

Feasibility of sensory, motor, and higher cognitive tasks. *Human Brain Mapping*, *12*(1), 25−41.

Posse, S., Fitzgerald, D., Gao, K., Habel, U., Rosenberg, D., Moore, G. J., et al. (2003). Real-time fMRI of temporolimbic regions detects amygdala activation during single-trial self-induced sadness. *Neuroimage*, *18*(3), 760−768.

Posse, S., Wiese, S., Gembris, D., Mathiak, K., Kessler, C., Grosse-Ruyken, B., et al. (1999). Enhancement of BOLD-contrast sensitivity by single-shot multi-echo functional MR imaging. *Magnetic Resonance in Medicine*, *42*(1), 87−97.

Rota, G., Sitaram, R., Veit, R., Erb, M., Weiskopf, N., Dogil, G., et al. (2009). Self-regulation of regional cortical activity using real-time fMRI: The right inferior frontal gyrus and linguistic processing. *Human Brain Mapping*, *30*, 1605−1614.

Ruiz, S., Sitaram, R., Sangyun, L., Caria, A., Soekadar, S., Veit, R., et al. (2008). Learned control of insular activity and functional connectivity changes using a fMRI Brain Computer Interface in Schizophrenia. 38th annual meeting of the Society for Neuroscience. Washington. *Schizophrenia Research* 102/1-3, 92 [full print version in press].

Seth, A. K. (2009). A MATLAB toolbox for Granger causal connectivity analysis. *Journal of Neuroscience Methods*, *186*(2), 262−273.

Sitaram, R., Lee, S., et al. (2010). Real-time support vector classification and feedback of multiple emotional brain states. *Neuroimage*, in press.

Skinner, B. F. (1938). *The behavior of organisms: An experimental analysis*. New York: Appleton-Century-Crofts.

Smyser, C., Grabowski, T. J., Frank, R. J., Haller, J. W., & Bolinger, L. (2001). Real-time multiple linear regression for fMRI supported by time-aware acquisition and processing. *Magnetic Resonance in Medicine*, *45*(2), 289−298.

Strehl, U., Leins, U., Goth, G., Klinger, C., Hinterberger, T., & Birbaumer, N. (2006). Self-regulation of slow cortical potentials: A new treatment for children with attention-deficit/hyperactivity disorder. *Pediatrics*, *118*, e1530−1540.

Studholme, C., Constable, R. T., & Duncan, J. S. (2000). Accurate alignment of functional EPI data to anatomical MRI using a physics-based distortion model. *IEEE Transactions on Medical Imaging*, *19*(11), 1115−1127.

Ture, U., Yasargil, D. C., Al-Mefty, O., & Yasargil, M. G. (1999). Topographic anatomy of the insular region. *Journal of Neurosurgery*, *90*, 720−733.

Veit, R., Flor, H., Erb, M., Hermann, C., Lotze, M., Grodd, W., et al. (2002). Brain circuits involved in emotional learning in antisocial behavior and social phobia in humans. *Neuroscience Letters*, *328*, 233−236.

Voyvodic, J. T. (1999). Real-time fMRI paradigm control, physiology, and behavior combined with near real-time statistical analysis. *Neuroimage*, *10*(2), 91−106.

Wager, T. D., Rilling, J. K., Smith, E. E., Sokolik, A., Casey, K. L., Davidson, R. J., et al. (2004). Placebo-induced changes in FMRI in the anticipation and experience of pain. *Science*, *303*, 1162−1167.

Weiskopf, N., Klose, U., Birbaumer, N., & Mathiak, K. (2005). Single-shot compensation of image distortions and BOLD contrast optimization using multi-echo EPI for real-time fMRI. *Neuroimage*, *24*(4), 1068−1079.

Weiskopf, N., Mathiak, K., Bock, S. W., Scharnowski, F., Veit, R., Grodd, W., et al. (2004). Principles of a brain-computer interface (BCI) based on real-time functional magnetic resonance imaging (fMRI). *IEEE Transactions on Biomedical Engineering*, *51*(6), 966−970.

Weiskopf, N., Scharnowski, F., Veit, R., Goebel, R., & Birbaumer, N. (2004). Self-regulation of local brain activity using real-time functional magnetic resonance imaging (fMRI). *Journal of Physiology Paris*, *98*(4-6), 357−373.

Weiskopf, N., Veit, R., Erb, M., Mathiak, K., Grodd, W., & Goebel, R. (2003). Physiological self-regulation of regional brain activity using real-time functional magnetic resonance imaging (fMRI), methodology and exemplary data. *Neuroimage, 19,* 577–586.

Yoo, S. S., Fairneny, T., Chen, N. K., Choo, S. E., Panych, L. P., Park, H., et al. (2004). Brain-computer interface using fMRI: Spatial navigation by thoughts. *Neuroreport, 15,* 1591–1595.

Yoo, S. S., Guttmann, C. R., Zhao, L., & Panych, L. P. (1999). Real-time adaptive functional MRI. *Neuroimage, 10*(5), 596–606.

Yoo, S. S., & Jolesz, F. A. (2002). Functional MRI for neurofeedback: Feasibility study on a hand motor task. *Neuroreport, 13,* 1377–1381.

Yoo, S. S., O'Leary, H. M., Fairneny, T., Chen, N. K., Panych, L. P., Park, H., et al. (2006). Increasing cortical activity in auditory areas through neurofeedback functional magnetic resonance imaging. *Neuroreport, 17,* 1273–1278.

Zaitsev, M., Hennig, J., Speck, O., et al. (2004). Point spread function mapping with parallel imaging techniques and high acceleration factors: Fast, robust, and flexible method for echo-planar imaging distortion correction. *Magnetic Resonance in Medicine, 52*(5), 1156–1166.

PART Three

Exogenous Neuromodulation Strategies

CHAPTER *10*

Repetitive Transcranial Magnetic Stimulation in Depression: Protocols, Mechanisms, and New Developments

Desirée Spronk[1], Martijn Arns[1,2], and Paul B. Fitzgerald[3]
[1]Research Institute Brainclinics, Nijmegen, The Netherlands
[2]Utrecht University, Department of Experimental Psychology, Utrecht, The Netherlands
[3]Monash Alfred Psychiatry Research Center (MAPrc), The Alfred and Monash University, School of Psychology and Psychiatry, Melbourne, Victoria, Australia

Contents

INTRODUCTION

TMS (transcranial magnetic stimulation) is a non-invasive neuromodulation technique. Nevertheless, it has a very direct influence on brain physiology. The basic principle of TMS is the application of short magnetic pulses over the scalp of a subject with the aim of inducing electrical currents in the neurons of the cortex. A typical TMS device consists of a stimulator that can

Neurofeedback and Neuromodulation Techniques and Applications
DOI: 10.1016/B978-0-12-382235-2.00010-X

257

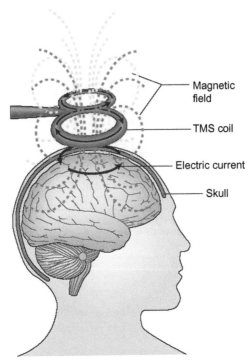

Figure 10.1 Visual illustration of the induction of electrical currents in the brain through the magnetic pulses (dashed lines) applied by means of the coil (8-shaped figure) positioned above the head. *(Adapted from Ridding and Rothwell, 2007.)*

generate a strong electrical current, and a coil in which the fluctuating electrical current generates magnetic pulses. If the magnetic pulses are delivered in the proximity of a conductive medium, e.g. the brain, a secondary current in the conductive material (e.g., neurons) is induced (Figure 10.1). In the practice of TMS, a subject is seated in a chair and an operator positions the coil above the scalp of the subject, tunes the stimulation parameters of the stimulator, and applies the TMS pulses.

Anthony Barker and his colleagues at the University of Sheffield were the first to develop a TMS device, introducing a new neuromodulatory technique in neuroscience. The first application, demonstrated first by these researchers, was the induction of a motor evoked potential (e.g., activating the muscles abducting the thumb) by means of applying a TMS pulse over the motor cortex (Barker, Jalinous, & Freeston, 1985).

Initially, TMS was used mainly in studies on motor conductivity through investigating the temporal aspects and amplitude of the evoked motor responses after stimulating the motor cortex. Continuing progress on the technical aspects of TMS devices soon made it possible to deliver *multiple* pulses within a short time period, i.e., repetitive TMS (rTMS). With the development of rTMS, researchers were able to induce changes that outlasted the stimulation period (Pascual-Leone et al., 1999). This has led to a considerable extension of the possible applications of TMS. Currently, rTMS is used for an increasing variety of applications such as the study of pathophysiology of diseases, the investigation of the contribution of certain brain regions to particular cognitive functions and, most relevant for this chapter, the treatment of psychiatric diseases.

The potential of repetitive TMS in the treatment of psychiatric disorders was suggested for the first time relatively soon after the development of the first TMS device in 1985. In a study on motor conductivity, changes in mood in several normal volunteers who received single pulses over the motor cortex were described (Bickford, Guidi, Fortesque, & Swenson, 1987). Following this initial observation, the technical progress and the increasing availability of TMS devices has led to the opportune investigation of rTMS in the treatment of depression. Apart from being the *first* investigated psychiatric application, it is also the *most* investigated psychiatric application in many centers all around the world. In addition, a TMS device has been approved by the FDA in late 2008, and a growing number of private outpatient as well as hospitalized patients with depression are treated in clinical settings (approximately 150 US centers in the middle of 2010).

Major depression is a common disorder, with millions of sufferers around the world and a lifetime prevalence of about 13% in men and 21% in women (Blazer et al., 1994). The World Health Organization has predicted that depression will globally become the second largest burden of disease by 2020, following cardiovascular conditions (Murray & Lopez, 1997). Individuals with depression experience a wide range of symptoms, including a loss of interest or pleasure, feelings of sadness, guilt, low self-esteem, disturbances in sleep and appetite, poor concentration and suicidal ideations (DSM-IV, American Psychiatric Association, 1994). It is obvious that major depression has a disabling effect on daily activity, indicating that effective treatment is crucial. Treatment with antidepressant medication is the most common and first line treatment for many individuals. However, a significant percentage of patients do not sufficiently respond to antidepressant medication (Keller et al., 2000; Kirsch et al., 2008; Rush et al., 2006) and some of the patients proceed to electroconvulsive therapy (ECT). Despite some remarkable clinical results (Husain et al., 2004), ECT is a controversial and unpopular treatment option due to the required induction of a seizure and associated side-effects such as memory loss (Robertson & Pryor, 2006). Following initial positive results with depression, and due to its painless and non-invasive administration, rTMS has been proposed as a "better" alternative to ECT (Paus & Barrett, 2004) or as an alternative for patients who may not be willing to undergo ECT, or for whom ECT may not be suitable. In order to compare efficacy of these treatments, rTMS and ECT have been jointly investigated in several studies (Eranti et al., 2007; Rosa et al., 2006). Of the several studies performed, Eranti et al., (2007) observed a great advantage for ECT. However, others (Grunhaus et al., 2003; Pridmore et al., 2000; Rosa et al., 2006) found comparable efficacy rates for ECT and rTMS in the treatment of depression. Notably, studies that have reported an advantage of ECT have compared an unlimited number of usually flexibly administered (unilateral or bilateral) ECT treatments to a fixed number of only one type of rTMS, potentially biasing the results of these studies. In addition, Eranti et al. (2007) included patients with psychotic depression whereas the other studies only involved non-psychotic depression (Grunhaus et al., 2003; Pridmore et al., 2000; Rosa et al., 2006), suggesting that rTMS might not be the best treatment option for the treatment of depression with psychotic features.

The early reports of rTMS as an antidepressant treatment modality consisted of pilot studies with a small number of subjects. In these early studies arbitrary stimulation parameters over various and non-specific brain regions were applied (Höflich et al., 1993; Kolbinger et al., 1995). A report by George et al. (1995) showed robust improvements in depressive symptoms in two out of six patients. This study marked the start of the serious pursuit of rTMS as a potential treatment option for depressed patients. Subsequently, a reasonably large number of open-label as well as randomized sham-controlled studies were performed. Most studies found a moderately favorable treatment effect for rTMS using various designs (Avery et al., 2006; Fitzgerald, Huntsman, Gunewardene, Kulkarni, & Daskalakis, 2006; Fitzgerald et al., 2003; George et al., 2010; Mogg et al., 2008; O'Reardon et al., 2007; Padberg et al., 1999; Rossini et al., 2005), which has recently been confirmed by several meta-analyses (Schutter, 2009; Schutter, 2010). However, some researchers could not replicate these findings and found no differences between sham and active treatment conditions (Loo et al., 2003; Nahas, Kozel, Li, Anderson, & George, 2003).

After 15 years of research, the general consensus is that rTMS treatment in depression *has* potential, but has not yet fully lived up to initial expectations. In large part this is due to limited understanding of the mechanisms underlying the clinical treatment effect. A substantial research effort, already in progress, may elucidate the mechanisms of the beneficial effects of rTMS in depressed patients. Hopefully, results of this effort will lead to continued improvements in treatment protocols, and provide patients with the best possible treatment of their depression.

In this chapter, a comprehensive overview of rTMS in the treatment of depression will be provided. In the first section various rTMS protocols will be reviewed in terms of the different stimulation parameters that are of interest. Subsequently, some potential physiological mechanisms that are associated with antidepressant outcome will be reviewed. In regard to this, we present an overview of rTMS-induced effects found in imaging studies, pharmacological studies, and genetic studies. Finally, we will address new developments in the field.

PROTOCOLS

The behavioral effects of rTMS have been found to depend on the frequency, intensity, and duration of stimulation (e.g. Avery et al., 2006; Fitzgerald et al., 2006b; O'Reardon et al., 2007; Padberg et al., 2002). The most important parameters that rTMS protocols in depression can be distinguished on are the stimulation frequency and the stimulation location. These will be discussed at length by reviewing literature that used diverse choices for these parameters. Some other relevant parameters (intensity, number of trains, inter-train interval, and number of sessions) will be briefly described. In Figure 10.2, some of the characteristics of an rTMS stimulation protocol are illustrated.

Progress in the development of technical aspects of TMS devices and advancing insights have led to a continuing progression of experimental and innovative protocols. Some more recently developed protocols investigated in the treatment of depression, such as theta burst stimulation and deep TMS stimulation, are discussed in the section "New Developments".

Stimulation Frequency

The stimulation frequency refers to the number of pulses delivered per second, as can be programmed on the TMS device. Examination of these rTMS studies in depression reveals that, at first glance, two types of studies

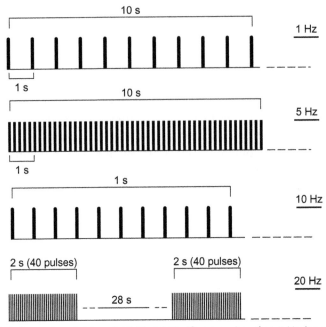

Figure 10.2 Examples of 10 s of rTMS at 1 Hz (first trace) and at 5 Hz (second trace); 1 s of rTMS at 10 Hz and an example of 20 Hz application (trains of 2 s interleaved by a pause of 28 s). *(Adapted from Rossi, Hallett, Rossini, Pascual-Leone, & The Safety of TMS Consensus Group, 2009.)*

can be discerned: studies performing high-frequency (also referred to as fast) rTMS (HF–rTMS) and studies in which low frequency (also referred to as slow) rTMS (LF–rTMS) parameters are applied. HF–rTMS usually includes frequency parameters of 5 Hz or above, whilst LF–rTMS incorporates stimulation frequencies of 1 Hz or below. HF–rTMS is usually applied over the left prefrontal cortex, whilst LF–rTMS is mostly applied over the right prefrontal cortex (see "Stimulation Location" below for a more elaborate review). In addition to studies applying solely HF–rTMS or LF–rTMS, combined approaches have been proposed.

High-Frequency rTMS

Most rTMS studies in depression to date have been performed by means of applying high-frequency stimulation (Avery et al., 2006; George et al., 2010; O'Reardon et al., 2007). HF–rTMS protocols have mostly used stimulation frequencies of 10 Hz (but this has varied from 5 to 20 Hz).

In the largest study to date, O'Reardon et al. (2007) reported significantly better clinical results in an active rTMS group in comparison to the sham group, as measured by the Hamilton Rating Scale for Depression (HAM-D) and the Montgomery Asberg Depression Rating Scale (MADRS). This was a randomized study in which 301 medication-free patients were treated with 10 Hz stimulation frequency. In a recent non-industry sponsored trial, George and colleagues (2010) demonstrated that 10 Hz HF-rTMS yielded a remission rate of 14% in the active group as compared to 5% in the sham. The total number of intention-to-treat patients was 190, a group that was characterized by a highly treatment-resistant depression. Apart from these large multi-center studies, numerous single site studies applying stimulation frequencies of 10 Hz have been performed. These have showed response (more than 50% decrease on the depression scale) rates between 30 and 50% (Avery et al., 2006; Garcia-Toro et al., 2001; George et al., 2010; Mogg et al., 2008; O'Reardon et al., 2007; Padberg et al., 1999; Rossini et al., 2005). Most of these studies have been performed in treatment-resistant patients. A few trials that have applied frequencies of 5, 17, or 20 Hz have been reported (Fitzgerald et al., 2006b; Luborzewski et al., 2007). In Fitzgerald's study (Fitzgerald et al., 2006b), patients who did not respond to a protocol with frequencies of 1 or 2 Hz (LF-rTMS see below) were assigned to either 5 Hz or 10 Hz HF-rTMS protocol. No significant differences in response to 5 or 10 Hz were shown. In addition, Luborzewski and colleagues (2007) have shown beneficial treatment effects in patients who had received 10 sessions of 20 Hz rTMS. Due to the limited number of studies no definitive conclusions can be drawn, but results suggest that 5, 17 or 20 Hz stimulation frequencies do at least have antidepressant effects. However, some reports have shown differential effects of different stimulation parameters, including a report of 9 Hz rTMS tending to be less beneficial than 10 Hz (Arns, Spronk, & Fitzgerald, 2010). To summarize, it is not yet known which exact frequencies appear to be the most beneficial in HF-rTMS, but 10 Hz rTMS has been investigated best and is often used.

Low-Frequency rTMS

In addition to the HF-rTMS studies in the treatment of depression, several LF-rTMS studies have been performed (Fitzgerald et al., 2003; Januel et al., 2006; Klein et al., 1999). For example, Klein et al. (1999) showed in a large sham-controlled study that 1 Hz rTMS, in which 70 patients were randomly assigned to sham or active treatment, yielded a response rate of 49% in the active treatment as compared to 25% in the sham. This study also showed a significant larger improvement in depression scores in the active as compared to the sham group. In the largest controlled study on LF-rTMS in depression, 130 patients were initially assigned to a stimulation protocol of either 1 or 2 Hz (Fitzgerald et al., 2006b). Of the 130 patients enrolled, approximately 51% could be classified as responders after 10 days of treatment. Interestingly the response rates between the 1 Hz and 2 Hz did not significantly differ. Although LF-rTMS is a more recently developed protocol and is less well studied, it appears to have beneficial effects comparable to HF-rTMS.

In order to systematically investigate if HF or LF-rTMS is more beneficial, protocols were directly compared (Fitzgerald et al., 2003; Fitzgerald, Hoy, Daskalakis, & Kulkarni, 2009; Isenberg et al., 2005). In a double-blind, randomized, sham-controlled study, 60 treatment-resistant patients were allocated into three groups; one received HF-rTMS trains to the left prefrontal cortex at 10 Hz, the second group received LF-rTMS trains at 1 Hz to the right prefrontal cortex and the third group received sham treatment. The clinical results showed that the groups treated with HF-rTMS and LF-rTMS had a similar reduction in depressive symptoms, and for both groups, treatment response was better than within the sham group (Fitzgerald et al., 2003). In another study with a similar aim, 27 subjects were assigned to either HF-rTMS (10Hz) or LF-rTMS (1Hz) rTMS. It was concluded that both treatment modalities appeared to be equally efficacious (Fitzgerald et al., 2009a). Schutter (2010), based on a meta-analysis of all randomized controlled LF-rTMS studies in depression, suggested that LF-rTMS might even be more beneficial than HF-rTMS. However, direct comparisons of the effect sizes of HF and LF-rTMS did not show a statistically significant difference. More research with larger samples is required to confirm these findings and demonstrate if LF-rTMS and HF-rTMS are similarly efficacious, or if LF-rTMS is more efficacious than HF-rTMS. Aside from the comparison of clinical effects, it appears that LF-rTMS is better tolerated, i.e., patients reported less headaches. It may also minimize the risk of inducing adverse events like seizures (Schutter, 2010).

Although the vast majority of studies have focused on low-frequency stimulation applied to the right and high-frequency stimulation applied to the left prefrontal cortex, it is to be noted that in a few studies parameters have varied from these traditional sites. Some have suggested that low frequency stimulation applied to the left may also have antidepressant effects, thus questioning the traditional model of laterality in depression.

Combined HF and LF-rTMS protocols

These aforementioned studies demonstrate evidence that active HF-rTMS and LF-rTMS are more effective in the treatment of depression as compared to sham. However, HF-rTMS and LF-rTMS are not necessarily incompatible with each other. In recent years, add-on, bilateral-sequential, and priming protocols have been postulated and investigated.

Add-on protocols concern the combination of one protocol with another protocol, e.g., when patients do not respond to LF-rTMS after several sessions, they can proceed to HF-rTMS treatment. In the aforementioned study by Fitzgerald et al. (2006b) in which LF-rTMS was investigated, non-responders to the low frequency protocol subsequently were treated with HF-rTMS. A subset of these LF-rTMS non-responders did respond to HF-rTMS. Hence, it is likely that different protocols act through different mechanisms and that different patient groups are susceptible to different approaches. It could also be argued that subjects in the add-on protocol received more sessions, and possibly needed longer to respond to treatment. Thus, the full extent of the increase in response rate might not solely be attributable to the change in stimulation frequency.

A second variant is the sequential stimulation protocol in which within one session both HF-rTMS and LF-rTMS are applied. This protocol was examined in a double-blind study that included 50 patients with depression. Half of the group received 1 Hz rTMS over the right prefrontal cortex, followed by HF-rTMS over the left prefrontal cortex in the same session, for a period of 4−6 weeks. The other half of the patients received sham stimulation in the same protocol. The higher response rates in the treatment group (44% vs. 8% in sham) suggested that a within-session LF/HF combination protocol might be more effective than applying either protocol alone (Fitzgerald et al., 2006a). However, this hypothesis could not be confirmed by a recent study by Pallanti et al. (2010) in which a sequential combination protocol was compared with unilateral LF-rTMS and sham. Of the three groups, patients who were treated with the unilateral LF-rTMS protocol benefited most from treatment. The authors propose that these results, in contrast to the findings of Fitzgerald et al. (2006a), suggest that a "simple" unilateral protocol is the first treatment of choice. Nevertheless, the authors believe that it remains relevant to further explore combination protocols and compare them to traditional unilateral protocols.

A third option is the unilateral combination of high and low frequency stimulation in a protocol referred to as "priming" stimulation. This involves the application of low intensity high-frequency trains (usually 6 Hz) followed by standard low frequency stimulation. Basic neurophysiological studies have shown that priming stimulation results in greater suppression of cortical excitability than low-frequency stimulation applied alone (Iyer, Schleper, & Wassermann, 2003). A single clinical study has compared such priming stimulation to 1 Hz TMS (both applied to the right side) and shown a greater clinical effect in the priming group compared to the sham group (Fitzgerald et al., 2008).

Stimulation Location

The dorsolateral prefrontal cortex (DLPFC) has been the primary area of interest for stimulation (see Figure 10.3). The motivation behind choosing this brain area stems from various imaging studies that indicated depression is associated with regional brain dysfunction in, among other regions, the DLPFC (Cummings, 1993). Other researchers have not only proposed an "underactivated" L-DLPFC, but suggested an imbalance between frontal regions. For example, the "frontal asymmetry hypothesis" of depression states that in depression there is an imbalance in left vs. right frontal brain activation (Henriques & Davidson, 1990; but also see Chapter 4 in this volume). In addition, of all brain regions known to be related to the pathophysiology of depression (e.g., prefrontal, cingulate, parietal, and temporal cortical regions, as well as parts of the striatum, thalamus, and hypothalamus) the DLPFC is regarded as most accessible for treatment with rTMS (Wassermann & Lisanby, 2001). On the basis of such previous theories and

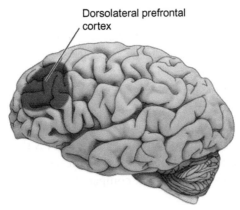

Figure 10.3 Image of the location of the (left) dorsolateral prefrontal cortex in the brain.

findings, the supposedly activating/HF-rTMS protocols are applied over the left DLPFC and supposedly inhibiting/LF-rTMS protocols are applied over the right DLPFC. The choice of the stimulation frequency is thus closely linked to the stimulation location.

In most studies, localizing the DLPFC has been performed by means of the "5 cm rule". The hand area of the primary motor cortex (M1) (which elicits a contralateral motor response of the thumb when stimulated), is taken as the detectable reference point. From there, the coil is moved 5 cm anteriorly, in a sagittal direction. Positioning the coil at that location during treatment is assumed to target the DLPFC. It can be argued that this literal "rule of thumb" has some flaws and may result in inconsistent results between sessions within subjects. Moreover, it may not target the DLPFC at all due to differences in head size and shape across individuals and — even more relevant — in the folding patterns of the cortex. In order to solve this problem, technical advances have enabled structural MRI-based neuronavigation systems. In neuronavigation, an MRI of a patient's brain is acquired before treatment. A series of software co-registrations are made between real anatomical points on the head (which are fixed in location) and the corresponding anatomical points in a three-dimensional reconstruction of the patient's MRI scan. This allows one to establish the scalp point that corresponds to a location on the brain scan that becomes the proposed target for TMS treatment. A more complicated process can also allow the position and orientation of the coil relative to the corresponding brain region to be monitored in real time. In a study by Herwig et al. (2001) the reliability of the "5 cm rule" was investigated by means of comparing the target area defined by the "5 cm rule" with the target defined by DLPFC neuronavigation. Of the total 22 subjects, the targets corresponded in only seven. In a similar study, it was found that the true DLPFC was in general located more anteriorly to the site traditionally identified by the "5 cm rule" (Fitzgerald et al., 2009b).

Together, these studies suggest that clinical efficacy may be improved by means of more precise targeting methods. This has been directly tested in one study with 52 patients who were randomized to stimulation localized by the "5 cm rule" or neuronavigation (Fitzgerald et al., 2009b). Neuronavigationally targeted treatment resulted in a statistically significant greater response in depression scores than treatment targeted by the traditional method.

Despite the fact that the majority of the studies target the DLPFC, some authors have argued that it has never been experimentally proven that the DLPFC is the most effective target for rTMS treatment of depression. In addition, the pathophysiology of depression is certainly not limited to the DLPFC (Drevets, Price, & Furey, 2008). Investigation of antidepressant effects of rTMS applied to other brain regions has therefore been explored (Schutter, Laan, van Honk, Vergouwen, & Koerselman, 2009). Schutter and colleagues (2009) applied 2 Hz rTMS at 90% of the motor threshold (see next section) to the right parietal cortex in a group of patients with depression for a period of 10 sessions. Their findings did not show statistically significant changes between the active and sham group. However, comparison of both groups on a partial response outcome (at least a 30% reduction in HAM-D score) showed a significantly higher response in the active rTMS group as compared to the sham group. This result suggests that targeting the right parietal cortex with 2 Hz rTMS may have antidepressant properties, although the effects were not as strong as compared to frontal HF or LF-rTMS. Although these findings need to be replicated in larger studies, they are encouraging regarding searching for other cortical targets in the treatment of depression with rTMS.

Stimulation Intensity, Trains, and Sessions

For rTMS to be effective, the magnetic field has to induce currents in the neurons of the cortex. The intensity of the magnetic field that induces this current is referred to as the stimulation intensity. This is usually expressed as a percentage of the motor threshold (MT). The MT is usually determined prior to each session by applying the TMS coil over the "thumb" area of the motor cortex. Single pulses are applied by stepwise variation of the output intensity of the device. The minimal output intensity which yields a motor response (moving of the thumb) in at least half of the applied trials is determined to be the MT. So if the intensity of a TMS protocol is 100% MT, then it is the same as the output intensity of the device which was determined to be MT. All other intensity values are reflected as a percentage of this MT, e.g., if the MT is at an output intensity of the device of 60%, then an intensity of 110% MT means that the output intensity is 66%. Although this determination of stimulation intensity may seem arbitrary, it takes individual differences in motor cortex excitability (and therefore excitability of other brain regions) into account. This contributes to a safer administration of TMS pulses to an individual. In depression protocols reported to date, the lowest stimulation intensity used was 80% MT (George et al., 1995) and the maximal intensity used was 120% MT (O'Reardon et al., 2007; Rumi et al., 2005). The majority of the depression protocols use stimulation intensities of 100% MT or 110% MT. In a study by Padberg et al. (2002), in which the relation between treatment efficacy and stimulation intensity was investigated, patients who were treated with a HF-rTMS (10 Hz) protocol at 100% MT showed a 30% decrease in depressive symptoms as measured by the HAM-D, as compared to a 15% decrease for patients who were treated with the same protocol but at 90% MT. This result, among others, suggests more beneficial outcomes for higher stimulation intensities. Therefore, more recent studies have used intensities of 110% and 120% MT (O'Reardon et al., 2007; Rumi et al., 2005), in contrast to earlier research where intensities between 80% and 100% MT were more common (George et al., 1997; Kimbrell et al., 1999).

In most rTMS protocols the stimulation is delivered in pulse trains (see Figure 10.2). That is, pulses are delivered in series separated by certain time intervals — the inter-train interval (ITI). This is done for two reasons. First, the effect of TMS pulses is cumulative in the brain (Hallett, 2007; Ridding & Rothwell, 2007), and this summation causes an increase of the likelihood of the induction of a seizure (the most serious potential side effect associated with rTMS). In several reports, safety guidelines in which maximum recommended values of stimulus parameters like stimulus intensity, train duration, number of trains, and ITI are provided for the safety of the patients (Rossi et al., 2009; Wassermann, 1998). Secondly, the repetitive release of strong electrical pulses causes heating of the electronics of the TMS device. The ITI between trains allows the device to partially cool down. Due to safety reasons for the subject and protection of the device, all devices are manufactured to automatically turn off as soon as a certain heat-limit has been reached. Newer TMS devices are designed with better cooling systems (e.g., air- or fluid-cooled coils), which reduce the likelihood of overheating. However, the overheating of the device is still possible when multiple sessions are performed within a short period, or if a highly demanding (e.g., high rate of pulse delivery) protocol is performed. Train durations in HF-rTMS protocols are usually between 2 and 10 seconds with an ITI between 20 and 60 seconds. In LF-rTMS protocols often continuous stimulation is used.

In studies performed thus far, the number of sessions applied has been highly variable, ranging from five sessions (Manes et al., 2001; Miniussi et al., 2005) to up to or greater than 30 sessions (Fitzgerald et al., 2006b; O'Reardon et al., 2007). However, to date, the majority of studies have involved a total of 10 sessions (for example, Fitzgerald et al., 2003; Garcia-Toro et al., 2001; Koerselman et al., 2004; Poulet et al., 2004). Based on more recent studies, a general trend towards a greater number of sessions (>10) is associated with continuing improvement in depression scores (Fitzgerald et al., 2006b; Rumi et al., 2005). Schutter (2009) suggested that similar to antidepressant medication, rTMS treatment may involve a delayed therapeutic onset. Investigation of the number of sessions optimally required is important for gaining information about the temporal course of the antidepressant effect.

The variety of protocols discussed above indicate that rTMS is an active field of research. Treatment outcome has been shown to vary with protocols, but some protocols have proven their efficacy. However, it has been argued that it is unlikely that the current combinations of stimulation parameters potentiate optimum clinical effects. It is likely that there is much room for improvement, and studies directly addressing the question of optimal stimulation parameters are urgently required. This statement is further supported by the finding that early rTMS depression protocols have shown less favorable results compared to relatively newer, more promising protocols (Gross et al., 2007). Increasing knowledge about the mechanisms underlying treatment efficacy — the topic of the next section — may result in new protocols with closer to optimal treatment effects.

MECHANISMS OF rTMS TREATMENT IN DEPRESSION

With rTMS the goal is to modulate brain activity, with a resultant reduction of depressive symptoms. Although clinical results appear promising, mechanisms explaining the symptomatic reduction are unknown. In order to optimize rTMS for therapeutic use, it is necessary to gain a better understanding of possible neurobiological mechanisms underlying the clinical response. This is currently a topic of active interdisciplinary research.

Knowledge of neurobiological mechanisms to date is derived from neuroimaging studies, studies on neurotransmitter and neuroendocrinologic systems, and from gene expression research. Together, these efforts will hopefully explain the substrate of the antidepressant effects of rTMS. In the following paragraphs, studies in each of the fields mentioned above on rTMS-induced changes will be reviewed. The neurophysiology of rTMS at the neuronal level in general is outside the scope of this review. However, the interested reader is referred to an excellent review by Wassermann and colleagues on this topic (Wassermann et al., 2008).

Neuroimaging

The combination of rTMS with neuroimaging research provides a unique opportunity to elucidate the underlying mechanisms of rTMS in the treatment of depression. Most imaging studies to date have used positron emission tomography (PET) or single-proton emission computed tomography (SPECT) to identify brain regions with altered blood flow or glucose metabolism as a result of rTMS. These modalities have lower temporal resolution compared to functional magnetic resonance imaging (fMRI), and therefore not much is known about the time course of brain activation in response to rTMS. Recently, however, some studies using near-infrared spectroscopy (NIRS) have been performed (Aoyama et al., 2009; Hanaoka, 2007; Kozel et al., 2009).

As discussed in the "Protocols" section, in most depression protocols rTMS is applied over the left or right DLPFC. Several neuroimaging studies have indeed demonstrated rTMS-induced changes within the DLPFC. HF-rTMS over the left DLPFC of depressed patients induces a local increase in regional cerebral blood flow (rCBF) as indicated by SPECT (Catafau et al., 2001; Loo et al., 2003; Kito et al., 2008a; Speer et al., 2000) and fMRI BOLD response (Cardoso et al., 2008). In contrast, imaging studies of LF-rTMS over the right DLPFC showed a local *decrease* in rCBF (Kito, Fujita, & Koga, 2008; Loo et al., 2003; Speer et al., 2000). It should be noted, however, that in an fMRI study Fitzgerald and colleagues (2007) could not replicate the local decrease in BOLD response following LF-rTMS. Instead, a bilateral frontal reduction in BOLD response was observed.

In early studies using PET/SPECT it was shown that changes in brain activation induced by rTMS were not limited to the stimulated area (Paus, Jech, Thompson, Comeau, Peters, & Evans, 1997). A single TMS pulse can lead to effects in more distal brain areas within the same network as the stimulated area (Siebner et al., 2009). In a similar vein, rTMS-induced changes in brain activity in depression may not necessarily be limited to the DLPFC; remote regions are often in good accordance with areas known to be associated with the pathophysiology of depression (reviewed in Fitzgerald et al., 2006c). In support of this theory, imaging studies cited above have also found changes in blood flow in remote/subcortical brain regions following rTMS (Baeken et al., 2009; Loo et al., 2003; Speer et al., 2000). Other brain regions that have been reported to show a change in rCBF after HF-rTMS over the left DLPFC are the ventrolateral prefrontal cortex, right-dominant orbitofrontal cortex, the anterior cingulate, the left subgenual cingulate, the anterior insula, and the right putamen/pallidum (Kito et al., 2008a). Of clinical relevance, it was demonstrated that increases in rCBF in the L–DLPFC are related to significant improvement in clinical outcomes, and that increases in the R–DLPFC and subcortical regions mentioned above are negatively correlated with the change in depressive symptoms (Kito et al., 2008b).

One neuroimaging study has directly compared the effects of high frequency stimulation applied to the left side with low frequency stimulation applied to the right (Fitzgerald et al., 2007). This study, using fMRI recordings during a cognitive task, found that low frequency stimulation produced a bilateral reduction in neural activity whereas high frequency stimulation had the opposite effect. The direction of these effects was in keeping with traditional models of the effect of low and high frequency TMS. However, the fact that changes were produced bilaterally when both groups improved clinically to a similar degree, is not consistent with laterality models of depression, such as that proposed by Henriques and Davison (1990).

Event-related potentials (ERPs), and especially late ERPs, are related to cognitive processes such as attention, stimulus evaluation, and early visual detection. Similar to other psychiatric disorders, a reduced P300 amplitude is often observed in depression (Blackwood, Whalley, Christie, Blackburn, St Clair, & McInnes, 1987; Himani, Tandon, & Bhatia, 1999). In a study by Möller et al. (Möller, Hjaltason, Ivarsson, Stefánsson, 2006) it was demonstrated that active TMS was associated with a significant increase in the P300 amplitude after 5 daily HF-rTMS sessions over the left DLPFC. In a study by our own group it was shown that using an auditory oddball paradigm, patients who were treated with HF-rTMS over left DLPFC showed localized changes on N1, P2, N2, and P300 amplitudes over left frontal areas, but not over the right frontal region. These results were interpreted as an increased positivity in the ERP which was localized to the stimulated area only (Spronk et al., 2008).

These findings demonstrate specific and selective alterations induced by repeated rTMS, which are distinct from those induced by other antidepressant treatments. The rTMS induced effects on neuroanatomical functions are commensurate with some known abnormalities in depression, e.g., decreased rCBF and metabolism values shown in a number of imaging studies (Baxter et al., 1989; Biver et al., 1994). Additionally, other research has shown similar changes in rCBF and metabolism relating to improvement of depression either after spontaneous recovery (Bench,

Frackowiak, & Dolan, 1995) or after treatment with antidepressant medication (Kennedy et al., 2001).

Neurochemical Effects: Neurotransmitters and Neuroendocrinology

Apart from altering rCBF in stimulated regions and connected networks, rTMS also has an effect on the neuroendocrinologic (Post & Keck, 2001) and neurotransmitter systems (Ben-Shachar, Belmaker, Grisaru & Klein, 1997; Strafella, Paus, Barrett & Dagher, 2001). Many lines of research on antidepressant mechanisms have focused on monoaminergic neurotransmission, i.e., through dopamine, norepinephrine and serotonin. Depression is thought to be associated with deficiencies in monoaminergic neurotransmission, and antidepressant medication is thought to act through enhancement of monoamines. These three neurotransmitter systems have also been investigated in relation to rTMS treatment (Ben-Shachar et al., 1997; Keck et al., 2000), and most studies support a role for the dopaminergic system. By means of microdialysis techniques in animal models, it was demonstrated that HF-rTMS induced an increase in the release of dopamine in the hippocampus (Ben-Shachar et al., 1997; Keck et al., 2000; Keck et al., 2002), the nucleus accumbens (Keck et al., 2002; Zangen & Hyodo, 2002) and dorsal striatum (Keck et al., 2002). It should be noted, however, that there are many methodological issues making interpretations from animal rTMS research difficult, such as the size of the head in relation to the coil size.

A few years later rTMS-induced changes in dopamine were investigated for the first time in human subjects. Strafella et al. (2001) found an increased dopamine release after HF-rTMS over the left DLPFC in the ipsilateral nucleus accumbens of healthy subjects by use of PET imaging (Strafella et al., 2001). The observation that increased dopamine levels were found only in the ipsilateral striatal area (site of stimulation) was particularly interesting, because it suggests that the increased release was exerted through cortico-striatal projections from the targeted DLPFC (Strafella et al., 2001). Taking this one step further, Pogarell and colleagues also found an increased striatal dopamine release in a small group of *depressive patients* after HF-rTMS over the left DLPFC by using SPECT (Pogarell et al., 2006; Pogarell et al., 2007). In these two studies, no correlation between the binding factors reflecting dopamine release and clinical outcome could be demonstrated. This needs to be investigated further in larger controlled studies (Pogarell et al., 2006).

In the study performed by Keck and colleagues (2002), a rTMS-induced effect on dopamine was found by using intracerebral microdialysis, but no effects on norepinephrine and serotonin were found. This finding suggests that rTMS mainly targets the dopamine system. Nevertheless, there are some indications that rTMS might modulate serotonergic neurotransmission. For instance, Juckel et al. (1999) showed that *electrical* stimulation of the prefrontal cortex of the rat resulted in an increased serotonin level in the amygdala and hippocampus; a similar pattern of release may occur after stimulation by rTMS. In addition, studies on serotonergic receptors and binding sites (which indirectly provide a measure of availability of certain neurotransmitters in the brain) after a single TMS session in a rat model showed an increase in serotonergic binding sites (Kole et al., 1999), and downregulation of receptors in cortical as well as subcortical areas (Ben-Shachar et al., 1999; Gur, Lerer, Dremencov, & Newman, 2000). With the exception of Keck et al. (2000) who found no effects on serotonin, no rTMS research has been conducted on the serotoninergic system in depression models, or in human depressed patients. This makes claims about TMS-induced changes on serotonin release highly speculative. Similarly speculative are claims regarding the effects of rTMS on the third member of the monoaminergic group, noradrenalin (norepinephrine). Limited studies are available and the findings are heterogeneous. Keck et al. (2000) found no changes on noradrenalin. Conversely, a study in mice found increased levels of monoaminergic transporter mRNA after a 20-day rTMS course. That was also associated with the binding and uptake of noradrenalin (Ikeda, Kurosawa, Uchikawa, Kitayama, & Nukina, 2005).

Another possible mechanism through which rTMS exerts its antidepressant effect involves the modulation of GABA and glutamate, which, respectively, are the main inhibitory and excitatory neurotransmitters. Both neurotransmitters are known to be associated with the pathology of depression and change with clinical improvement in depression (Petty et al., 1992). So far, only a few studies have directly addressed rTMS-induced changes in GABAergic neurotransmission. In an animal model, GABAergic levels were increased in hippocampal regions and striatum, and reduced in hypothalamic regions after 15 days of LF-rTMS stimulation (Yue, Xiao-Lin, & Tao, 2009). The same authors looked at glutamatergic changes and found similar results: an increase in glutamate in striatal and hippocampal regions, but a decrease in the hypothalamus (Yue et al., 2009). Additionally, in an *in vivo* study of depressed patients with a specific focus on the nucleus accumbens, changes in glutamate levels were observed after successful treatment of 10 HF–rTMS sessions (Luborzewski et al., 2007). Interestingly, the pre-treatment baseline level was related to treatment effects. Responders showed lower pre-treatment glutamate levels, and showed the highest increase in glutamate after successful treatment (see also later section on "Optimizing Treatment"). This suggests that in at least some of the patients, a reduction of depressive symptoms may happen through a restoration of relative gluta-mate levels (Luborzewski et al., 2007).

Repetitive TMS is known to exert changes in excitability thresholds on a neuronal level. It is known that LF–rTMS in particular induces pro-longed *decreases* in motor cortex excitability (Chen et al., 1997), while HF–rTMS induces an *increase* in motor cortex excitability (Pascual-Leone, Valls-Solé, Wassermann, & Hallett, 1994). Cortical excitability is thought to be maintained by a balance of neurotransmitter levels of GABA and glutamate. It can be hypothesized that glutamate and GABA in this animal model is mediated by excitability levels. To the best of the author's knowledge, only Luborzewski's study (2007) investigated rTMS-induced changes in levels of glutamate in depressed patients. More research on the release of GABA and glutamate by means of using *in vivo* techniques is needed to better specify the involvement of these neurotransmitters. In addition, future studies should specifically address the relationships between GABA/glutamate, treatment, and outcome.

Neurotrophins

Another candidate as a mechanism for the rTMS treatment effect in depression is the modulation and release of neurotrophins. BDNF is a neurotrophin, which plays a role in survival of neuronal cells and in syn-aptic plasticity and connectivity (Bath & Lee, 2006). In patients with depression, abnormal expression of BDNF has been observed (Shimizu et al., 2003) and, moreover, an upregulation as a result of antidepressant medication (Angelucci, Brenè, & Mathé, 2005; Shimizu et al., 2003) has been demonstrated. Since there is extensive literature that indicates a rela-tion between BDNF and depression (and related outcomes), BDNF became another likely candidate to investigate in relation to the antide-pressant treatment response to rTMS.

BDNF serum and plasma levels have, in fact, been investigated in sev-eral rTMS studies (Angelucci et al., 2004; Yukimasa et al., 2006; Zanardini et al., 2006). In a preliminary study by Lang et al. (2006) no changes in

BDNF serum level were observed after 10 sessions of HF–rTMS treatment. However, other studies on HF–rTMS-induced effects in treatment of depression yielded different findings (Yukimasa et al., 2006; Zanardini et al., 2006). In one study, BDNF serum levels were assessed before and after a series of five rTMS sessions and considered in relation to treatment outcome as rated by the HAM-D. Half of the participants (N = 8) were treated with a LF–rTMS design, while the other half (N = 8) were treated with a HF–rTMS design. Results showed that BDNF serum levels significantly increased over the treatment period. Interestingly, no changes between the HF and LF group were found, i.e. both showed equal increases in BDNF levels (Zanardini et al., 2006). In a study by Yukimasa et al. (2006) a similar relationship between treatment response and BDNF plasma levels was observed in a group of 26 patients who were treated with HF–rTMS. BDNF plasma levels increased at the end of the treatment period, but solely in patients who could be classified as responders (>50% decrease in depressive symptoms as measured on the HAM-D scale) or partial responders (>25% decrease in depressive symptoms). Together, these findings suggest that rTMS is indeed able to induce effects on BDNF levels. The finding that BDNF levels were changed only in the responder group suggests that the BDNF level is related to the *clinical* outcome, rather than simply a physiological effect. This is further supported by the finding that responses to HF and LF–rTMS appear to be similar.

Genetics

In the above-mentioned studies, several likely candidates associated with (and perhaps responsible for) an rTMS-induced antidepressant response were discussed. Another group of candidates includes genetic effects. As discussed in the "Neurotrophin" section, the modulation of the expression of brain-derived neurotrophic factors (BDNF) is a likely modulating factor through which treatment response is exerted. Hence, it is not surprising, that some of the *genetic* studies have focused on BDNF mRNA expression (Müller, Toschi, Kresse, Post, & Keck, 2000). Müller and colleagues investigated BDNF mRNA expression in an animal model involving applying 55 HF–rTMS sessions over a period of 11 weeks. They found significant increases in BDNF mRNA expression in the hippocampus (CA3 region) and parietal and piriform cortices. In addition, in an animal model of vascular dementia, mRNA expression in the hippocampal CA1 area was investigated in two groups of rats; one group received LF–rTMS and the other group received HF–rTMS for a period of six weeks. Both groups showed an increase in mRNA protein expressions of BDNF (Wang et al., 2010). However, in yet another genetics study, no rTMS induced effects on BDNF mRNA expression could be demonstrated (Hausmann, Weis, Marksteiner, Hinterhuber, & Humpel, 2000), possibly due to a relatively small number of sessions. Further limitations are that effects were not shown in a specific animal model of depression in any of these three studies. Also, the number of studies in this area is limited. For a discussion on genetic polymorphisms and treatment outcome in human patients see the section on "Optimizing Treatment".

NEW DEVELOPMENTS

As a new and dynamic field, rTMS is the topic of a considerable research and innovative developments are numerous. These developments are of a diverse nature, including technological progress in equipment and software, protocol innovations and optimizations, and advances in the understanding of long-term effects. Some examples are the investigation of applicability of theta burst stimulation (the delivery of bursts of 50 Hz pulses usually at a rate of 5 Hz) and new equipment such as the H-coil for deeper brain stimulation.

Progress in Protocols

In addition to the "traditional" LF and HF frequency studies, a newly developed theta-burst stimulation (TBS) protocol has been proposed; referred to as "patterned TMS". This has been put forward as a technique that could have important implications for the treatment of conditions such as epilepsy, depression, and Parkinson's disease (Paulus, 2005). TBS usually involves short bursts of 50 Hz rTMS applied at a rate of 5 Hz (hence the name *theta* burst stimulation). In fact there are two frequencies within one train of stimuli; the inter-burst frequency of 50 Hz (e.g., 3 pulses at a rate of 50 Hz) and the frequency of delivery of the number of bursts within one second which is at a rate of 5 per second (5 Hz). TBS can be applied as either a continuous (cTBS), or intermittent (iTBS) train (Huang, Edwards, Rounis, Bhatia, & Rothwell, 2005). See Figure 10.4 for an illustration of both types of TBS protocols.

Until recently, this rapid delivery of pulses as happens in a TBS protocol was not possible due to technical limitations of older stimulators. TBS has therefore only been investigated since 2005 (Huang et al., 2005).

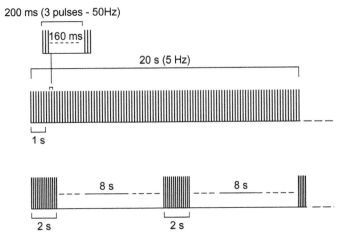

Figure 10.4 Examples of the two most common TBS protocols: continuous TBS (first trace) and intermittent TBS (second trace). *(Adapted from Rossi et al., 2009.)*

In the years after its introduction, it has been shown that TBS induces changes in cortical excitability that may last longer than traditional TMS protocols (Huang et al., 2009; Ishikawa et al., 2007). In regard to the observation of the more sustained effect, Chistyakov, Rubicsek, Kaplan, Zaaroor, & Klein (2010) suggested that TBS might be more effective than traditional HF and LF-rTMS in the treatment of depression. They assigned 33 patients to different types of TBS-TMS treatment protocols over either left or right DLPFC. Despite the relatively high response rate, these findings should be regarded as preliminary and non-specific since no changes between different types of protocols were observed. To the authors' knowledge, this is the only study that has investigated the antidepressant effect of TBS-TMS in the treatment of depression. However, since the TBS protocols are assumed to be more capable of inducing long-lasting effects, it is likely that their application in rTMS depression treatment will increase in coming years.

Technical Progress

In response to limitations of currently used coils, a new type of coil "the H-coil" (Brainsway) was developed. The coils that are in current use (figure of eight/circular coils) are thought to penetrate underlying brain tissue only to a depth of 1.5—2 cm and are not capable of directly targeting deeper brain regions (Zangen et al., 2005). H-coils, on the other hand, are capable of stimulating deeper brain regions (Zangen et al., 2005). To date, there are several reports in which it has been presented that brain stimulation by means of the H-coil is safe and that there is potential for use of the coil in clinical applications (Levkovitz et al., 2007; Zangen et al., 2005). The application of the H-coil in the treatment of depression is currently under investigation in a multi-site trial.

Optimizing Treatment

A better understanding of the neurophysiological and clinical features of depressed patients who respond to rTMS, together with clarity on the neurobiological mechanisms of the induced effect of rTMS treatment in depression, will contribute to the development of more effective forms of rTMS. The field involved in identifying such features is referred to as Personalized Medicine: a research towards establishing patient's characteristics (clinical, physiological or parametric variables) related to (better) clinical outcome. Especially relevant to the rTMS area is the research on identifying objective markers of clinical response. Several studies have focused on addressing this question by investigating specific clinical features. Negative predictors for treatment outcome identified so far are age (Brakemeier, Luborzewski, Danker-Hopfe, Kathmann, & Bajbouj, 2007; Fregni et al., 2006) and therapy resistance (Brakemeier et al., 2007; Brakemeier et al., 2008; Fregni et al., 2006). These results suggest that elderly patients and patients with a greater number of prior treatment failures are less likely to benefit from rTMS. However, this has not been confirmed by all studies in this area (Fitzgerald et al., 2006b). In contrast, a shorter duration of the depressive episode and a high severity of sleep disturbance are predictive of better treatment outcome (Brakemeier et al., 2007).

A different group of potential predictors can be obtained from the neurophysiological data. One study indicated that some patients with depression responded better to LF-rTMS, while others improved only after treatment with HF-rTMS (Kimbrell et al., 1999). These two patient groups differed on pre-treatment baseline regional cerebral blood flow. Patients with a relatively low level of rCBF generally responded better to HF-rTMS (20 Hz), whereas patients displaying relatively high baseline rCBF levels showed a better response to LF-rTMS (Kimbrell et al., 1999). Baeken et al. (2009) showed that higher *bilateral* baseline metabolic activity in the DLPFC and anterior cingulate cortex correlated with better treatment outcome.

In addition, Speer et al. (2009) correlated treatment outcome after 2 weeks of LF or HF-rTMS with pre-treatment baseline baseline perfusion measures. Baseline hypo-perfusion was associated with a more beneficial effect of HF-rTMS compared to LF-rTMS (Speer et al., 2009).

While EEG measures have been relatively well studied in the prediction of treatment response to antidepressant medication (Bruder et al., 2008; Cook et al., 1999; Spronk et al., 2010), their potential in predicting response to rTMS treatment is generally considered limited but promising. In the search for physiological markers for treatment response to rTMS, Price and colleagues (Price, Lee, Garvey, & Gibson, 2008) investigated alpha EEG activity measures, i.e., individual alpha power and frequency, and asymmetry index in 39 patients with treatment resistant depression. None of the measures was found to be a promising candidate for response prediction. Recently Daskalakis, Fitzgerald, Greenwald, and Devlin (2008) were the first to report the potential predictive value of an EEG biomarker initially developed for prediction of treatment response to antidepressant medication. This biomarker (labeled antidepressant treatment response (ATR) index) is measured from frontal electrode positions and is based on the proportion of relative and absolute theta power. In Daskalakis' study it was shown that subjects who could be classified as "responders" after 6 weeks of treatment scored higher on this ATR index. As these early reports indicate, current knowledge of the utility of EEG in the prediction of antidepressant treatment outcome is limited. It has, however, been proposed as having great potential for predicting response to rTMS in the treatment of depression. For example, it has been suggested that rTMS can potentially interact with specific EEG frequency patterns (Funk & George, 2008). In accordance with this notion, Jin, O'Halloran, Plon, Sandman, and Potkin (2006) compared different rTMS stimulation frequencies in the treatment of patients suffering from schizophrenia; two groups received treatment with conventional frequencies, but one group was treated with a stimulation frequency identical to their individualized frontal alpha peak frequency. The group who received the individualized frequency showed a higher reduction in negative symptoms in comparison to the patients who were treated with standard stimulation frequencies. In a report by Arns et al. (2010) a similar approach was taken in the treatment of depression. However, in this study subjects were treated with a stimulation frequency of one Hz above their individualized alpha peak frequency. The results demonstrated this type of individualized stimulation frequency was not beneficial. In contrast, this study suggested that there could be differential effects of different TMS stimulation frequencies; more specifically, 9 Hz yielded different effects compared to 10 Hz TMS. Furthermore, the study by Arns et al. (2010) demonstrated a clear relation of an individual alpha peak frequency to clinical outcome, where a low alpha peak frequency (7–8 Hz) was associated with lower clinical efficacy. This was also shown in a study by Conca and colleagues (2000) who found that non-responders to rTMS had a slower alpha peak frequency. Clearly, more studies are needed to further explore this.

In addition to demographical and physiological markers, genetic markers may have potential in the prediction of treatment outcome. Several genetic polymorphisms have been investigated in relation to antidepressant treatment outcome in medication studies, for example, BDNF, COMT, and serotonin-related candidate genes (Benedetti, Colombo, Pirovano, Marino & Smeraldi, 2009; Peters et al., 2009; Zou, Ye, Feng, Su, Pan, & Liao, 2010). However, genetics as potential biomarkers for susceptibility to antidepressant medications is still a relatively novel concept, and only a limited amount of research has been conducted. This holds also for the investigation of genetic predictors of rTMS treatment outcome. As discussed previously in this chapter, several studies show treatment-induced changes on BDNF. To date, in respect to the rTMS treatment of depression several genetic polymorphisms have been proposed to be related to treatment outcome. Among them are the genetic polymorphisms associated with BDNF expression, the BDNF Val66Met (Bocchio-Chiavetto et al., 2008; Cheeran et al., 2008) and candidate genes related to expression of serotonin (Bocchio-Chiavetto et al., 2008; Zanardi et al., 2007) (for a discussion of BDNF and serotonin release, see "Mechanisms" above).

Bocchio-Chiabetto and colleagues (2008) demonstrated in their study that carriers of the LL variant of the 5-HTTLPR gene showed significantly greater decreases in depressive symptoms following rTMS (as reflected by percentage decrease on the HAM-D), in comparison to carriers of the S allele. The serotonin-related polymorphisms SERTPR and 5-HT(1A) have also been investigated in relation to depression treatment outcome (Zanardi et al., 2007). Results indicated that polymorphisms related to both genes were to some extent related to treatment outcome, but carriers of the 5HT(1A) C/C gene specifically received more benefit from active rTMS than sham rTMS. This was in contrast to polymorphism carriers of the SERTPR gene, who showed response to treatment outcome regardless of the treatment condition (active or sham).

In addition to their finding on the relation of the 5-HTTLPR with treatment outcome, Bocchio-Chiabetto and colleagues (2008) demonstrated in the same study that BDNF Val/Val homozygotes were better responders than carriers of the Met allele (carriers of MET/MET or MET/VAL). These outcomes can be linked to the study results of Cheeran et al. (2008), who compared differences in excitability measures between Val/Val carriers and carriers of the Met allele. Subjects were investigated using two TBS protocols; a cTBS protocol which is thought to suppress excitability and an iTBS protocol which is known to generally cause an increase in excitability. Change in amplitude measures of the motor evoked potential was taken as an outcome measure reflecting excitability. The results showed that Met allele carriers had less (or no) rTMS-induced changes in excitability; in both TBS protocols no changes in excitability in either direction were evident. Highly speculatively, it can be argued that these results potentially indicate that this same group of Met carriers are less receptive to rTMS-induced clinical improvement. However, it must be emphasized that iTBS and cTBS TMS protocols are very different from traditional HF and LF rTMS depression protocols.

In summary, although rTMS is a relative newcomer among the treatment options for depression, the investigation of "individual characteristics" related to treatment response appears to be progressing rather rapidly. Developments to date seem to mainly focus on fMRI and PET imaging studies and to a lesser extent on genetic polymorphism and EEG parameters. Possibly this is due to the observed direct and indirect interactions with underlying brain regions, and the fact that PET and fMRI imaging are especially effective for highlighting induced changes in regional blood flow and metabolism. The utility of genetic polymorphism in relation to predicting treatment response, in particular the BDNF gene, has potential. TMS devices now allow for a fairly extended choice in treatment parameters (e.g., stimulation intensity, location, frequency etc.). The application of physiological predictors may better guide the parameters to be selected in the future. Evidence for considerable clinical efficacy is required if rTMS is to become accepted as a regular treatment option for depression.

ACKNOWLEDGMENTS

The authors would like to thank Michiel Kleinnijenhuis for reading the manuscript and providing valuable comments.

REFERENCES

American Psychiatric Association. (1994). *Diagnostic and statistical manual of mental disorders* (4th ed.) (DSM-IV). Washington, DC: Author.

Angelucci, F., Brenè, S., & Mathé, A. A. (2005). BDNF in schizophrenia, depression and corresponding animal models. *Molecular Psychiatry, 10*(4), 345−352.

Angelucci, F., Oliviero, A., Pilato, F., Saturno, E., Dileone, M., Versace, V., et al. (2004). Transcranial magnetic stimulation and BDNF plasma levels in amyotrophic lateral sclerosis. *Neuroreport, 15*(4), 717−720.

Aoyama, Y., Hanaoka, N., Kameyama, M., Suda, M., Sato, T., Song, M., et al. (2009). Stimulus intensity dependence of cerebral blood volume changes in left frontal lobe by low-frequency rtms to right frontal lobe: A near-infrared spectroscopy study. *Neuroscience Research, 63*(1), 47−51.

Arns, M., Spronk, D., & Fitzgerald, P. B. (2010). Potential differential effects of 9 Hz rTMS and 10 Hz rTMS in the treatment of depression. *Brain Stimulation, 3,* 124−126.

Avery, D. H., Holtzheimer, P. E., Fawaz, W., Russo, J., Neumaier, J., Dunner, D. L., et al. (2006). A controlled study of repetitive transcranial magnetic stimulation in medication-resistant major depression. *Biological Psychiatry, 59*(2), 187−194.

Baeken, C., De Raedt, R., Van Hove, C., Clerinx, P., De Mey, J., & Bossuyt, A. (2009). HF-rTMS treatment in medication-resistant melancholic depression: Results from 18FDG-PET brain imaging. *CNS Spectrums, 14*(8), 439−448.

Barker, A. T., Jalinous, R., & Freeston, I. L. (1985). Non-invasive magnetic stimulation of human motor cortex. *Lancet, 1*(8437), 1106−1107.

Bath, K. G., & Lee, F. S. (2006). Variant BDNF (Val66Met) impact on brain structure and function. *Cognitive and Affective Behavioral Neuroscience, 6*(1), 79−85.

Baxter, L. R., Schwartz, J. M., Phelps, M. E., Mazziotta, J. C., Guze, B. H., Selin, C. E., et al. (1989). Reduction of prefrontal cortex glucose metabolism common to three types of depression. *Archives of General Psychiatry, 46*(3), 243−250.

Ben-Shachar, D., Belmaker, R. H., Grisaru, N., & Klein, E. (1997). Transcranial magnetic stimulation induces alterations in brain monoamines. *Journal of Neural Transmission (Vienna, Austria), 104*(2−3), 191−197.

Ben-Shachar, D., Gazawi, H., Riboyad-Levin, J., & Klein, E. (1999). Chronic repetitive transcranial magnetic stimulation alters beta-adrenergic and 5-HT2 receptor characteristics in rat brain. *Brain Research, 816*(1), 78−83.

Bench, C. J., Frackowiak, R. S., & Dolan, R. J. (1995). Changes in regional cerebral blood flow on recovery from depression. *Psychological Medicine, 25*(2), 247−261.

Benedetti, F., Colombo, C., Pirovano, A., Marino, E., & Smeraldi, E. (2009). The catechol-o-methyltransferase val(108/158)met polymorphism affects antidepressant response to paroxetine in a naturalistic setting. *Psychopharmacology, 203*(1), 155−160.

Bickford, R. G., Guidi, M., Fortesque, P., & Swenson, M. (1987). Magnetic stimulation of human peripheral nerve and brain: Response enhancement by combined magnetoelectrical technique. *Neurosurgery, 20*(1), 110−116.

Biver, F., Goldman, S., Delvenne, V., Luxen, A., De Maertelaer, V., Hubain, P., et al. (1994). Frontal and parietal metabolic disturbances in unipolar depression. *Biological Psychiatry, 36*(6), 381−388.

Blackwood, D. H., Whalley, L. J., Christie, J. E., Blackburn, I. M., St, Clair, D. M., & McInnes, A. (1987). Changes in auditory P3 event-related potential in schizophrenia and depression. *British Journal of Psychiatry: Journal of Mental Science, 150,* 154−160.

Blazer, D. G., Kessler, R. C., McGonagle, K. A., & Swartz, M. S. (1994). The prevalence and distribution of major depression in a national community sample: The national comorbidity survey. *American Journal of Psychiatry, 151*(7), 979−986.

Bocchio-Chiavetto, L., Miniussi, C., Zanardini, R., Gazzoli, A., Bignotti, S., Specchia, C., et al. (2008). 5-HTTLPR and BDNF val66met polymorphisms and response to rTMS treatment in drug resistant depression. *Neuroscience Letters*, *437*(2), 130–134.

Brakemeier, E. L., Luborzewski, A., Danker-Hopfe, H., Kathmann, N., & Bajbouj, M. (2007). Positive predictors for antidepressive response to prefrontal repetitive transcranial magnetic stimulation (rtms). *Journal of Psychiatric Research*, *41*(5), 395–403.

Brakemeier, E. L., Wilbertz, G., Rodax, S., Danker-Hopfe, H., Zinka, B., Zwanzger, P., et al. (2008). Patterns of response to repetitive transcranial magnetic stimulation (rTMS) in major depression: Replication study in drug-free patients. *Journal of Affective Disorders*, *108*(1-2), 59–70.

Bruder, G. E., Sedoruk, J. P., Stewart, J. W., McGrath, P. J., Quitkin, F. M., & Tenke, C. E. (2008). EEG alpha measures predict therapeutic response to an SSRI antidepressant: Pre and post treatment findings. *Biological Psychiatry*, *63*(12), 1171.

Cardoso, E. F., Fregni, F., Martins Maia, F., Boggio, P. S., Luis Myczkowski, M., Coracini, K., et al. (2008). rTMS treatment for depression in Parkinson's Disease increases BOLD responses in the left prefrontal cortex. *International Journal of Neuropsychopharmacology/Official Scientific Journal of the Collegium Internationale Neuropsychopharmacologicum (CINP)*, *11*(2), 173–183.

Catafau, A. M., Perez, V., Gironell, A., Martin, J. C., Kulisevsky, J., Estorch, M., et al. (2001). SPECT mapping of cerebral activity changes induced by repetitive transcranial magnetic stimulation in depressed patients. A pilot study. *Psychiatry Research*, *106*(3), 151–160.

Cheeran, B., Talelli, P., Mori, F., Koch, G., Suppa, A., Edwards, M., et al. (2008). A common polymorphism in the brain-derived neurotrophic factor gene (BDNF) modulates human cortical plasticity and the response to rTMS. *Journal of Physiology*, *586*(Pt 23), 5717–5725.

Chen, R., Gerloff, C., Classen, J., Wassermann, E. M., Hallett, M., & Cohen, L. G. (1997). Safety of different inter-train intervals for repetitive transcranial magnetic stimulation and recommendations for safe ranges of stimulation parameters. *Electroencephalography and Clinical Neurophysiology*, *105*(6), 415–421.

Chistyakov, A. V., Rubicsek, O., Kaplan, B., Zaaroor, M., & Klein, E. (2010). Safety, tolerability and preliminary evidence for antidepressant efficacy of theta-burst transcranial magnetic stimulation in patients with major depression. *International Journal of Neuropsychopharmacology/Official Scientific Journal of the Collegium Internationale Neuropsychopharmacologicum (CINP)*, 1–7.

Conca, A., Swoboda, E., König, P., Koppi, S., Beraus, W., Künz, A., et al. (2000). Clinical impacts of single transcranial magnetic stimulation (sTMS) as an add-on therapy in severely depressed patients under SSRI treatment. *Human Psychopharmacology*, *15*(6), 429–438.

Cook, I. A., Leuchter, A. F., Witte, E., Abrams, M., Uijtdehaage, S. H., Stubbeman, W., et al. (1999). Neurophysiologic predictors of treatment response to fluoxetine in major depression. *Psychiatry Research*, *85*(3), 263–273.

Cummings, J. L. (1993). The neuroanatomy of depression. *Journal of Clinical Psychiatry*, *54* (Suppl), 14–20.

Daskalakis, Z., Fitzgerald, P., Greenwald, S., & Devlin, P. (2008). EEG ATR measures clinical response to rTMS treatment in MDD. *Brain Stimulation*, *1*(3), 268.

Drevets, W. C., Price, J. L., & Furey, M. L. (2008). Brain structural and functional abnormalities in mood disorders: Implications for neurocircuitry models of depression. *Brain Structure & Function*, *213*(1–2), 93–118.

Eranti, S., Mogg, A., Pluck, G., Landau, S., Purvis, R., Brown, R. G., et al. (2007). A randomized, controlled trial with 6-month follow-up of repetitive transcranial magnetic stimulation and electroconvulsive therapy for severe depression. *American Journal of Psychiatry, 164*(1), 73–81.

Fitzgerald, P. B., Benitez, J., de Castella, A., Daskalakis, Z. J., Brown, T. L., & Kulkarni, J. (2006a). A randomized, controlled trial of sequential bilateral repetitive transcranial magnetic stimulation for treatment-resistant depression. *American Journal of Psychiatry, 163*(1), 88–94.

Fitzgerald, P. B., Brown, T. L., Marston, N. A. U., Daskalakis, Z. J., de Castella, A., & Kulkarni, J. (2003). Transcranial magnetic stimulation in the treatment of depression: A double-blind, placebo-controlled trial. *Archives of General Psychiatry, 60*(10), 1002.

Fitzgerald, P. B., Hoy, K., Daskalakis, Z. J., & Kulkarni, J. (2009a). A randomized trial of the anti-depressant effects of low- and high-frequency transcranial magnetic stimulation in treatment-resistant depression. *Depression and Anxiety, 26*(3), 229–234.

Fitzgerald, P. B., Hoy, K., McQueen, S., Herring, S., Segrave, R., Been, G., et al. (2008). Priming stimulation enhances the effectiveness of low-frequency right prefrontal cortex transcranial magnetic stimulation in major depression. *Journal of Clinical Psychopharmacology, 28*(1), 52–58.

Fitzgerald, P. B., Hoy, K., McQueen, S., Maller, J. J., Herring, S., Segrave, R., et al. (2009b). A randomized trial of rTMS targeted with MRI based neuro-navigation in treatment-resistant depression. *Neuropsychopharmacology, 34*(5), 1255–1262.

Fitzgerald, P. B., Huntsman, S., Gunewardene, R., Kulkarni, J., & Daskalakis, Z. J. (2006b). A randomized trial of low-frequency right-prefrontal-cortex transcranial magnetic stimulation as augmentation in treatment-resistant major depression. *International Journal of Neuropsychopharmacology/Official Scientific Journal of the Collegium Internationale Neuropsychopharmacologicum (CINP), 9*(6), 655–666.

Fitzgerald, P. B., Oxley, T. J., Laird, A. R., Kulkarni, J., Egan, G. F., & Daskalakis, Z. J. (2006c). An analysis of functional neuroimaging studies of dorsolateral prefrontal cortical activity in depression. *Psychiatry Research, 148*(1), 33–45.

Fitzgerald, P. B., Sritharan, A., Daskalakis, Z. J., de Castella, A. R., Kulkarni, J., & Egan, G. (2007). A functional magnetic resonance imaging study of the effects of low frequency right prefrontal transcranial magnetic stimulation in depression. *Journal of Clinical Psychopharmacology, 27*(5), 488–492.

Fregni, F., Marcolin, M. A., Myczkowski, M., Amiaz, R., Hasey, G., Rumi, D. O., et al. (2006). Predictors of antidepressant response in clinical trials of transcranial magnetic stimulation. *International Journal of Neuropsychopharmacology/Official Scientific Journal of the Collegium Internationale Neuropsychopharmacologicum (CINP), 9*(6), 641–654.

Funk, A. P., & George, M. S. (2008). Prefrontal EEG asymmetry as a potential biomarker of antidepressant treatment response with transcranial magnetic stimulation (TMS): A case series. *Clinics in EEG Neuroscience, 39*(3), 125–130.

Garcia-Toro, M., Pascual-Leone, A., Romera, M., Gonzalez, A., Mico, J., Ibarra, O., et al. (2001). *Journal of Neurology, Neurosurgery, and Psychiatry, 71*(4), 546–548.

George, M. S., Wassermann, E. M., Kimbrell, T. A., Little, J. T., Williams, W. E., Danielson, A. L., et al. (1997). Mood improvement following daily left prefrontal repetitive transcranial magnetic stimulation in patients with depression: A placebo-controlled crossover trial. *American Journal of Psychiatry, 154*(12), 1752–1756.

George, M. S., Wassermann, E. M., Williams, W. A., Callahan, A., Ketter, T. A., Basser, P., et al. (1995). Daily repetitive transcranial magnetic stimulation (rTMS) improves mood in depression. *Neuroreport, 6*(14), 1853–1856.

George, M. S., Lisanby, S. H., Avery, D., McDonald, W. M., Durkalski, V., Pavlicova, M., et al. (2010). Daily left prefrontal transcranial magnetic stimulation therapy for major depressive disorder: A sham-controlled randomized trial. *Archives of General Psychiatry, 67*(5), 507–516.

Gross, M., Nakamura, L., Pascual-Leone, A., & Fregni, F. (2007). Has repetitive transcranial magnetic stimulation (rTMS) treatment for depression improved? A systematic review and meta-analysis comparing the recent vs. the earlier rTMS studies. *Acta Psychiatrica Scandinavica, 116*(3), 165–173.

Grunhaus, L., Schreiber, S., Dolberg, O. T., Polak, D., & Dannon, P. N. (2003). A randomized controlled comparison of electroconvulsive therapy and repetitive transcranial magnetic stimulation in severe and resistant nonpsychotic major depression. *Biological Psychiatry, 53*(4), 324–331.

Gur, E., Lerer, B., Dremencov, E., & Newman, M. E. (2000). Chronic repetitive transcranial magnetic stimulation induces subsensitivity of presynaptic serotonergic autoreceptor activity in rat brain. *Neuroreport, 11*(13), 2925–2929.

Hallett, M. (2007). Transcranial magnetic stimulation: A primer. *Neuron, 55*(2), 187–199.

Hanaoka, N., Aoyama, Y., Kameyama, M., Fukuda, M., & Mikuni, M. (2007). Deactivation and activation of left frontal lobe during and after low-frequency repetitive transcranial magnetic stimulation over right prefrontal cortex: A near-infrared spectroscopy study. *Neuroscience Letters, 414*(2), 99–104.

Hausmann, A., Weis, C., Marksteiner, J., Hinterhuber, H., & Humpel, C. (2000). Chronic repetitive transcranial magnetic stimulation enhances c-Fos in the parietal cortex and hippocampus. *Brain Research Molecular Brain Research, 76*(2), 355–362.

Henriques, J. B., & Davidson, R. J. (1990). Regional brain electrical asymmetries discriminate between previously depressed and healthy control subjects. *Journal of Abnormal Psychology, 99*(1), 22–31.

Herwig, U., Padberg, F., Unger, J., Spitzer, M., & Schönfeldt-Lecuona, C. (2001). Transcranial magnetic stimulation in therapy studies: Examination of the reliability of "standard" coil positioning by neuronavigation. *Biological Psychiatry, 50*(1), 58–61.

Himani, A., Tandon, O. P., & Bhatia, M. S. (1999). A study of p300-event related evoked potential in the patients of major depression. *Indian Journal of Physiology and Pharmacology, 43*(3), 367–372.

Höflich, G., Kasper, S., Hufnagel, A., Ruhrmann, S., & Moller, H. J. (1993). Application of transcranial magnetic stimulation in the treatment of drug-resistant major depression: A report of two cases. *Human Psychopharmacology, 8*, 361–365.

Huang, Y. Z., Edwards, M. J., Rounis, E., Bhatia, K. P., & Rothwell, J. C. (2005). Theta burst stimulation of the human motor cortex. *Neuron, 45*(2), 201–206.

Huang, Y. Z., Rothwell, J. C., Lu, C. S., Wang, J., Weng, Y. H., Lai, S. C., et al. (2009). The effect of continuous theta burst stimulation over premotor cortex on circuits in primary motor cortex and spinal cord. *Clinical Neurophysiology, 120*(4), 796–801.

Husain, M. M., Rush, A. J., Fink, M., Knapp, R., Petrides, G., Rummans, T., et al. (2004). Speed of response and remission in major depressive disorder with acute electroconvulsive therapy (ECT): A consortium for research in ECT (CORE) report. *Journal of Clinical Psychiatry, 65*(4), 485–491.

Ikeda, T., Kurosawa, M., Uchikawa, C., Kitayama, S., & Nukina, N. (2005). Modulation of monoamine transporter expression and function by repetitive transcranial magnetic stimulation. *Biochemical and Biophysical Research Communications, 327*(1), 218–224.

Isenberg, K., Downs, D., Pierce, K., Svarakic, D., Garcia, K., Jarvis, M., et al. (2005). Low frequency rTMS stimulation of the right frontal cortex is as effective as high frequency rTMS stimulation of the left frontal cortex for antidepressant-free, treatment-resistant depressed patients. *Annals of Clinical Psychiatry, 17*(3), 153–159.

Ishikawa, S., Matsunaga, K., Nakanishi, R., Kawahira, K., Murayama, N., Tsuji, S., et al. (2007). Effect of theta burst stimulation over the human sensorimotor cortex on motor and somatosensory evoked potentials. *Clinical Neurophysiology, 118*(5), 1033–1043.

Iyer, M. B., Schleper, N., & Wassermann, E. M. (2003). Priming stimulation enhances the depressant effect of low-frequency repetitive transcranial magnetic stimulation. *Journal of Neuroscience, 23*(34), 10867–10872.

Januel, D., Dumortier, G., Verdon, C. M., Stamatiadis, L., Saba, G., Cabaret, W., et al. (2006). A double-blind sham controlled study of right prefrontal repetitive transcranial magnetic stimulation (rTMS): Therapeutic and cognitive effect in medication free unipolar depression during 4 weeks. *Progress in Neuro-Psychopharmacology & Biological Psychiatry, 30*(1), 126–130.

Jin, Y., O'Halloran, J. P., Plon, L., Sandman, C. A., & Potkin, S. G. (2006). Alpha EEG predicts visual reaction time. *International Journal of Neuroscience, 116*(9), 1035–1044.

Juckel, G., Mendlin, A., & Jacobs, B. L. (1999). Electrical stimulation of rat medial prefrontal cortex enhances forebrain serotonin output: Implications for electroconvulsive therapy and transcranial magnetic stimulation in depression. *Neuropsychopharmacology, 21*(3), 391–398.

Keck, M. E., Sillaber, I., Ebner, K., Welt, T., Toschi, N., Kaehler, S. T., et al. (2000). Acute transcranial magnetic stimulation of frontal brain regions selectively modulates the release of vasopressin, biogenic amines and amino acids in the rat brain. *European Journal of Neuroscience, 12*(10), 3713–3720.

Keck, M. E., Welt, T., Müller, M. B., Erhardt, A., Ohl, F., Toschi, N., et al. (2002). Repetitive transcranial magnetic stimulation increases the release of dopamine in the mesolimbic and mesostriatal system. *Neuropharmacology, 43*(1), 101–109.

Keller, M. B., McCullough, J. P., Klein, D. N., Arnow, B., Dunner, D. L., Gelenberg, A. J., et al. (2000). A comparison of nefazodone, the cognitive behavioral-analysis system of psychotherapy, and their combination for the treatment of chronic depression. *New England Journal of Medicine, 342*(20), 1462–1470.

Kennedy, S. H., Evans, K. R., Krüger, S., Mayberg, H. S., Meyer, J. H., McCann, S., et al. (2001). Changes in regional brain glucose metabolism measured with positron emission tomography after paroxetine treatment of major depression. *American Journal of Psychiatry, 158*(6), 899–905.

Kimbrell, T. A., Little, J. T., Dunn, R. T., Frye, M. A., Greenberg, B. D., Wassermann, E. M., et al. (1999). Frequency dependence of antidepressant response to left prefrontal repetitive transcranial magnetic stimulation (rTMS) as a function of baseline cerebral glucose metabolism. *Biological Psychiatry, 46*(12), 1603–1613.

Kirsch, I., Deacon, B. J., Huedo-Medina, T. B., Scoboria, A., Moore, T. J., & Johnson, B. T. (2008). Initial severity and antidepressant benefits: A meta-analysis of data submitted to the food and drug administration. *PLoS Med, 5*(2), e45.

Kito, S., Fujita, K., & Koga, Y. (2008a). Changes in regional cerebral blood flow after repetitive transcranial magnetic stimulation of the left dorsolateral prefrontal cortex in treatment-resistant depression. *Journal of Neuropsychiatry and Clinical Neurosciences, 20*(1), 74–80.

Kito, S., Fujita, K., & Koga, Y. (2008b). Regional cerebral blood flow changes after low-frequency transcranial magnetic stimulation of the right dorsolateral prefrontal cortex in treatment-resistant depression. *Neuropsychobiology, 58*(1), 29–36.

Klein, E., Kreinin, I., Chistyakov, A., Koren, D., Mecz, L., Marmur, S., et al. (1999). Therapeutic efficacy of right prefrontal slow repetitive transcranial magnetic stimulation in major depression: A double-blind controlled study. *Archives of General Psychiatry, 56*(4), 315–320.

Koerselman, F., Laman, D. M., van Duijn, H., van Duijn, M. A., & Willems, M. A. (2004). A 3-month, follow-up, randomized, placebo-controlled study of repetitive transcranial magnetic stimulation in depression. *Journal of Clinical Psychiatry, 65*(10), 1323–1328.

Kolbinger, H. M., Höflich, G., Hufnagel, A., Möller, H. J., & Kasper, S. (1995). Transcranial magnetic stimulation (TMS) in the treatment of major depression—a pilot study. *Human Psychopharmacology, 10,* 305—310.

Kole, M. H., Fuchs, E., Ziemann, U., Paulus, W., & Ebert, U. (1999). Changes in 5-HT1A and NMDA binding sites by a single rapid transcranial magnetic stimulation procedure in rats. *Brain Research, 826*(2), 309—312.

Kozel, F. A., Tian, F., Dhamne, S., Croarkin, P. E., McClintock, S. M., Elliott, A., et al. (2009). Using simultaneous repetitive transcranial magnetic stimulation/functional near infrared spectroscopy (rTMS/fNIRS) to measure brain activation and connectivity. *Neuroimage, 47*(4), 1177—1184.

Lang, U. E., Bajbouj, M., Gallinat, J., & Hellweg, R. (2006). Brain-derived neurotrophic factor serum concentrations in depressive patients during vagus nerve stimulation and repetitive transcranial magnetic stimulation. *Psychopharmacology, 187*(1), 56—59.

Levkovitz, Y., Roth, Y., Harel, E. V., Braw, Y., Sheer, A., & Zangen, A. (2007). A randomized controlled feasibility and safety study of deep transcranial magnetic stimulation. *Clinical Neurophysiology, 118*(12), 2730—2744.

Loo, C. K., Sachdev, P. S., Haindl, W., Wen, W., Mitchell, P. B., Croker, V. M., et al. (2003). High (15 Hz) and low (1 Hz) frequency transcranial magnetic stimulation have different acute effects on regional cerebral blood flow in depressed patients. *Psychological Medicine, 33*(06), 997—1006.

Luborzewski, A., Schubert, F., Seifert, F., Danker-Hopfe, H., Brakemeier, E. L., Schlattmann, P., et al. (2007). Metabolic alterations in the dorsolateral prefrontal cortex after treatment with high-frequency repetitive transcranial magnetic stimulation in patients with unipolar major depression. *Journal of Psychiatric Research, 41*(7), 606—615.

Manes, F., Jorge, R., Morcuende, M., Yamada, T., Paradiso, S., & Robinson, R. G. (2001). A controlled study of repetitive transcranial magnetic stimulation as a treatment of depression in the elderly. *International Psychogeriatrics, 13*(2), 225—231.

Miniussi, C., Bonato, C., Bignotti, S., Gazzoli, A., Gennarelli, M., Pasqualetti, P., et al. (2005). Repetitive transcranial magnetic stimulation (rTMS) at high and low frequency: An efficacious therapy for major drug-resistant depression? *Clinical Neurophysiology, 116* (5), 1062—1071.

Mogg, A., Pluck, G., Eranti, S. V., Landau, S., Purvis, R., Brown, R. G., et al. (2008). A randomized controlled trial with 4-month follow-up of adjunctive repetitive transcranial magnetic stimulation of the left prefrontal cortex for depression. *Psychological Medicine, 38*(3), 323—333.

Möller, A. L., Hjaltason, O., Ivarsson, O., & Stefánsson, S. B. (2006). The effects of repetitive transcranial magnetic stimulation on depressive symptoms and the P(300) event-related potential. *Nordic Journal of Psychiatry, 60*(4), 282—285.

Murray, C. J., & Lopez, A. D. (1997). Global mortality, disability, and the contribution of risk factors: Global burden of disease study. *Lancet, 349*(9063), 1436—1442.

Müller, M. B., Toschi, N., Kresse, A. E., Post, A., & Keck, M. E. (2000). Long-term repetitive transcranial magnetic stimulation increases the expression of brain-derived neurotrophic factor and cholecystokinin mRNA, but not neuropeptide tyrosine mRNA in specific areas of rat brain. *Neuropsychopharmacology, 23*(2), 205—215.

Nahas, Z., Kozel, F. A., Li, X., Anderson, B., & George, M. S. (2003). Left prefrontal transcranial magnetic stimulation (TMS) treatment of depression in bipolar affective disorder: A pilot study of acute safety and efficacy. *Bipolar Disorders, 5*(1), 40—47.

O'Reardon, J. P., Solvason, H. B., Janicak, P. G., Sampson, S., Isenberg, K. E., Nahas, Z., et al. (2007). Efficacy and safety of transcranial magnetic stimulation in the acute treatment of major depression: A multisite randomized controlled trial. *Biological Psychiatry, 62*(11), 1208—1216.

Padberg, F., di Michele, F., Zwanzger, P., Romeo, E., Bernardi, G., Schüle, C., et al. (2002). Plasma concentrations of neuroactive steroids before and after repetitive transcranial magnetic stimulation (rTMS) in major depression. *Neuropsychopharmacology, 27* (5), 874−878.

Padberg, F., Zwanzger, P., Thoma, H., Kathmann, N., Haag, C., Greenberg, B. D., et al. (1999). Repetitive transcranial magnetic stimulation (rTMS) in pharmacotherapy-refractory major depression: Comparative study of fast, slow and sham rTMS. *Psychiatry Research, 88*(3), 163−171.

Padberg, F., Zwanzger, P., Keck, M. E., Kathmann, N., Mikhaiel, P., Ella, R., et al. (2002). Repetitive transcranial magnetic stimulation (rTMS) in major depression: Relation between efficacy and stimulation intensity. *Neuropsychopharmacology, 27*(4), 638−645.

Pallanti, S., Bernardi, S., Rollo, A. D., Antonini, S., & Quercioli, L. (2010). Unilateral low frequency versus sequential bilateral repetitive transcranial magnetic stimulation: Is simpler better for treatment of resistant depression? *Neuroscience, 167*(2), 323−328.

Pascual-Leone, A., Tarazona, F., Keenan, J., Tormos, J. M., Hamilton, R., & Catala, M. D. (1999). Transcranial magnetic stimulation and neuroplasticity. *Neuropsychologia, 37*(2), 207−217.

Pascual-Leone, A., Valls-Solé, J., Wassermann, E. M., & Hallett, M. (1994). Responses to rapid-rate transcranial magnetic stimulation of the human motor cortex. *Brain, 117*(4), 847−858.

Paulus, W. (2005). Toward establishing a therapeutic window for rTMS by theta burst stimulation. *Neuron, 45*(2), 181−183.

Paus, T., & Barrett, J. (2004). Transcranial magnetic stimulation (TMS) of the human frontal cortex: Implications for repetitive TMS treatment of depression. *Journal of Psychiatry and Neuroscience, 29*(4), 268.

Paus, T., Jech, R., Thompson, C. J., Comeau, R., Peters, T., & Evans, A. C. (1997). Transcranial magnetic stimulation during positron emission tomography: A new method for studying connectivity of the human cerebral cortex. *Journal of Neuroscience, 17*(9), 3178−3184.

Peters, E. J., Slager, S. L., Jenkins, G. D., Reinalda, M. S., Garriock, H. A., Shyn, S. I., et al. (2009). Resequencing of serotonin-related genes and association of tagging SNPS to citalopram response. *Pharmacogenetics and Genomics, 19*(1), 1−10.

Petty, F., Kramer, G. L., Gullion, C. M., & Rush, A. J. (1992). Low plasma gamma-aminobutyric acid levels in male patients with depression. *Biological Psychiatry, 32*(4), 354−363.

Pogarell, O., Koch, W., Pöpperl, G., Tatsch, K., Jakob, F., Mulert, C., et al. (2007). Acute prefrontal rTMS increases striatal dopamine to a similar degree as d-amphetamine. *Psychiatry Research, 156*(3), 251−255.

Pogarell, O., Koch, W., Pöpperl, G., Tatsch, K., Jakob, F., Zwanzger, P., et al. (2006). Striatal dopamine release after prefrontal repetitive transcranial magnetic stimulation in major depression: Preliminary results of a dynamic [123I] IBZM SPECT study. *Journal of Psychiatric Research, 40*(4), 307−314.

Post, A., & Keck, M. E. (2001). Transcranial magnetic stimulation as a therapeutic tool in psychiatry: What do we know about the neurobiological mechanisms? *Journal of Psychiatric Research, 35*(4), 193−215.

Poulet, E., Brunelin, J., Boeuve, C., Lerond, J., D'Amato, T., Dalery, J., et al. (2004). Repetitive transcranial magnetic stimulation does not potentiate antidepressant treatment. *European Psychiatry, 19*(6), 382−383.

Price, G. W., Lee, J. W., Garvey, C., & Gibson, N. (2008). Appraisal of sessional EEG features as a correlate of clinical changes in an rTMS treatment of depression. *Clinical EEG and Neuroscience, 39*(3), 131−138.

Pridmore, S., Bruno, R., Turnier-Shea, Y., Reid, P., & Rybak, M. (2000). Comparison of unlimited numbers of rapid transcranial magnetic stimulation (rTMS) and ECT treatment sessions in major depressive episode. *International Journal of Neuropsychopharmacology/Official Scientific Journal of the Collegium Internationale Neuropsychopharmacologicum (CINP)*, *3*(2), 129–134.

Ridding, M. C., & Rothwell, J. C. (2007). Is there a future for therapeutic use of transcranial magnetic stimulation? *Nature Reviews Neuroscience*, *8*(7), 559–567.

Robertson, H., & Pryor, R. (2006). Memory and cognitive effects of ECT: Informing and assessing patients. *Advances in Psychiatric Treatment*, *12*(3), 228–237.

Rosa, M. A., Gattaz, W. F., Pascual-Leone, A., Fregni, F., Rosa, M. O., Rumi, D. O., et al. (2006). Comparison of repetitive transcranial magnetic stimulation and electroconvulsive therapy in unipolar non-psychotic refractory depression: A randomized, single-blind study. *International Journal of Neuropsychopharmacology/Official Scientific Journal of the Collegium Internationale Neuropsychopharmacologicum (CINP)*, *9*(6), 667–676.

Rossi, S., Hallett, M., Rossini, P. M., & Pascual-Leone, A. The Safety of TMS Consensus Group. (2009). Safety, ethical considerations, and application guidelines for the use of transcranial magnetic stimulation in clinical practice and research. *Clinical Neurophysiology*, *120*(12), 2008–2039.

Rossini, D., Lucca, A., Zanardi, R., Magri, L., & Smeraldi, E. (2005). Transcranial magnetic stimulation in treatment-resistant depressed patients: A double-blind, placebo-controlled trial. *Psychiatry Research*, *137*(1–2), 1–10.

Rumi, D. O., Gattaz, W. F., Rigonatti, S. P., Rosa, M. A., Fregni, F., Rosa, M. O., et al. (2005). Transcranial magnetic stimulation accelerates the antidepressant effect of amitriptyline in severe depression: A double-blind placebo-controlled study. *Biological Psychiatry*, *57*(2), 162–166.

Rush, A. J., Trivedi, M. H., Wisniewski, S. R., Nierenberg, A. A., Stewart, J. W., Warden, D., et al. (2006). Acute and longer-term outcomes in depressed outpatients requiring one or several treatment steps: A STAR*D report. *American Journal of Psychiatry*, *163*(11), 1905–1917.

Schutter, D. J. (2009). Antidepressant efficacy of high-frequency transcranial magnetic stimulation over the left dorsolateral prefrontal cortex in double-blind sham-controlled designs: a meta-analysis. *Psychological Medicine*, *39*(1), 65–75.

Schutter, D. J. (2010). Quantitative review of the efficacy of slow-frequency magnetic brain stimulation in major depressive disorder. *Psychological Medicine*, doi: 7,10.1017/S003329171000005X.

Schutter, D. J., Laman, D. M., van Honk, J., Vergouwen, A. C., & Koerselman, G. F. (2009). Partial clinical response to 2 weeks of 2 Hz repetitive transcranial magnetic stimulation to the right parietal cortex in depression. *International Journal of Neuropsychopharmacology*, *12*(5), 643–650.

Shimizu, E., Hashimoto, K., Okamura, N., Koike, K., Komatsu, N., Kumakiri, C., et al. (2003). Alterations of serum levels of brain-derived neurotrophic factor (BDNF) in depressed patients with or without antidepressants. *Biological Psychiatry*, *54*(1), 70–75.

Siebner, H. R., Bergmann, T. O., Bestmann, S., Massimini, M., Johansen-Berg, H., Mochizuki, H., et al. (2009). Consensus paper: Combining transcranial stimulation with neuroimaging. *Brain Stimulation*, *2*(2), 58–80.

Speer, A. M., Benson, B. E., Kimbrell, T. K., Wassermann, E. M., Willis, M. W., Herscovitch, P., et al. (2009). Opposite effects of high and low frequency rTMS on mood in depressed patients: Relationship to baseline cerebral activity on PET. *Journal of Affective Disorders*, *115*(3), 386–394.

Speer, A. M., Kimbrell, T. A., Wassermann, E. M., D'Repella, J., Willis, M. W., Herscovitch, P., et al. (2000). Opposite effects of high and low frequency rTMS on regional brain activity in depressed patients. *Biological Psychiatry*, *48*(12), 1133–1141.

Spronk, D., Arns, M., Barnett, K. J., Cooper, N. J., & Gordon, E. (2010). An investigation of EEG, genetic and cognitive markers of treatment response to antidepressant medication in patients with major depressive disorder: A pilot study. *Journal of Affective Disorders*, doi:10.1016/j.jad.2010.06.021.

Spronk, D., Arns, M., Bootsma, A., van Ruth, R., & Fitzgerald, P. B. (2008). Long-term effects of left frontal rTMS on EEG and ERPs in patients with depression. *Clinical EEG and Neuroscience*, *39*(3), 118−124.

Strafella, A. P., Paus, T., Barrett, J., & Dagher, A. (2001). Repetitive transcranial magnetic stimulation of the human prefrontal cortex induces dopamine release in the caudate nucleus. *Journal of Neuroscience*, *21*(15), RC157.

Wassermann, E. M. (1998). Risk and safety of repetitive transcranial magnetic stimulation: Report and suggested guidelines from the international workshop on the safety of repetitive transcranial magnetic stimulation. *Electroencephalography and Clinical Neurophysiology*, *108*(1), 1−16.

Wassermann, E. M., Epstein, C. M., & Ziemann, U. (2008). *The Oxford handbook of transcranial stimulation*. New York: Oxford University Press.

Wassermann, E. M., & Lisanby, S. H. (2001). Therapeutic application of repetitive transcranial magnetic stimulation: A review. *Clinical Neurophysiology*, *112*(8), 1367−1377.

Yue, L., Xiao-Lin, H., & Tao, S. (2009). The effects of chronic repetitive transcranial magnetic stimulation on glutamate and gamma-aminobutyric acid in rat brain. *Brain Research*, *1260*(C), 94−99.

Yukimasa, T., Yoshimura, R., Tamagawa, A., Uozumi, T., Shinkai, K., Ueda, N., et al. (2006). High-frequency repetitive transcranial magnetic stimulation improves refractory depression by influencing catecholamine and brain-derived neurotrophic factors. *Pharmacopsychiatry*, *39*(2), 52−59.

Zanardi, R., Magri, L., Rossini, D., Malaguti, A., Giordani, S., Lorenzi, C., et al. (2007). Role of serotonergic gene polymorphisms on response to transcranial magnetic stimulation in depression. *European Neuropsychopharmacology*, *17*(10), 651−657.

Zanardini, R., Gazzoli, A., Ventriglia, M., Perez, J., Bignotti, S., Rossini, P. M., et al. (2006). Effect of repetitive transcranial magnetic stimulation on serum brain derived neurotrophic factor in drug resistant depressed patients. *Journal of Affective Disorders*, *91*(1), 83−86.

Zangen, A., & Hyodo, K. (2002). Transcranial magnetic stimulation induces increases in extracellular levels of dopamine and glutamate in the nucleus accumbens. *Neuroreport*, *13*(18), 2401−2405.

Zangen, A., Roth, Y., Voller, B., & Hallett, M. (2005). Transcranial magnetic stimulation of deep brain regions: Evidence for efficacy of the H-coil. *Clinical Neurophysiology*, *116*(4), 775−779.

Zou, Y. F., Ye, D. Q., Feng, X. L., Su, H., Pan, F. M., & Liao, F. F. (2010). Meta-analysis of BDNF val66met polymorphism association with treatment response in patients with major depressive disorder. *European Neuropsychopharmacology*, *20*(8), 535−544.

CHAPTER 11

Transcranial Magnetic Stimulation for Tinnitus

Berthold Langguth[1] and Dirk de Ridder[2]

[1]Department of Psychiatry and Psychotherapy and Tinnitus Clinic, University of Regensburg, Regensburg, Germany
[2]TRI Tinnitus Clinic, BRAI²N and Department of Neurosurgery, University of Antwerp, Antwerp, Belgium

Contents

TINNITUS: INTRODUCTION

Tinnitus refers to a condition in which a patient has a hearing percept that can take the form of ringing, buzzing, roaring or hissing (among others) in the absence of an external sound (Eggermont, 2007; A. R. Moller, 2007b). Tinnitus can be classified as being either objective or subjective. In the objective form, which is rare, a real sound is generated by an internal biological source, reaching the ear through conduction in body tissues. The source can be vascular turbulence, pulsations or spasm of the muscles in the middle ear, Eustachian tube or soft palate. Unlike subjective tinnitus, an observer, using a stethoscope, can often hear objective tinnitus. Subjective tinnitus refers to a phantom auditory sensation for which no objective sound can be identified and only the person who has the tinnitus can hear it. Some patients perceive the phantom sound as

Neurofeedback and Neuromodulation Techniques and Applications
DOI: 10.1016/B978-0-12-382235-2.00011-1
293

coming from inside the ear, others report that the phantom sound is located inside the head, while a few perceive the phantom sound as coming from outside the head. Some patients experience bilateral tinnitus, while others hear it in just one ear. Subjective tinnitus is by far more prevalent than objective tinnitus and is the subject of this present chapter.

Subjective tinnitus is often associated with a lesion of the peripheral auditory system, such as presbyacusis, Menière's disease, noise trauma, sudden deafness or drug-related ototoxicity (Eggermont, 2007). However these pathologies are not directly causing tinnitus. Rather the neuroplastic changes that occur in the brain as reaction to sensory deafferentation represent the neural correlate of tinnitus (A. R. Moller, 2007a). Thus, the mechanisms involved in tinnitus generation share similarities with those responsible for phantom pain after limb amputation (A. R. Moller, 2007a).

With a prevalence of 10% in the adult population, tinnitus is a very common symptom (Axelsson & Ringdahl, 1989). Approximately 1 percent of the population is severely affected by tinnitus with major negative impacts on quality of life (Axelsson & Ringdahl, 1989). Severe tinnitus is frequently associated with depression, anxiety, and insomnia (Cronlein, Langguth, Geisler, & Hajak, 2007; Dobie, 2003; Langguth et al., 2007) and is very difficult to treat (Dobie, 1999). The most frequently used therapy techniques consist of auditory stimulation and cognitive behavioral treatment that improve habituation and coping strategies. However, more causally oriented treatment strategies are missing. Therefore, new treatment strategies need to be developed, which directly act on the pathophysiological mechanisms that cause the auditory phantom perception phenomenon.

Even if the pathophysiology of the different forms of tinnitus is still incompletely understood, there is growing consensus in the neuroscientific community that chronic tinnitus as an auditory phantom perception might be the correlate of maladaptive attempts of the brain at reorganization due to distorted sensory input (A. R. Moller, 2007a).

In animal models a large variety of neuroplastic changes have been demonstrated after sensory deafferentation, including an increased neuronal firing rate, increased neural synchronicity, and alterations of the tonotopic map (Eggermont, 2007). These findings are paralleled by results from functional imaging and electrophysiological studies in tinnitus patients where functional and structural alterations in the central auditory system have been observed. Both positron emission tomography (PET) (Arnold, Bartenstein, Oestreicher, Romer, & Schwaiger, 1996; Giraud et al., 1999; Lanting, de Kleine, & van Dijk, 2009; Lockwood et al.,

1999; Lockwood et al., 2000) and functional magnetic resonance imaging (fMRI) (Lanting et al., 2009; Melcher, Sigalovsky, Guinan, & Levine, 2000; Smits et al., 2007) have demonstrated changes of neuronal activity in central auditory pathways in tinnitus patients. Electroencephalography (EEG) and magnetoencephalography (MEG) data have shown a reduction of alpha power and an increase in slow waves and in gamma activity in auditory areas (Llinas, Ribary, Jeanmonod, Kronberg, & Mitra, 1999; Lorenz, Muller, Schlee, Hartmann, & Weisz, 2009; van der Loo et al., 2009; Weisz et al., 2007). The model of thalamocortical dysrhythmia, which has been elaborated by Llinas and colleagues (Llinas, Urbano, Leznik, Ramirez, & van Marle, 2005; Llinas et al., 1999), provides an explanation for the findings in tinnitus patients. According to this model, thalamic deafferentiation from auditory input, e.g. due to hearing loss, may produce slow theta-frequency oscillations in thalamocortical ensembles due to changes in firing patterns of thalamic relay cells. As a consequence, reduced lateral inhibition at the cortical level is thought to generate high-frequency activity in the gamma band that could be the neuronal correlate of the tinnitus percept (Llinas et al., 2005, 2009). This increased synchronized firing in the gamma band together with decreased lateral inhibition after deafferentation may induce cortical reorganization via a simple Hebbian mechanisms (Eggermont & Roberts, 2004) and neural plasticity which finally results in alterations of the tonotopic map. Such a shift in the tonotopic map has been demonstrated at the tinnitus frequency by magnetic source imaging (Muhlnickel, Elbert, Taub, & Flor, 1998).

However, imaging studies in patients with impaired consciousness clearly demonstrate that activity in the auditory cortex is not sufficient for conscious auditory perception (Boly et al., 2004). Persisting connectivity with frontal and temporoparietal areas is required for conscious auditory processing. Increased activity in frontal and temporoparietal areas has been identified by functional imaging studies in tinnitus patients (Andersson et al., 2000; Giraud et al., 1999; Lockwood et al., 1998; Mirz et al., 2000; Plewnia, Reimold, Najib, Brehm et al., 2007). Based on the clinical analogies between tinnitus distress and pain distress and based on neuroimaging data it is tempting to speculate that the tinnitus distress network and the pain matrix involve similar brain structures (Moisset & Bouhassira, 2007). Unpleasantness of pain activates the anterior cingulate (Price, 2000) and orbitofrontal cortices, amygdala, hypothalamus, posterior insula, primary motor cortex, and frontal pole (Kulkarni et al., 2005). One may further speculate that the perception of tinnitus and pain intensity could be related to auditory and somatosensory cortex activation, respectively, but that the distress associated with its perception might be related to activation of a common general non-specific "distress network". This notion is supported by a recent study which demonstrates activation of this distress network during unpleasant symptoms in a somatoform disorder, even in the absence of a real physical stimulus (Landgrebe, Barta et al., 2008). Furthermore, distress due to dyspnoea in asthma activates the same network (von Leupoldt et al., 2009).

Even though no specific studies have been performed for selectively identifying neural activation underlying tinnitus distress, PET studies comparing tinnitus patients and healthy controls have demonstrated activation of brain areas such as anterior cingulate (ACC) (Plewnia, Reimold, Najib, Reischl, Plontke, & Gerloff, 2007) or the anterior insula (Lockwood et al., 1998).

Synchronization analysis based on MEG data has shown that functional connectivity between ACC and right frontal lobe is correlated to tinnitus intrusiveness, a measure of tinnitus distress (Schlee, Weisz, Bertrand, Hartmann, & Elbert, 2008). A recent MEG study looking at phase-locked connectivity in the tinnitus network suggests that the tinnitus network changes over time (Schlee, Hartmann, Langguth, & Weisz, 2009). In patients with a tinnitus history of less than 4 years, the left temporal cortex was predominant in the gamma network whereas in patients with tinnitus duration of more than 4 years the gamma network was more widely distributed, including more frontal and parietal regions (Schlee, Hartmann et al., 2009).

Even if the central auditory system has been the primary focus of interest of neurobiological tinnitus research, theoretical considerations, pathophysiological models of tinnitus (Jastreboff, 1990; Jastreboff, Brennan, & Sasaki, 1988; Moller, 1994, 2003) and neuroimaging data (Giraud et al., 1999; Lockwood et al., 1998, 1999; Mirz et al., 2000; Plewnia, Reimold, Najib, Brehm et al., 2007) all support critical involvement of non-auditory brain areas in the pathophysiology of chronic tinnitus.

TRANSCRANIAL MAGNETIC STIMULATION

In 1985 Barker and colleagues demonstrated that it is possible to depolarize neurons in the brain using external magnetic stimulation (Barker, Jalinous, & Freeston, 1985).

The stimulator delivers a short-lasting (100–300 μs) high current pulse in an insulated coil of wire, which is placed above the skull over the region of particular interest. This induces a magnetic field (1.5–2 Tesla) perpendicular to the coil which penetrates the scalp and brain with little impedance. An electrical field is induced perpendicular to the magnetic field resulting in neuronal depolarization of the underlying brain area. Magnetic coils can have different shapes. Round coils are relatively powerful. Figure-eight-shaped coils are more focal with a maximal current at the intersection of the two round components (Ridding & Rothwell, 1997). Due to the strong decline of the magnetic field with increasing distance from the coil, direct stimulation effects are limited to superficial cortical areas. However, stimulation effects can be propagated to functionally connected remote areas.

Whereas single magnetic pulses do not seem to have longer-lasting effects, the application of multiple pulses in rhythmic sessions, called repetitive transcranial magnetic stimulation (rTMS), can have effects that outlast the stimulation period. These effects resemble those seen in animal experiments where repeated stimulation of many pathways has been shown to produce changes in the effectiveness of synapses in the same circuits (Post & Keck, 2001). Low frequency (≤ 1 Hz) rTMS has been repeatedly shown to result in a decrease in cortical excitability (Hallett, 2000; Hoffman & Cavus, 2002), whereas high-frequency (5–20 Hz) rTMS results in an increase in excitability (Pascual-Leone, Grafman, & Hallett, 1994). Low-frequency and high-frequency TMS of the auditory cortex have been linked to long-term potentiation and long-term depression (LTP and LTD) respectively (Wang, Wang, & Scheich, 1996), which are thought to be important in learning and memory (Wang et al., 1996).

rTMS can also be used to transiently disturb on-going neural activity in the stimulated cortical area, thus creating a transient functional lesion. Such an approach can help to identify whether a given brain area is critically involved in a specific behavioral task.

Because of these unique and powerful features, rTMS became increasingly popular in various fields, including cognitive neuroscience and clinical application (for review see Simons & Dierick, 2005; Walsh & Rushworth, 1999). However, despite its utility, the exact mechanisms of how rTMS stimulates neurons and interferes with neural functions are still incompletely understood (Ridding & Rothwell, 1997).

Rationale for the Use of Neuromodulation in Investigation, Diagnosis, and Treatment of Tinnitus

As described before, the phantom perception of sound seems to be a consequence of altered activity in the central nervous system. An increasing number of animal and human studies have contributed to a more and more detailed identification of the neural correlate of tinnitus. In short, alterations of neural firing and oscillatory activity (Llinas et al., 1999, 2005; van der Loo et al., 2009; Weisz et al., 2007), alterations of neural synchrony (Seki & Eggermont, 2003) and changes in the tonotopic maps (Muhlnickel et al., 1998) have been observed. These changes are not restricted to one specific brain area. Rather they can be conceived as alterations of a network involving auditory and non-auditory brain areas (Schlee et al., 2008; Schlee, Hartmann et al., 2009; Schlee, Mueller, Hartmann, Keil, Lorenz, & Weisz, 2009). These changes of neural activity seem to arise from dysfunctional plastic responses to altered sensory input, which is auditory deprivation in most cases (Norena, Micheyl, Chery-Croze, & Collet, 2002; Norena & Eggermont, 2005, 2006). Frontal and parietal brain areas seem to have an important modulatory role (Lockwood et al., 1998; Schlee, Hartmann et al., 2009). However, neuroimaging studies represent only a correlative approach with its inherent limitations. Thus it remains unclear whether the observed alterations are critically involved in the pathophysiology or whether they represent epiphenomena. Interfering with neural activity in these regions with single sessions of rTMS can be used as a non-invasive test to probe their relevance for the pathophysiology of tinnitus (Plewnia, Bartels, & Gerloff, 2003). This method can potentially also be further developed as a diagnostic test to differentiate pathophysiologically distinct forms of tinnitus.

Any causally oriented therapy of tinnitus should aim at normalizing the tinnitus-related disturbed neuronal network activity. In principle there are two possibilities. The first approach consists of restoring the disturbed auditory input to the auditory cortex. This can be done indirectly by hearing aids (Moffat et al., 2009), cochlear (Brackmann, 1981; Van de Heyning et al., 2008), auditory nerve (Holm, Staal, Mooij, & Albers, 2005), and brainstem implants (Soussi & Otto, 1994) which have all been shown to improve tinnitus in selected patients. Another option is to supply the missing information directly to the auditory cortex (De Ridder & Van de Heyning, 2007) or to interfere with the distributed "tinnitus network" directly. This can be done at the auditory cortex by implanted electrodes (De Ridder, De Mulder, Menovsky, Sunaert, & Kovacs, 2007; De Ridder, De Mulder, Verstraeten et al., 2007; De Ridder et al., 2006; De Ridder et al., 2004; Friedland et al., 2007; Seidman et al., 2008), tDCS (Fregni et al., 2006; Vanneste et al., 2010) or rTMS (De Ridder et al., 2005; Khedr, Rothwell, & El-Atar, 2009; Kleinjung et al., 2005;

Londero, Langguth, De Ridder, Bonfils, & Lefaucheur, 2006) or potentially at other hubs of the distributed "tinnitus network" (Schlee, Hartmann et al., 2009; Schlee, Mueller et al., 2009), or combined (Kleinjung, Vielsmeier, Landgrebe, Hajak, & Langguth, 2008). Also neurofeedback has been proposed to normalize pathological oscillatory activity directly (EEG-based) (Dohrmann, Weisz, Schlee, Hartmann, & Elbert, 2007) or indirectly (fMRI-based) (Haller, Birbaumer, & Veit, 2010). Whereas stimulation by implanted electrodes or pharmacotherapy can be performed permanently, rTMS, tDCS or neurofeedback can only be applied for a limited amount of time. Nevertheless these methods hold therapeutic potential, since all of them can induce plastic changes which outlast the treatment period (Allen, Pasley, Duong, & Freeman, 2007; Wang et al., 1996). These long-lasting effects with limited treatment time can be either explained by learning-like effects, or by the disruption of dysfunctional networks, which then allow the re-establishment of a more physiological state.

Single Sessions of rTMS

Within the last years several studies with single sessions of rTMS have been performed with the goal to transiently reduce tinnitus perception (see Table 11.1). In these types of studies, results were largely based on the administration of high-frequency rTMS (10—20 Hz). In a pilot trial, stimulation of the left temporoparietal cortex with high-frequency rTMS (10 Hz) resulted in a transient reduction of tinnitus in 57% of the participants (Plewnia et al., 2003). This result has been confirmed in a large series of 114 patients with unilateral tinnitus (De Ridder et al., 2005). rTMS at frequencies between 1 and 20 Hz was applied over the auditory cortex contralateral to the site of tinnitus perception. Better tinnitus suppression was achieved with higher stimulation frequencies and shorter tinnitus duration, indicating the potential of TMS as a diagnostic tool for differentiating different forms of chronic tinnitus. Single TMS sessions have also been used as a screening method to select patients for surgical implantation of cortical electrodes (De Ridder, De Mulder, Menovsky et al., 2007; De Ridder et al., 2006; De Ridder, De Mulder, Verstraeten et al., 2007).

Two studies (Folmer, Carroll, Rahim, Shi, & Hal Martin, 2006; Fregni et al., 2006) confirmed the result of transient tinnitus reduction after high-frequency stimulation of the left temporoparietal cortex,

Table 11.1 Effects of single sessions of rTMS on tinnitus

Authors	Stimulation site	Coil positioning	Frequency	Intensity	Pulses/ session	Control condition	Results
Plewnia et al., 2003	Various scalp positions	10–20 EEG system	10 Hz	120% MT	30	Stimulation of non-auditory cortical areas	In 8 patients (58%) tinnitus suppression after left temporal/ temporoparietal stimulation
De Ridder et al., 2005	Auditory cortex contralateral to tinnitus site	Anatomical landmarks	1, 5, 10, 20 Hz	90% MT	200	Coil angulation	In 60 patients (53%) good or partial tinnitus suppression after active rTMS, in 33% suppression after sham rTMS
Fregni et al., 2006	Left temporoparietal areas	10–20 EEG system	10 Hz	120% MT	30	Sham coil and active stimulation of mesial parietal cortex	In 3 patients (42%) tinnitus suppression after left temporoparietal stimulation, no effect for both control rTMS conditions
Folmer et al., 2006	Left and right temporal cortex	10–20 EEG system	10 Hz	100% MT	150	Sham coil	In 6 patients (40%) tinnitus suppression after active rTMS, in four of the patients after contralateral rTMS in two patient after ipsilateral TMS; in

Study	Target	Navigation	Frequency	Intensity	Pulses	Control	Results
							2 patients suppression after sham rTMS
Londero et al., 2006	Contralateral auditory cortex	fMRI-guided neuronavigation	1, 10 Hz	120% MT	30	Stimulation over non-auditory cortical areas	8 patients were stimulated over the auditory cortex with 1 Hz ; in 5 of them (62.5%) tinnitus suppression; no suppression after 1 Hz rTMS of non-auditory targets; no suppression after 10 Hz, in 2 patients suppression after stimulation of a control position
Plewnia et al., 2007	Area of maximum tinnitus-related PET activation (temporoparietal cortex),	Neuronavigational system, based on H_2O PET with and without lidocaine	1 Hz	120% MT	300, 900, 1800	Control position (occipital cortex)	In 6 patients (75%) tinnitus reduction after active rTMS, better suppression with more pulses
De Ridder et al., 2007	Auditory cortex contralateral to tinnitus site	Anatomical landmarks	5, 10, 20 Hz tonic; 5, 10, 20 Hz burst	90% MT	200	Coil angulation	14 placebo-negative patients were analyzed: In those with narrow band/white noise tinnitus burst TMS was more effective in tinnitus suppression as compared to tonic

(Continued)

Table 11.1 (Continued)

Authors	Stimulation site	Coil positioning	Frequency	Intensity	Pulses/ session	Control condition	Results
							TMS, whereas for pure tone tinnitus no difference was found between burst and tonic
Poreisz et al., 2009	Inferior temporal cortex	10–20 EEG electrode system, T3	Continuous theta burst, intermittent theta burst, immediate theta burst	80% MT	600	No placebo condition	Significant tinnitus reduction only for continuous theta burst immediately after stimulation
Meeus et al., 2009	Auditory cortex contralateral to tinnitus site	Anatomical landmarks	1, 5, 10, 20 Hz tonic; 5, 10, 20 Hz burst	50% maximal stimulator output (independently of individual MT)	200	Coil angulation	No difference between tonic and burst rTMS in pure tone tinnitus (about 50% average suppression in unilateral and 30% in bilateral tinnitus). For bilateral narrow band tinnitus superiority of burst stimulation compared to tonic stimulation; better effects in patients with lower MT

MT = Motor threshold.

whereas one study (Londero et al., 2006) demonstrated reliable tinnitus suppression in only 1 out of 13 subjects after a single session of high frequency rTMS. Additionally, in one small study it has been shown that the participants with significant tinnitus reduction after rTMS also had good response to anodal transcranial direct current stimulation (tDCS) (Fregni et al., 2006). In order to try to improve TMS results, PET scans have been used to determine the stimulation target, based on changes of cerebral blood flow before and after lidocaine injection (Plewnia, Reimold, Najib, Brehm et al., 2007): single sessions of low frequency (1 Hz) rTMS with the coil navigated to the individually determined areas in the temporoparietal cortex resulted in tinnitus reduction in 6 out of 8 patients lasting up to 30 minutes.

Repeated Sessions of rTMS in Tinnitus

The application of low-frequency rTMS in repeated sessions was motivated by positive results of 1 Hz rTMS in the treatment of auditory hallucinations and other neuropsychiatric disorders characterized by focal hyperexcitability (Hoffman & Cavus, 2002). In the temporal cortex of rodents the induction of LTD- and LTP-like effects had been demonstrated (Wang et al., 1996) and in humans low-frequency rTMS reliably reduced cortical excitability in the motor cortex (Chen et al., 1997) and in the frontal cortex (Speer et al., 2001). Based on these data, low-frequency rTMS has been proposed for achieving longer-lasting improvement of tinnitus complaints by reducing auditory cortex hyperactivity (Eichhammer, Langguth, Marienhagen, Kleinjung, & Hajak, 2003; Langguth et al., 2003). An increasing amount of studies using this approach as a treatment for tinnitus have been published (Table 11.2). Most rTMS treatment studies applied low-frequency rTMS in long trains of 1200−2000 pulses repeatedly over 5−10 days. In all controlled studies a statistically significant improvement of tinnitus complaints has been documented. However, the quantity of improvement and also the duration of treatment effects varied across studies, probably due to differences in study design, stimulation parameters and patient populations.

Repetitive TMS has been applied over temporal or temporoparietal areas. In the first clinical study to verify whether low-frequency rTMS could induce long-lasting effects, [18F]deoxyglucose (FDG) PET was performed in 14 patients and a neuronavigational system allowed the positioning of the TMS coil exactly over the site of maximum activation in

Table 11.2 Effects of repeated sessions of rTMS in tinnitus patients

Authors	Stimulation site	Coil positioning	Frequency	Intensity	Sessions	Pulses/ session	Design	Control condition	Results
Kleinjung et al., 2005	Area of maximum PET activation in the temporal cortex (12 left, 2 right)	Neuro-navigational system, based on FDG-PET	1 Hz	110% MT	5	2000	Sham-controlled, crossover	Sham coil	Significant reduction of tinnitus after active rTMS as compared to sham rTMS; lasting tinnitus reduction (6 months)
Langguth et al., 2006	Left auditory cortex,	10–20 EEG system	1 Hz	110% MT	10	2000	Open	No control condition	Significant reduction of tinnitus until end of follow-up (3 months)
Plewnia et al., 2007	Area of maximum tinnitus related PET activation (temporoparietal cortex; 3 left, 3 right)	Neuro-navigational system, based on H_2O PET with and without lidocaine	1 Hz	120% MT	10	1800	Sham-controlled, crossover	Occipital cortex	Significant reduction of tinnitus after active rTMS, as compared to the control condition; no lasting effects
Kleinjung et al., 2007	Left auditory cortex	Neuro-navigational system, based on structural MRI	1 Hz	110% MT	10	2000	Open	No control condition	Significant tinnitus reduction after rTMS, lasting up during follow-up period (3 months) responders were characterized by shorter tinnitus duration and less hearing impairment
Rossi et al., 2007	Left secondary auditory cortex	8 patients: neuronavigational system 8 patients: according to 10–20 EEG system, halfway	1 Hz	120% MT	5	1200	Sham-controlled, crossover	Coil angulation + electrical stimulation of facial nerve	Significant reduction of tinnitus after active rTMS, as compared to the control condition, no lasting effects

Study	Coil localization	Stimulation frequency	Intensity	Sessions	Pulses	Study design	Control/comment	Outcome
Smith et al., 2007	Area of maximal PET activation in the temporal cortex, neuronavigational system	Neuro-navigational system, based on FDG-PET	1 Hz	110% MT	5	1800	Sham-controlled, crossover	Coil angulation between T3 and C3/T5	Modest response to active treatment in 3 patients (75%)
Khedr et al., 2008	Left temporoparietal cortex	10–20 EEG system	1 Hz, 10 Hz, 25 Hz	100% MT	10	1500	Sham-controlled, parallel group design	Occipital cortex	Significant reduction of tinnitus after all three active rTMS conditions, as compared to the control condition; tinnitus reduction lasting during follow-up period (4 months and 12 months)
Langguth et al., 2008	Left auditory cortex	Neuro-navigational system, based on structural MRI	1 Hz, 6 Hz + 1 Hz	110% MT (90% MT for 6 Hz rTMS)	10	2000	Randomization between two active treatment conditions, parallel group design	No sham control condition	Significant improvement for both stimulation conditions, no difference between conditions, no lasting effects
Lee et al., 2008	Left temporoparietal cortex	??	0.5 Hz	100% MT	5	600	Open study	No control condition	No significant reduction of tinnitus
				10	2000			

(Continued)

Table 11.2 (Continued)

Authors	Stimulation site	Coil positioning	Frequency	Intensity	Sessions	Pulses/ session	Design	Control condition	Results
Kleinjung et al., 2008	Left auditory cortex; left dorsolateral prefrontal cortex	Neuro-navigational system, based on structural MRI	1 Hz, 20 Hz (DLPFC) + 1 Hz	110% MT			Two active treatment conditions, parallel group design	No sham control condition	Directly after stimulation significant improvement for both stimulation conditions, at 3 month follow-up significantly better results for the combined frontal and temporal stimulation
Kleinjung et al., 2009	Left auditory cortex	Neuro-navigational system, based on structural MRI	1 Hz, 1 Hz + Levodopa	110% MT	10	2000	Randomization between two active treatment conditions, parallel group design	No sham control condition	Significant improvement for both stimulation conditions, no difference between conditions, no lasting effects
Marcondes et al., 2010	Left temporoparietal cortex	10–20 EEG system	1 Hz	110% MT	5	1020	Sham controlled, parallel group design	Sham coil	Significant improvement after active rTMS but not after sham rTMS, beneficial treatment effects still detectable at 6 months follow-up
Frank et al., 2010	Left temporal	10–20 EEG system	1 Hz	110% MT	10	2000	Open	No control condition	Significant tinnitus reduction after rTMS in patients with unilateral leftsided and bilateral tinnitus, but not in rightsided tinnitus, effects lasting up during follow-up period (3 months)

MT = Motor threshold.

the auditory cortex (Kleinjung et al., 2005). After active treatment, a significant decrease in the score of the Tinnitus Questionnaire was observed, whereas sham treatment showed no effect. Treatment effects were still detectable 6 months after treatment. Another study investigated the effects of 2 weeks of rTMS applied over the area of maximum lidocaine-related activity change as determined by $[^{15}O]H_2O$ PET (Plewnia, Reimold, Najib, Brehm et al., 2007). This approach also resulted in moderate, but significant effects after active stimulation. Since PET scans are not readily available, easier applicable techniques have been proposed for determining coil localization, based on the 10−20 EEG coordinate system. This approach also has resulted in a significant reduction of tinnitus severity after 10 sessions of 1 Hz rTMS (Langguth et al., 2006). Beneficial effects of low frequency rTMS have been confirmed by several further controlled studies (Marcondes et al., 2010; Rossi et al., 2007; Smith et al., 2007). One study (Rossi et al., 2007) used peripheral electrical stimulation as a control condition and thus demonstrated that the reduction of tinnitus is not mediated by somatosensory afferents, but by cortical stimulation. Subsequently a study was performed using functional imaging (FDG PET) before and after rTMS (Smith et al., 2007). They demonstrated in their small sample that a clinical reduction after rTMS was paralleled by reduced metabolic activity in the stimulated area. Changes of brain activity also were demonstrated after rTMS in another study (Marcondes et al., 2010), but these changes were not exactly in the stimulated area, rather in the left inferior temporal lobe, a sensory integration area. Interestingly, this study revealed 6 months' long-lasting effects after only five stimulation sessions, which might be due to the fact that only tinnitus patients with normal audiograms were included, as it has been demonstrated that severe hearing loss worsens rTMS results (Kleinjung et al., 2007).

While some studies demonstrated effects that outlasted the stimulation period up to 6 or 12 months (Khedr et al., 2009; Kleinjung et al., 2005; Marcondes et al., 2010), others were not able to observe prolonged effects (Plewnia, Reimold, Najib, Reischl et al., 2007; Smith et al., 2007). The total amount of rTMS sessions may be an important variable in achieving long-term effects in tinnitus patients (Langguth et al., 2003), analogous to what has been observed in other rTMS applications such as depression (Gershon, Dannon, & Grunhaus, 2003) and auditory hallucinations (Hoffman et al., 2005).

A recent case report showed that it is possible to use maintenance rTMS to manage chronic tinnitus (Mennemeier et al., 2008). In this patient, tinnitus could be improved each time it re-occurred, by applying one to three maintenance rTMS sessions. After three maintenance rTMS sessions it finally stabilized on a low level. The positive effect of this maintenance stimulation could also be confirmed by reduced cerebral metabolism in PET imaging after treatment. The rationale for using rTMS for maintenance treatment of tinnitus relies on the fact that those patients who respond once to rTMS treatment also experience positive effects from a second series of rTMS (Langguth, Landgrebe, Hajak, & Kleinjung, 2008).

The concept of specific effects of low-frequency rTMS for reducing focal hyperexcitability has been challenged by a recent study which compared effects of 1 Hz, 10 Hz, and 25 Hz rTMS (Khedr, Rothwell, Ahmed, & El-Atar, 2008). Whereas sham rTMS treatment had no effect, active stimulation over the left temporoparietal cortex resulted in a reduction of tinnitus irrespective of the stimulation frequency. Follow-up assessment one year after treatment demonstrated a trend for higher efficiency of 10 and 25 Hz as compared to 1 Hz (Khedr et al., 2009). Experimental data from motor cortex stimulation in healthy subjects indicates that LTD-like effects induced by low-frequency rTMS can be enhanced by high-frequency priming stimulation (Iyer, Schleper, & Wassermann, 2003). However, in a clinical study high-frequency priming stimulation failed to enhance the therapeutic efficacy of low-frequency rTMS for the treatment of tinnitus (Langguth, Kleinjung et al., 2008), further indicating that the mechanisms by which rTMS affects tinnitus differ from those LTD-like effects observed after motor cortex stimulation.

Repetitive TMS can be applied in a tonic and a burst mode. The burst stimulation technique has been proposed for enhancing rTMS effects. It consists of bursts of three pulses at a frequency of 50 Hz, applied every 200 ms (5 Hz, theta burst) (Huang, Edwards, Rounis, Bhatia, & Rothwell, 2005). Burst TMS has been shown to induce more pronounced and longer-lasting effects on human motor cortex than tonic stimulation (Huang et al., 2005). Single sessions of continuous theta burst stimulation over the temporal cortex in tinnitus patients resulted in short-lasting reduction of tinnitus loudness compared to effects achieved with single sessions of tonic stimulation and other theta burst protocols had no effect at all (Poreisz, Paulus, Moser, & Lang, 2009). In two other studies single sessions of burst stimulation were compared with tonic stimulation (De Ridder, van der Loo et al., 2007a, 2007b). Burst stimulation yielded similar efficacy as tonic stimulation in patients with pure tone tinnitus, but was superior in patients with noise-like tinnitus. A possible explanation for this finding is that pure tone tinnitus may be related to increased neuronal activity in the classical (lemniscal) auditory pathways, which mainly fire tonically, whereas noise-like tinnitus may be the result of increased activity in the non-classical (extra-lemniscal) pathways, which is characterized by burst firing. A follow-up study of the same group replicated this result for bilateral tinnitus, but not for unilateral tinnitus (Meeus, Blaivie, Ost, De Ridder, & Van de Heyning, 2009). Furthermore, results of this study suggested that higher stimulation intensity may result in slightly better tinnitus suppression.

The neurobiology of chronic tinnitus suggests that neuronal changes are not limited to the auditory pathways (Lockwood et al., 1998; Schlee, Hartmann et al., 2009; Schlee, Mueller et al., 2009). Recent progress in consciousness research has demonstrated that hyperactivity within primary sensory areas alone is not sufficient for conscious tinnitus perception. Rather, synchronized co-activation of frontal and parietal areas seems to be necessary (Boly et al., 2004). This suggests that tinnitus might be an emergent property of a network, rather than just an expression of hyperactivity in the auditory cortex. Therefore it may be better to modulate more than one area involved in the tinnitus network. In one pilot study 32 patients received either low-frequency temporal rTMS or a combination of high-frequency prefrontal and low-frequency temporal rTMS (Kleinjung, Eichhammer et al., 2008). Immediately after therapy there was an improvement of the Tinnitus Questionnaire score for both groups but no differences between groups. However, after 3 months a remarkable advantage for combined prefrontal and temporal rTMS treatment was noted. These data indicate that modulation of both frontal and temporal cortex activity might represent a promising enhancement strategy for improving TMS effects in tinnitus patients.

Combination of rTMS with pharmacologic intervention also has been suggested for potentiating rTMS effects, analogous to what has been described for tDCS (Nitsche et al., 2006; Terney et al., 2008). It is known from animal experiments that neuronal plasticity can be enhanced by dopaminergic receptor activation (Otani, Blond, Desce, & Crepel, 1998). However, in a clinical pilot study the administration of 100 mg Levodopa before rTMS was not successful in enhancing rTMS effects in tinnitus patients (Kleinjung et al., 2009).

There are few prognostic factors that determine the rTMS outcome for tinnitus. Several studies reported that shorter tinnitus duration was related to better treatment outcome (De Ridder et al., 2005; Khedr et al., 2008; Kleinjung et al., 2007; Plewnia, Reimold, Najib, Brehm et al., 2007). Normal hearing was also suggested as a positive clinical predictor for good treatment response (Kleinjung et al., 2007; Marcondes et al., 2010). Interestingly, short tinnitus duration and normal hearing have been demonstrated to be positive predictors in other treatment options for tinnitus as well (De Ridder et al., 2010; M. B. Moller, Moller, Jannetta, & Jho, 1993; Ryu, Yamamoto, Sugiyama, & Nozue, 1998).

Methodological Considerations

Evaluation of treatment efficacy requires adequate methodology for control of unspecific treatment and placebo effects. The majority of controlled studies published to date have used placebo treatment in cross-over designs. Potential shortcomings of this approach include carry-over effects and missed long-term effects due to limited observation periods. Different methods have been reported to control for placebo effects. Besides the sham coil system (Kleinjung et al., 2005), which mimics the sound of the active coil without generating a magnetic field, an angulation of an active coil tilted 45° (Smith et al., 2007) or 90° (De Ridder et al., 2005; Rossi et al., 2007) to the skull surface, and stimulation of non-auditory brain areas (Plewnia, Reimold, Najib, Brehm et al., 2007) have been described. Another option is to use two coils, with the inactive coil positioned on the target and the active coil 90° perpendicular to and on top of it (Meeus, De Ridder, & Van de Heyning, 2009). This has the advantage that the sensory perception of the coil is the same (apart from the muscle contractions). Finding an optimal control condition for treatment studies is difficult due to limitations in blinding of patient and operator to different stimulus conditions, and due to the fact that TMS itself results in auditory and somatosensory stimulation in addition to its brain stimulation activity. One possible solution is a control condition that involves electrical stimulation of the facial nerve (Rossi et al., 2007). But even this method has to be considered with care as modulating the motor system can alter tinnitus perception. This has become clear with the tinnitus modulating effects of ventral intermedius nucleus stimulation performed in the setting of movement disorders (Shi, Burchiel, Anderson, & Martin, 2009).

In most studies validated tinnitus questionnaires and visual analogue scales serve as primary outcome measurements due to the lack of objective parameters. The improvement in tinnitus rating after stimulation is associated with a reduction of metabolic activity on PET scan (Smith et al., 2007). Therefore functional imaging might evolve as an objective marker of treatment effects in the future.

Safety Aspects

An extensive body of literature demonstrates that rTMS is a safe and well tolerated technique (Rossi, Hallett, Rossini, & Pascual-Leone, 2009), at least if stimulation is performed according to published safety guidelines (Rossi et al., 2009; Wassermann, 1998). Most data are available from rTMS studies in depressed subjects. In an analysis of 10 000 cumulative rTMS sessions performed for depression no deaths or seizures were encountered (Janicak et al., 2008). Most adverse events in this analysis were mild to moderate in intensity. Transient headaches and scalp discomfort were the most common adverse events. Auditory threshold and cognitive function did not change. There was a low discontinuation rate (4.5%) due to adverse events during acute treatment (Janicak et al., 2008). Another study demonstrated that after 2—4 weeks of daily prefrontal rTMS there was no sign of structural MRI changes (Nahas et al., 2000), no significant changes in auditory thresholds and no significant electroencephalogram abnormalities (Loo et al., 2001). It is essential that contraindications such as electronic implants (e.g. cardiac pacemakers, cochlea implants), intracranial pieces of metal or previous epileptic seizures are considered.

CONCLUSION

Available literature converges in the finding that rTMS seems to be a promising tool for investigating the pathophysiology of tinnitus. Data also indicate its diagnostic potential for differentiating pathophysiologically distinct forms of tinnitus.

An increasing number of clinical studies also suggest a therapeutic potential for rTMS. Even though there are now six placebo-controlled studies from six different centers, all demonstrating a beneficial effect of rTMS in equal percentages of responders, these results must be considered preliminary, due to small sample sizes, methodological hetereogeneity, and high inter-subject variability. The duration of treatment effects remains inconclusive. Effects outlasted the stimulation period up to 12 months in some studies whereas others could not demonstrate any after-effects. Replication in multicenter trials with a large number of patients and long-term follow-up are needed before further conclusions can be drawn (Landgrebe, Binder et al., 2008). Further clinical research is needed to define those subgroups of patients which benefit most from rTMS. Better understanding of the pathophysiology of the different forms of tinnitus on one side and the neurobiological effects of rTMS on the other side will be critical for optimizing and individualizing treatment protocols.

REFERENCES

Allen, E. A., Pasley, B. N., Duong, T., & Freeman, R. D. (2007). Transcranial magnetic stimulation elicits coupled neural and hemodynamic consequences. *Science*, *317*(5846), 1918−1921.

Andersson, G., Lyttkens, L., Hirvela, C., Furmark, T., Tillfors, M., & Fredrikson, M. (2000). Regional cerebral blood flow during tinnitus: A PET case study with lidocaine and auditory stimulation. *Acta Otolaryngology*, *120*(8), 967−972.

Arnold, W., Bartenstein, P., Oestreicher, E., Romer, W., & Schwaiger, M. (1996). Focal metabolic activation in the predominant left auditory cortex in patients suffering from tinnitus: A PET study with [18F]deoxyglucose. *ORL: Journal of Otorhinolaryngology and Related Specialties*, *58*(4), 195−199.

Axelsson, A., & Ringdahl, A. (1989). Tinnitus − a study of its prevalence and characteristics. *British Journal of Audiology*, *23*(1), 53−62.

Barker, A. T., Jalinous, R., & Freeston, I. L. (1985). Non-invasive magnetic stimulation of human motor cortex. *Lancet*, *1*(8437), 1106−1107.

Boly, M., Faymonville, M. E., Peigneux, P., Lambermont, B., Damas, P., Del Fiore, G., et al. (2004). Auditory processing in severely brain injured patients: Differences between the minimally conscious state and the persistent vegetative state. *Archives of Neurology*, *61*(2), 233−238.

Brackmann, D. E. (1981). Reduction of tinnitus in cochlear-implant patients. *Journal of Laryngology and Otology*, *4*(Suppl), 163−165.

Chen, R., Classen, J., Gerloff, C., Celnik, P., Wassermann, E. M., Hallett, M., et al. (1997). Depression of motor cortex excitability by low-frequency transcranial magnetic stimulation. *Neurology*, *48*(5), 1398−1403.

Cronlein, T., Langguth, B., Geisler, P., & Hajak, G. (2007). Tinnitus and insomnia. *Progress in Brain Research*, *166*, 227−233.

De Ridder, D., De Mulder, G., Menovsky, T., Sunaert, S., & Kovacs, S. (2007). Electrical stimulation of auditory and somatosensory cortices for treatment of tinnitus and pain. *Progress in Brain Research*, *166*, 377−388.

De Ridder, D., De Mulder, G., Verstraeten, E., Seidman, M., Elisevich, K., Sunaert, S., et al. (2007). Auditory cortex stimulation for tinnitus. *Acta Neurochirurgica*, *Suppl 97* (Pt 2), 451−462.

De Ridder, D., De Mulder, G., Verstraeten, E., Van der Kelen, K., Sunaert, S., Smits, M., et al. (2006). Primary and secondary auditory cortex stimulation for intractable tinnitus. *ORL: Journal of Otorhinolaryngology and Related Specialties*, *68*(1), 48−54, discussion 54-45

De Ridder, D., De Mulder, G., Walsh, V., Muggleton, N., Sunaert, S., & Moller, A. (2004). Magnetic and electrical stimulation of the auditory cortex for intractable tinnitus. Case report. *Journal of Neurosurgery*, *100*(3), 560−564.

De Ridder, D., & Van de Heyning, P. (2007). The Darwinian plasticity hypothesis for tinnitus and pain. *Progress in Brain Research*, *166*, 55−60.

De Ridder, D., van der Loo, E., Van der Kelen, K., Menovsky, T., van de Heyning, P., & Moller, A. (2007a). Do tonic and burst TMS modulate the lemniscal and extralemniscal system differentially? *International Journal of Medical Science, 4*(5), 242–246.

De Ridder, D., van der Loo, E., Van der Kelen, K., Menovsky, T., van de Heyning, P., & Moller, A. (2007b). Theta, alpha and beta burst transcranial magnetic stimulation: Brain modulation in tinnitus. *International Journal of Medical Science, 4*(5), 237–241.

De Ridder, D., Vanneste, S., Adriaenssens, I., Lee, A. P., Plazier, M., Menovsky, T., et al. (2010). Microvascular decompression for tinnitus: Significant improvement for tinnitus intensity without improvement for distress. A 4-year limit. *Neurosurgery, 66*(4), 656–660.

De Ridder, D., Verstraeten, E., Van der Kelen, K., De Mulder, G., Sunaert, S., Verlooy, J., et al. (2005). Transcranial magnetic stimulation for tinnitus: Influence of tinnitus duration on stimulation parameter choice and maximal tinnitus suppression. *Otology and Neurotology, 26*(4), 616–619.

Dobie, R. A. (1999). A review of randomized clinical trials in tinnitus. *Laryngoscope, 109*(8), 1202–1211.

Dobie, R. A. (2003). Depression and tinnitus. *Otolaryngology Clinics of North America, 36*(2), 383–388.

Dohrmann, K., Weisz, N., Schlee, W., Hartmann, T., & Elbert, T. (2007). Neurofeedback for treating tinnitus. *Progress in Brain Research, 166,* 473–485.

Eggermont, J. J. (2007). Pathophysiology of tinnitus. *Progress in Brain Research, 166,* 19–35.

Eggermont, J. J., & Roberts, L. E. (2004). The neuroscience of tinnitus. *Trends in Neuroscience, 27*(11), 676–682.

Eichhammer, P., Langguth, B., Marienhagen, J., Kleinjung, T., & Hajak, G. (2003). Neuronavigated repetitive transcranial magnetic stimulation in patients with tinnitus: A short case series. *Biological Psychiatry, 54*(8), 862–865.

Folmer, R. L., Carroll, J. R., Rahim, A., Shi, Y., & Hal Martin, W. (2006). Effects of repetitive transcranial magnetic stimulation (rTMS) on chronic tinnitus. *Acta Otolaryngology, 556*(Suppl), 96–101.

Fregni, F., Marcondes, R., Boggio, P. S., Marcolin, M. A., Rigonatti, S. P., Sanchez, T. G., et al. (2006). Transient tinnitus suppression induced by repetitive transcranial magnetic stimulation and transcranial direct current stimulation. *European Journal of Neurology, 13*(9), 996–1001.

Friedland, D. R., Gaggl, W., Runge-Samuelson, C., Ulmer, J. L., & Kopell, B. H. (2007). Feasibility of auditory cortical stimulation for the treatment of tinnitus. *Otology and Neurotology, 28*(8), 1005–1012.

Gershon, A. A., Dannon, P. N., & Grunhaus, L. (2003). Transcranial magnetic stimulation in the treatment of depression. *American Journal of Psychiatry, 160*(5), 835–845.

Giraud, A. L., Chery-Croze, S., Fischer, G., Fischer, C., Vighetto, A., Gregoire, M. C., et al. (1999). A selective imaging of tinnitus. *Neuroreport, 10*(1), 1–5.

Haller, S., Birbaumer, N., & Veit, R. (2010). Real-time fMRI feedback training may improve chronic tinnitus. *European Radiology, 20*(3), 696–703.

Hallett, M. (2000). Transcranial magnetic stimulation and the human brain. *Nature, 406*(6792), 147–150.

Hoffman, R. E., & Cavus, I. (2002). Slow transcranial magnetic stimulation, long-term depotentiation, and brain hyperexcitability disorders. *American Journal of Psychiatry, 159*(7), 1093–1102.

Hoffman, R. E., Gueorguieva, R., Hawkins, K. A., Varanko, M., Boutros, N. N., Wu, Y. T., et al. (2005). Temporoparietal transcranial magnetic stimulation for auditory hallucinations: Safety, efficacy and moderators in a fifty patient sample. *Biological Psychiatry, 58* (2), 97–104.

Holm, A. F., Staal, M. J., Mooij, J. J., & Albers, F. W. (2005). Neurostimulation as a new treatment for severe tinnitus: A pilot study. *Otology and Neurotology, 26*(3), 425–428; discussion 428.

Huang, Y. Z., Edwards, M. J., Rounis, E., Bhatia, K. P., & Rothwell, J. C. (2005). Theta burst stimulation of the human motor cortex. *Neuron, 45*(2), 201–206.

Iyer, M. B., Schleper, N., & Wassermann, E. M. (2003). Priming stimulation enhances the depressant effect of low-frequency repetitive transcranial magnetic stimulation. *Journal of Neuroscience, 23*(34), 10867–10872.

Janicak, P. G., O'Reardon, J. P., Sampson, S. M., Husain, M. M., Lisanby, S. H., Rado, J. T., et al. (2008). Transcranial magnetic stimulation in the treatment of major depressive disorder: A comprehensive summary of safety experience from acute exposure, extended exposure, and during reintroduction treatment. *Journal of Clinical Psychiatry, 69*(2), 222–232.

Jastreboff, P. J. (1990). Phantom auditory perception (tinnitus): Mechanisms of generation and perception. *Neuroscience Research, 8*(4), 221–254.

Jastreboff, P. J., Brennan, J. F., & Sasaki, C. T. (1988). An animal model for tinnitus. *Laryngoscope, 98*(3), 280–286.

Khedr, E. M., Rothwell, J. C., Ahmed, M. A., & El-Atar, A. (2008). Effect of daily repetitive transcranial magnetic stimulation for treatment of tinnitus: Comparison of different stimulus frequencies. *Journal of Neurology, Neurosurgery and Psychiatry, 79*(2), 212–215.

Khedr, E. M., Rothwell, J. C., & El-Atar, A. (2009). One-year follow up of patients with chronic tinnitus treated with left temporoparietal rTMS. *European Journal of Neurology, 16*(3), 404–408.

Kleinjung, T., Eichhammer, P., Landgrebe, M., Sand, P., Hajak, G., Steffens, T., et al. (2008). Combined temporal and prefrontal transcranial magnetic stimulation for tinnitus treatment: A pilot study. *Otolaryngology, Head and Neck Surgery, 138*(4), 497–501.

Kleinjung, T., Eichhammer, P., Langguth, B., Jacob, P., Marienhagen, J., Hajak, G., et al. (2005). Long-term effects of repetitive transcranial magnetic stimulation (rTMS) in patients with chronic tinnitus. *Otolaryngology, Head and Neck Surgery, 132*(4), 566–569.

Kleinjung, T., Steffens, T., Landgrebe, M., Vielsmeier, V., Frank, E., Hajak, G., et al. (2009). Levodopa does not enhance the effect of low-frequency repetitive transcranial magnetic stimulation in tinnitus treatment. *Otolaryngology Head and Neck Surgery, 140* (1), 92–95.

Kleinjung, T., Steffens, T., Sand, P., Murthum, T., Hajak, G., Strutz, J., et al. (2007). Which tinnitus patients benefit from transcranial magnetic stimulation? *Otolaryngology, Head and Neck Surgery, 137*(4), 589–595.

Kleinjung, T., Vielsmeier, V., Landgrebe, M., Hajak, G., & Langguth, B. (2008). Transcranial magnetic stimulation: A new diagnostic and therapeutic tool for tinnitus patients. *International Tinnitus Journal, 14*(2), 112–118.

Kulkarni, B., Bentley, D. E., Elliott, R., Youell, P., Watson, A., Derbyshire, S. W., et al. (2005). Attention to pain localization and unpleasantness discriminates the functions of the medial and lateral pain systems. *European Journal of Neuroscience, 21*(11), 3133–3142.

Landgrebe, M., Barta, W., Rosengarth, K., Frick, U., Hauser, S., Langguth, B., et al. (2008). Neuronal correlates of symptom formation in functional somatic syndromes: A fMRI study. *Neuroimage, 41*(4), 1336–1344.

Landgrebe, M., Binder, H., Koller, M., Eberl, Y., Kleinjung, T., Eichhammer, P., et al. (2008). Design of a placebo-controlled, randomized study of the efficacy of repetitive transcranial magnetic stimulation for the treatment of chronic tinntius. *BMC Psychiatry, 8,* 23.

Langguth, B., Eichhammer, P., Wiegand, R., Marienhegen, J., Maenner, P., Jacob, P., et al. (2003). Neuronavigated rTMS in a patient with chronic tinnitus. Effects of 4 weeks treatment. *Neuroreport, 14*(7), 977—980.

Langguth, B., Kleinjung, T., Fischer, B., Hajak, G., Eichhammer, P., & Sand, P. G. (2007). Tinnitus severity, depression, and the big five personality traits. *Progress in Brain Research, 166,* 221—225.

Langguth, B., Kleinjung, T., Frank, E., Landgrebe, M., Sand, P., Dvorakova, J., et al. (2008). High-frequency priming stimulation does not enhance the effect of low-frequency rTMS in the treatment of tinnitus. *Experimental Brain Research, 184*(4), 587—591.

Langguth, B., Landgrebe, M., Hajak, G., & Kleinjung, T. (2008). Re: Maintenance repetitive transcranial magnetic stimulation can inhibit the return of tinnitus. *Laryngoscope, 118*(12), 2264; author reply 2264-2265.

Langguth, B., Zowe, M., Landgrebe, M., Sand, P., Kleinjung, T., Binder, H., et al. (2006). Transcranial magnetic stimulation for the treatment of tinnitus: A new coil positioning method and first results. *Brain Topography, 18*(4), 241—247.

Lanting, C. P., de Kleine, E., & van Dijk, P. (2009). Neural activity underlying tinnitus generation: Results from PET and fMRI. *Hearing Research, 255*(1-2), 1—13.

Llinas, R., Urbano, F. J., Leznik, E., Ramirez, R. R., & van Marle, H. J. (2005). Rhythmic and dysrhythmic thalamocortical dynamics: GABA systems and the edge effect. *Trends in Neuroscience, 28*(6), 325—333.

Llinas, R. R., Ribary, U., Jeanmonod, D., Kronberg, E., & Mitra, P. P. (1999). Thalamocortical dysrhythmia: A neurological and neuropsychiatric syndrome characterized by magnetoencephalography. *Proceedings of the National Academy of Sciences of the U S A, 96*(26), 15 222—15 227.

Lockwood, A. H., Salvi, R. J., Burkard, R. F., Galantowicz, P. J., Coad, M. L., & Wack, D. S. (1999). Neuroanatomy of tinnitus. *Scandinavian Audiology, 51*(Suppl), 47—52.

Lockwood, A. H., Salvi, R. J., Coad, M. L., Towsley, M. L., Wack, D. S., & Murphy, B. W. (1998). The functional neuroanatomy of tinnitus: Evidence for limbic system links and neural plasticity. *Neurology, 50*(1), 114—120.

Londero, A., Langguth, B., De Ridder, D., Bonfils, P., & Lefaucheur, J. P. (2006). Repetitive transcranial magnetic stimulation (rTMS): A new therapeutic approach in subjective tinnitus? *Neurophysiology Clinics, 36*(3), 145—155.

Loo, C., Sachdev, P., Elsayed, H., McDarmont, B., Mitchell, P., Wilkinson, M., et al. (2001). Effects of a 2- to 4-week course of repetitive transcranial magnetic stimulation (rTMS) on neuropsychologic functioning, electroencephalogram, and auditory threshold in depressed patients. *Biological Psychiatry, 49*(7), 615—623.

Lorenz, I., Muller, N., Schlee, W., Hartmann, T., & Weisz, N. (2009). Loss of alpha power is related to increased gamma synchronization-A marker of reduced inhibition in tinnitus? *Neuroscience Letters, 453*(3), 225—228.

Marcondes, R. A., Sanchez, T. G., Kii, M. A., Ono, C. R., Buchpiguel, C. A., Langguth, B., et al. (2010). Repetitive transcranial magnetic stimulation improve tinnitus in normal hearing patients: A double-blind controlled, clinical and neuroimaging outcome study. *European Journal of Neurology, 17*(1), 38—44.

Meeus, O., Blaivie, C., Ost, J., De Ridder, D., & Van de Heyning, P. (2009). Influence of tonic and burst transcranial magnetic stimulation characteristics on acute inhibition of subjective tinnitus. *Otology and Neurotology, 30*(6), 697—703.

Meeus, O. M., De Ridder, D., & Van de Heyning, P. H. (2009). Transcranial magnetic stimulation (TMS) in tinnitus patients. *B-ENT, 5*(2), 89—100.

Melcher, J. R., Sigalovsky, I. S., Guinan, J. J., Jr., & Levine, R. A. (2000). Lateralized tinnitus studied with functional magnetic resonance imaging: Abnormal inferior colliculus activation. *Journal of Neurophysiology, 83*(2), 1058—1072.

Mennemeier, M., Chelette, K. C., Myhill, J., Taylor-Cooke, P., Bartel, T., Triggs, W., et al. (2008). Maintenance repetitive transcranial magnetic stimulation can inhibit the return of tinnitus. *Laryngoscope, 118*(7), 1228–1232.

Mirz, F., Gjedde, A., Ishizu, K., & Pedersen, C. B. (2000). Cortical networks subserving the perception of tinnitus – a PET study. *Acta Otolaryngology, 543*(Suppl), 241–243.

Moffat, G., Adjout, K., Gallego, S., Thai-Van, H., Collet, L., & Norena, A. J. (2009). Effects of hearing aid fitting on the perceptual characteristics of tinnitus. *Hearing Research, 254*(1-2), 82–91.

Moisset, X., & Bouhassira, D. (2007). Brain imaging of neuropathic pain. *Neuroimage, 37*(Suppl 1), S80–88.

Moller, A. (1994). Tinnitus. In R. Jackler, & D. Brackmann (Eds.), *Neurotology* (pp. 153–166). St Louis, MO: Mosby.

Moller, A. R. (2003). Pathophysiology of tinnitus. *Otolaryngology Clinics of North America, 36*(2), 249–266, v-vi

Moller, A. R. (2007a). The role of neural plasticity in tinnitus. *Progress in Brain Research, 166*, 37–45.

Moller, A. R. (2007b). Tinnitus: Presence and future. *Progress in Brain Research, 166*, 3–16.

Moller, M. B., Moller, A. R., Jannetta, P. J., & Jho, H. D. (1993). Vascular decompression surgery for severe tinnitus: Selection criteria and results. *Laryngoscope, 103*(4 Pt 1), 421–427.

Muhlnickel, W., Elbert, T., Taub, E., & Flor, H. (1998). Reorganization of auditory cortex in tinnitus. *Proceedings of the National Academy of Sciences of the U S A, 95*(17), 10 340–10 343.

Nahas, Z., DeBrux, C., Chandler, V., Lorberbaum, J. P., Speer, A. M., Molloy, M. A., et al. (2000). Lack of significant changes on magnetic resonance scans before and after 2 weeks of daily left prefrontal repetitive transcranial magnetic stimulation for depression. *Journal of ECT, 16*(4), 380–390.

Nitsche, M. A., Lampe, C., Antal, A., Liebetanz, D., Lang, N., Tergau, F., et al. (2006). Dopaminergic modulation of long-lasting direct current-induced cortical excitability changes in the human motor cortex. *European Journal of Neuroscience, 23*(6), 1651–1657.

Norena, A. J., & Eggermont, J. J. (2005). Enriched acoustic environment after noise trauma reduces hearing loss and prevents cortical map reorganization. *Journal of Neuroscience, 25*(3), 699–705.

Norena, A. J., & Eggermont, J. J. (2006). Enriched acoustic environment after noise trauma abolishes neural signs of tinnitus. *Neuroreport, 17*(6), 559–563.

Norena, A., Micheyl, C., Chery-Croze, S., & Collet, L. (2002). Psychoacoustic characterization of the tinnitus spectrum: Implications for the underlying mechanisms of tinnitus. *Audiology and Neurootology, 7*(6), 358–369.

Otani, S., Blond, O., Desce, J. M., & Crepel, F. (1998). Dopamine facilitates long-term depression of glutamatergic transmission in rat prefrontal cortex. *Neuroscience, 85*(3), 669–676.

Pascual-Leone, A., Grafman, J., & Hallett, M. (1994). Modulation of cortical motor output maps during development of implicit and explicit knowledge. *Science, 263*(5151), 1287–1289.

Plewnia, C., Bartels, M., & Gerloff, C. (2003). Transient suppression of tinnitus by transcranial magnetic stimulation. *Annals of Neurology, 53*(2), 263–266.

Plewnia, C., Reimold, M., Najib, A., Brehm, B., Reischl, G., Plontke, S. K., et al. (2007). Dose-dependent attenuation of auditory phantom perception (tinnitus) by PET-guided repetitive transcranial magnetic stimulation. *Human Brain Mapping, 28*(3), 238–246.

Plewnia, C., Reimold, M., Najib, A., Reischl, G., Plontke, S. K., & Gerloff, C. (2007). Moderate therapeutic efficacy of positron emission tomography-navigated repetitive transcranial magnetic stimulation for chronic tinnitus: A randomised, controlled pilot study. *Journal of Neurology, Neurosurgery and Psychiatry, 78*(2), 152–156.

Poreisz, C., Paulus, W., Moser, T., & Lang, N. (2009). Does a single session of theta-burst transcranial magnetic stimulation of inferior temporal cortex affect tinnitus perception? *BMC Neuroscience, 10,* 54.

Post, A., & Keck, M. E. (2001). Transcranial magnetic stimulation as a therapeutic tool in psychiatry: What do we know about the neurobiological mechanisms? *Journal of Psychiatric Research, 35*(4), 193–215.

Price, D. D. (2000). Psychological and neural mechanisms of the affective dimension of pain. *Science, 288*(5472), 1769–1772.

Ridding, M. C., & Rothwell, J. C. (1997). Stimulus/response curves as a method of measuring motor cortical excitability in man. *Electroencephalography Clinics of Neurophysiology, 105*(5), 340–344.

Rossi, S., De Capua, A., Ulivelli, M., Bartalini, S., Falzarano, V., Filippone, G., et al. (2007). Effects of repetitive transcranial magnetic stimulation on chronic tinnitus: A randomised, crossover, double blind, placebo controlled study. *Journal of Neurology, Neurosurgery and Psychiatry, 78*(8), 857–863.

Rossi, S., Hallett, M., Rossini, P. M., & Pascual-Leone, A. (2009). Safety, ethical considerations, and application guidelines for the use of transcranial magnetic stimulation in clinical practice and research. *Clinical Neurophysiology, 120*(12), 2008–2039.

Ryu, H., Yamamoto, S., Sugiyama, K., & Nozue, M. (1998). Neurovascular compression syndrome of the eighth cranial nerve. What are the most reliable diagnostic signs? *Acta Neurochirurgica (Wien), 140*(12), 1279–1286.

Schlee, W., Hartmann, T., Langguth, B., & Weisz, N. (2009). Abnormal resting-state cortical coupling in chronic tinnitus. *BMC Neuroscience, 10,* 11.

Schlee, W., Mueller, N., Hartmann, T., Keil, J., Lorenz, I., & Weisz, N. (2009). Mapping cortical hubs in tinnitus. *BMC Biology, 7,* 80.

Schlee, W., Weisz, N., Bertrand, O., Hartmann, T., & Elbert, T. (2008). Using auditory steady state responses to outline the functional connectivity in the tinnitus brain. *PLoS ONE, 3*(11), e3720.

Seidman, M. D., Ridder, D. D., Elisevich, K., Bowyer, S. M., Darrat, I., Dria, J., et al. (2008). Direct electrical stimulation of Heschl's gyrus for tinnitus treatment. *Laryngoscope, 118*(3), 491–500.

Seki, S., & Eggermont, J. J. (2003). Changes in spontaneous firing rate and neural synchrony in cat primary auditory cortex after localized tone-induced hearing loss. *Hearing Research, 180*(1-2), 28–38.

Shi, Y., Burchiel, K. J., Anderson, V. C., & Martin, W. H. (2009). Deep brain stimulation effects in patients with tinnitus. *Otolaryngology Head and Neck Surgery, 141*(2), 285–287.

Simons, W., & Dierick, M. (2005). Transcranial magnetic stimulation as a therapeutic tool in psychiatry. *World Journal of Biology and Psychiatry, 6*(1), 6–25.

Smith, J. A., Mennemeier, M., Bartel, T., Chelette, K. C., Kimbrell, T., Triggs, W., et al. (2007). Repetitive transcranial magnetic stimulation for tinnitus: A pilot study. *Laryngoscope, 117*(3), 529–534.

Smits, M., Kovacs, S., de Ridder, D., Peeters, R. R., van Hecke, P., & Sunaert, S. (2007). Lateralization of functional magnetic resonance imaging (fMRI) activation in the auditory pathway of patients with lateralized tinnitus. *Neuroradiology, 49*(8), 669–679.

Soussi, T., & Otto, S. R. (1994). Effects of electrical brainstem stimulation on tinnitus. *Acta Oto-Laryngologica, 114*(2), 135–140.

Speer, A. M., Repella, J. D., Figueras, S., Demian, N. K., Kimbrell, T. A., Wasserman, E. M., et al. (2001). Lack of adverse cognitive effects of 1 Hz and 20 Hz repetitive transcranial magnetic stimulation at 100% of motor threshold over left prefrontal cortex in depression. *J ECT, 17*(4), 259–263.

Terney, D., Bergmann, I., Poreisz, C., Chaieb, L., Boros, K., Nitsche, M. A., et al. (2008). Pergolide increases the efficacy of cathodal direct current stimulation to reduce the amplitude of laser-evoked potentials in humans. *Journal of Pain Symptom Management, 36*(1), 79–91.

Van de Heyning, P., Vermeire, K., Diebl, M., Nopp, P., Anderson, I., & De Ridder, D. (2008). Incapacitating unilateral tinnitus in single-sided deafness treated by cochlear implantation. *Annals of Otology, Rhinology and Laryngology, 117*(9), 645–652.

van der Loo, E., Gais, S., Congedo, M., Vanneste, S., Plazier, M., Menovsky, T., et al. (2009). Tinnitus intensity dependent gamma oscillations of the contralateral auditory cortex. *PLoS ONE, 4*(10), e7396: 7391-7395.

Vanneste, S., Plazier, M., Ost, J., van der Loo, E., Van de Heyning, P., & De Ridder, D. (2010). Bilateral dorsolateral prefrontal cortex modulation for tinnitus by transcranial direct current stimulation: A preliminary clinical study. *Experimental Brain Research, 204*(2), 283–287.

von Leupoldt, A., Sommer, T., Kegat, S., Baumann, H. J., Klose, H., Dahme, B., et al. (2009). Dyspnea and pain share emotion-related brain network. *Neuroimage, 48*(1), 200–206.

Walsh, V., & Rushworth, M. (1999). A primer of magnetic stimulation as a tool for neuropsychology. *Neuropsychologia, 37*(2), 125–135.

Wang, H., Wang, X., & Scheich, H. (1996). LTD and LTP induced by transcranial magnetic stimulation in auditory cortex. *Neuroreport, 7*(2), 521–525.

Wassermann, E. M. (1998). Risk and safety of repetitive transcranial magnetic stimulation: Report and suggested guidelines from the International Workshop on the Safety of Repetitive Transcranial Magnetic Stimulation. *Electroencephalography and Clinical Neurophysiology, 108*(1), 1–16.

Weisz, N., Muller, S., Schlee, W., Dohrmann, K., Hartmann, T., & Elbert, T. (2007). The neural code of auditory phantom perception. *Journal of Neuroscience, 27*(6), 1479–1484.

CHAPTER 12

Neurophysiological Effects of Transcranial Direct Current Stimulation

Jay S. Reidler[1], Soroush Zaghi[1,2], and Felipe Fregni[1,2]
[1]Laboratory of Neuromodulation, Spaulding Rehabilitation Hospital, Harvard Medical School, Boston, Massachusetts, USA
[2]Berenson-Allen Center for Noninvasive Brain Stimulation, Beth Israel Deaconess Medical Center, Harvard Medical School, Boston, Massachusetts, USA

Contents

INTRODUCTION

Transcranial direct current stimulation (tDCS) is a technique of brain stimulation that has been increasingly investigated as a clinical tool for the treatment of neuropsychiatric disorders. The growing interest in this technique underscores the importance of elucidating its underlying neurophysiology. Here we provide a review of research on the neurophysiological effects of tDCS. Studies from electrophysiology and transcranial magnetic stimulation have shown that tDCS can modulate cortical-excitability in a polarity-dependent fashion. Generally, anodal stimulation increases cortical excitability, while cathodal stimulation decreases it. Furthermore, these changes in cortical excitability are dependent on current density and stimulation duration. tDCS has been shown to modulate activity in both the motor and visual cortices, and more recently has been shown to directly influence excitability of the spinal cord. Anodal tDCS has been shown to increase intracortical facilitation and diminish intracortical inhibition, while cathodal tDCS has been shown to have the reverse effect. tDCS has also been shown to modulate transcallosal inhibition and may be a promising tool for enhancing the effects of paired-associative stimulation. Neuropharmacological studies suggest that the immediate effects of tDCS are due to modulation of neuronal membrane potentials at subthreshold levels, thus increasing or decreasing the rate of action potential firing. Long-term effects, lasting for periods well beyond the time of stimulation, likely involve NMDA-receptor dependent mechanisms. Future research should utilize alternative experimental techniques, study the neurophysiology underlying the clinical effects of tDCS, investigate improved tDCS technology and parameters of stimulation, and examine whether the neurophysiological effects of tDCS vary in populations with neuropsychiatric conditions.

THE GROWING FIELD OF BRAIN STIMULATION

Applications of brain stimulation have been rapidly growing in the neurological sciences. Deep brain stimulation allows for the precise stimulation of deep neural structures such as thalamic, subthalamic, and pallidal nuclei. Such interventions are used clinically, for example, in the treatment of advanced Parkinson's disease, providing excellent results in controlling dystonias and tremors (Limousin & Martinez-Torres, 2008) and holding some promise for the treatment of mood disorders (Mayberg et al., 2005) and obsessive—compulsive disorder (Lakhan & Callaway, 2010). At the level of the cortex, electrodes placed in the epidural area above the motor cortex are used for motor cortex stimulation, a clinical treatment shown to assuage many forms of chronic neuropathic pain (Lima & Fregni, 2008).

While these methods of brain stimulation have demonstrated remarkable progress, one limitation is the need for surgical penetration of the skull and brain, an expensive procedure that carries considerable risk.

Due to the downsides of surgical approaches, methods of neurofeedback and transcranial brain stimulation have become substantially more appealing for their capacity to safely modulate brain activity in a manner that is both more accessible and affordable. Neurofeedback is a method of endogenous neuromodulation in which the subject responds to real-time measurements of brain activity such as electroencephalography (Egner & Sterman, 2006; Gevensleben et al., 2010). In recent years, two external neuromodulatory techniques have been revisited that stimulate the human brain through the intact scalp: transcranial magnetic stimulation (TMS) and low-intensity transcranial electrical stimulation. Substantial research has been devoted to TMS, a method of brain stimulation that involves using a large, rapidly changing magnetic field to induce electrical stimulating currents in the brain. However, growing evidence suggests that transcranial electrical stimulation, which has different mechanisms of action, may also be a powerful and cost-effective approach to neuromodulation (Priori, Hallett, & Rothwell, 2009; Zaghi, Heine, & Fregni, 2009). Increased understanding of the neurophysiology underlying transcranial direct current stimulation (tDCS), a form of low-intensity transcranial electrical stimulation, has further stimulated research into clinical applications of this technology.

Among the various techniques of brain stimulation, tDCS stands out as one of the simplest in design. tDCS involves the administration of direct current through the scalp. A battery-powered current generator capable of delivering small currents (usually less than 10 mA) is attached to two sponge-based electrodes. The sponge electrodes are soaked, applied over the hair to the scalp, and held in place by a non-conducting rubber band affixed around the head. Current is injected through the scalp and skull to change the membrane potentials of neurons in the underlying cortex, resulting in real-time neurophysiological effects (see Figure 12.1). Importantly, tDCS only modulates neuronal activity and does not actually stimulate action potentials.

tDCS has been valuable in exploring the effects of cortical modulation on various neural networks implicated in language (Floel, Rosser, Michka, Knecht, & Breitenstein, 2008), sensory perception (Boggio, Zaghi, Lopes, & Fregni, 2008), decision-making (Fecteau et al., 2007), memory (Fregni, Boggio, Nitsche et al., 2005), and emotional pain (Boggio, Zaghi, &

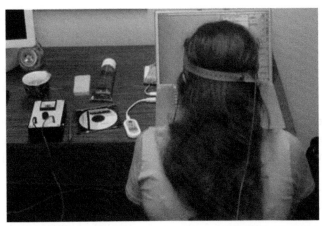

Figure 12.1 Transcranial direct current stimulation. In tDCS, two sponge-enclosed rubber electrodes are soaked in saline and applied to the scalp. Small wires attach the electrodes to a battery-powered direct current (DC) generator. In series with the DC generator, there is an amperemeter, which allows the tDCS operator to alter the internal resistance of the device with a dial to reach a target current ranging from 0.5 mA to 2.0 mA. Stimulation diffuses through the scalp and skull, resulting in real-time neurophysiological effects.

Fregni, 2009), among other cognitive processes. tDCS has also been introduced as an effective tool to alleviate chronic pain. Preliminary small sample-size studies and case reports with tDCS have shown initial positive results in modulating chronic pain in patients with terminal cancer (Silva et al., 2007), fibromyalgia (Fregni, Gimenes et al., 2006), and traumatic spinal cord injury (Fregni, Boggio, Lima et al., 2006). Recent studies suggest that tDCS may also facilitate motor and working memory rehabilitation following stroke, showing significant effects lasting two weeks (Boggio, Nunes et al., 2007; Jo et al., 2009; Nowak, Grefkes, Ameli, & Fink, 2009). Additionally, tDCS might be an interesting tool for modulating mood and other cognitive processes such as craving in substance abuse (Boggio, Bermpohl et al., 2007; Boggio, Sultani et al., 2008; Fregni et al., 2008). (For review of clinical applications of tDCS, see Zaghi, Acar, Hultgren, Boggio, & Fregni, 2010.)

Although these recent studies show encouraging results in the clinical arena, it is critical that we understand the underlying neurophysiology of tDCS so that we can optimize the parameters of stimulation and use of this technique. The field of neurophysiology includes the study of nervous system function with a scope that ranges from effects on membranes and cells to systems and behavior. Here we provide an up-to-date review of current research on the neurophysiological effects of tDCS and provide directions for future research in the field.

ELECTROPHYSIOLOGY OF tDCS

Historical Perspective

The utilization of low-intensity electrical stimulation likely had its origins in the eighteenth century, with studies of galvanic (i.e., direct) current in animals and humans by Giovanni Aldini and Alexandre Volta (Goldensohn, 1998; Priori, 2003). Yet because such stimulation induced variable results, or sometimes none at all, the use of low-intensity direct current was progressively abandoned in the first half of the 20th century with the introduction of neuropsychiatric drugs and other forms of brain stimulation such as electroconvulsive therapy (Priori, 2003), which involves transcranial stimulation at substantially higher intensities (>500 mA).

At the turn of the millennium, increasing interest in TMS, which was first developed in 1985 (Barker, Jalinous, & Freeston, 1985), revitalized interest in other forms of transcranial brain stimulation such as tDCS. Using TMS-induced motor evoked potentials as a marker of motor cortex excitability, Nitsche and Paulus (2000) demonstrated the possibility of modulating cortical excitability with tDCS. They found that weak direct current applied to the scalp was associated with excitability changes of up to 40% that lasted several minutes to hours after the end of stimulation (Nitsche & Paulus, 2000). Importantly, in this initial seminal study, they showed that electrode montage was essential for determining the effects of tDCS. A mathematical model then showed that while around half of the tDCS current diffuses across the scalp, the current distribution penetrating the scalp and skull is indeed sufficient to modify the transmembrane neuronal potential and influence the excitability of individual neurons without actually eliciting an action potential (Miranda, Lomarev, & Hallett, 2006; Wagner, Valero-Cabre, & Pascual-Leone, 2007). As our understanding of the neurophysiology of tDCS has improved over the past decade, we can now in hindsight appreciate the mixed results produced in studies on the effects of tDCS that took place in the mid-twentieth century (Murphy, Boggio, & Fregni, 2009).

TMS is a method of neurostimulation and neuromodulation that has been central to the investigation of the neurophysiological effects of tDCS, as it provides a measure of cortical excitability. We therefore begin our discussion of the electrophysiology of tDCS with a brief discussion of TMS.

TMS as a Tool for Measuring the Effects of tDCS

TMS was introduced about 25 years ago by Barker et al. (1985) who showed that it is possible to activate the corticospinal tract by applying a short-lasting magnetic field over the intact scalp in awake human subjects (Barker et al., 1985). TMS is a technique of brain stimulation that uses the principle of electromagnetic induction to induce currents in the brain. A coil of copper wire encased in plastic is placed on the subject's scalp overlying the region of the brain to be stimulated. As current passes through the coil, a magnetic field is generated in a plane perpendicular to the coil. The current passed is strong but extremely brief, producing a magnetic field that changes rapidly in time, reaching 2 Tesla in about 50 μs and decaying back to 0 Tesla in the same amount of time. For single pulse stimulators, magnetic fields of 1-4 Tesla in strength and durations of approximately 1 millisecond are typically used. The quickly changing magnetic field penetrates the skin and skull of the subject unimpeded, without causing discomfort, and induces a secondary electrical current in the subject's brain that is strong enough to depolarize cellular membranes and induce neuronal activity (Fregni, Boggio, Valle et al., 2006; Zaghi et al., 2009) (see Figure 12.2).

When TMS is applied to the motor cortex at suprathreshold intensity, it generates electrical currents in the motor cortex, which are observed as a contraction of muscles on the contralateral side of the body. TMS does not activate corticospinal neurons directly, but instead activates interneurons as demonstrated by research showing that TMS induces a corticospinal volley with indirect waves rather than direct waves. It is possible then to measure the latency and amplitude of the evoked potentials in electromyographic (EMG) signal recordings from the muscles, referred to as motor evoked potentials or MEPs as a measure of general corticospinal excitability. Since MEPs measure cortical excitability at any given moment in time, valuable information about the electrophysiology of the corticospinal tract can be acquired using this method (Ilmoniemi et al., 1997; Petersen, Pyndt, & Nielsen, 2003). Similarly, TMS can be employed to evoke the perception of visual phosphenes (sensation of light due to a stimulus other than light rays) when pulses are applied to the occipital cortex.

TMS can be used to study other aspects of motor cortex function such as intracortical facilitation and inhibition (ICF and ICI, respectively) and bihemispheric interactions via transcallosal inhibition using paired pulse

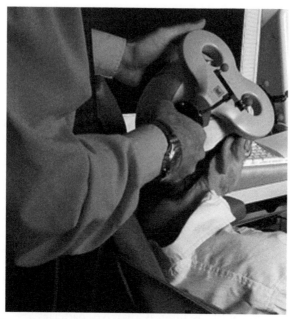

Figure 12.2 Transcranial magnetic stimulation. In TMS, a coil of copper wire encased in plastic is rested on the subject's scalp overlying the area of the brain to be stimulated. As current is delivered through the coil, a magnetic field reaching 2 Tesla is generated in a plane perpendicular to the coil. This rapidly changing magnetic field penetrates the skin and skull of the subject unimpeded and induces a secondary electrical current in the subject's brain that is strong enough to depolarize cellular membranes and induce neuronal activity.

TMS. Paired–pulse stimulation involves administration of two consecutive stimuli using the same coil for ICF and ICI, or two coils for transcallosal inhibition. Additionally, when a TMS pulse is administered to the occipital cortex during the presentation of a visual stimulus, it is possible to record changes in the waveform and topography of visual evoked potentials (VEP) in electroencephalography (EEG) recordings. It is also possible to measure cortical potentials induced by TMS using EEG (Miniussi & Thut, 2010). This combination of TMS and high-resolution EEG provides a remarkably powerful tool for the assessment of corticocortical and interhemispheric functional connections (Thut, Ives, Kampmann, Pastor, & Pascual-Leone, 2005). Moreover, the mapping and localization of neuronal responses to TMS stimulation of motor and visual cortices are substantially affected by baseline cortical excitability, execution of neuropsychological tasks, and medication use (Fregni, Boggio, Valle et al., 2006). Thus, TMS can be used to study the electrophysiological properties of transcranial direct current stimulation (Fregni, Boggio, Valle et al., 2006; Thut et al., 2005).

Transcranial Delivery of Current

The first consideration in understanding the neurophysiology of tDCS is to appreciate how currents applied with tDCS might affect neuronal activity. That is, how does direct current applied at the scalp translate into modulation of neuronal excitability? The central idea is that the current applied at the scalp produces an extracellular voltage gradient at the level of the cortex that alters the potential difference across neuronal membranes. A step-by-step, detailed explanation follows.

In tDCS, two (or more) relatively large anode and cathode sponge-enclosed rubber electrodes are applied to the scalp. The sponge electrodes usually measure about $20-35 \text{ cm}^2$ in area. Small wires attach the electrodes to a battery-powered direct current (DC) generator. The DC generator can be powered with as little as two AA batteries (~ 3 volts) or a single 9-volt battery. In series with the DC generator, there is an ampere-meter, which allows the tDCS operator to alter the internal resistance of the device with a dial to reach a target current. In tDCS, target currents usually range from 0.5 mA to 2.0 mA.

The objective of tDCS is for low amplitude direct currents to penetrate the skull and enter the brain. However, because current will flow in the path of least resistance, there is substantial shunting of current at the scalp. In this context, the current density plays an important role in determining the extent to which the applied current actually penetrates the skull to enter the brain.

By means of a magnetic resonance imaging (MRI)-derived finite element model specific to tDCS, Wagner et al. (2007) tested various electrode montages to analyze the role that tissue heterogeneity and anatomical variations played on the final current density distribution along the scalp and at the cortex (Wagner, Fregni et al., 2007). In one modeling experiment, the electrode area was varied from 1 to 49 cm^2 while maintaining fixed electrode placement (anode over the right M1 and cathode over the left supraorbital area) and non-variable constant current flow of 1 mA. Although the applied current densities (i.e. current intensity/electrode size) ranged from 10 A/m^2 (for the 1 cm^2 electrode) to 0.21 A/m^2 (for the 49 cm^2 electrodes), the shunting (i.e., the flow of current along the scalp surface as opposed to the cortex) effects were considerably larger for the 1 cm^2 electrodes compared to the other montages. Current densities in the skin were as much as 86 times greater than those seen in the cortex for the 1 cm^2 electrodes compared to a factor of approximately 9 for the 49 cm^2 electrodes. In other terms, 98.8% of the current was shunted through the skin vs. the cortex with use of the small 1 cm^2, but only 89.5% of the current was shunted through the skin with use of the larger 49 cm^2 electrodes. This shows that roughly 1.2% of the 10 A/m^2 (or 0.12 A/m^2) and 10.5% of the 0.21 A/m^2 current density (or 0.021 A/m^2) does penetrate to the level of the cortex with the use of small and large electrodes, respectively. Essentially, greater shunting occurs with smaller electrode areas, although a greater final cortical current density can be achieved. According to the study, the maximum local cortical current densities in this experiment ranged from 0.081 to 0.141 A/m^2, which were distributed in a non-linear fashion reflective of the relative heterogeneous anatomical and geometrical properties of the brain tissue. With varying electrode placement and constant current source (1 mA/35 cm^2 surface electrode area, or 0.29 A/m^2), the maximum local cortical current densities ranged from 0.077 to 0.20 A/m^2, with current densities of opposite polarity underlying the cathode and anode electrodes. Scalp current densities ranged from 8.85 to 17.25 times larger in magnitude than the cortical current densities (89.8% to 94.5% shunting rate).

The above discussion underscores the fact that low amplitude current applied at the scalp can indeed penetrate to the level of the cortex. It is important to keep in mind that this current flow is reflective of an electric potential (or voltage gradient) which allows for the flow of ions between the two electrodes. On a cellular level, the voltage gradient establishes opposing polarities at either end of the neurons affected by the electric field. This creates a difference in the transmembrane potential along the neuronal membrane and so causes current to flow across the membrane and along the inside of the neuron according to the resistances presented by properties of the neuronal membrane and intracellular space (Jefferys, Deans, Bikson, & Fox, 2003). This current flow modulates the neuronal membrane potential and therefore results in changes to spontaneous neuronal activity.

Current Density

Neurons and other excitable cells produce two types of electrical potential. The first is a non-propagated local potential called an electrotonic potential, which is due to a local change in ionic conductance (e.g., synaptic activity that engenders a local current). When it spreads along a stretch of membrane, the electrotonic potential decrements to become exponentially smaller. The second form of electric potential is a propagated impulse called an action potential. Electrotonic potentials represent changes to the neuron's membrane potential that do not lead directly to the generation of new current by action potentials. Neurons that are small in relation to their length (such as some neurons in the brain) have only electrotonic potentials; longer neurons utilize electrotonic potentials to trigger the action potential.

This discussion becomes important as we continue to appreciate how tDCS affects neuronal excitability. In contrast to TMS, which can both induce action potentials (neurostimulation) and modulate neuronal activity by influencing electrotonic potentials (neuromodulation) or inducing secondary synaptic changes, tDCS is strictly a neuromodulatory technique. tDCS does not induce action potentials because of limitations in cortical current density. As a reference point, cortical current density magnitudes are far lower than action potential thresholds: 0.079 to 0.20 A/m^2 induced by tDCS as compared to 22 to 275 A/m^2 required to trigger an action potential (Tehovnik, 1996). Thus, the effects of tDCS on cortical neurons are transmitted as electrotonic potentials only, which spread along the neuron, altering the likelihood with which that neuron may reach an action potential via temporal and spatial summation with other electrotonic synaptic inputs. This underscores the point that the magnitude of the current density has important implications in the neuromodulatory outcome of stimulation. Indeed, it has been shown that larger current densities result in stronger effects of tDCS (Boggio et al., 2006; Iyer et al., 2005; Nitsche & Paulus, 2000), while lower current densities (less than 0.24 A/m^2) for a few minutes do not induce any significant biological changes (Paulus, 2004).

Stimulation Duration

Interestingly, depending on the duration of stimulation, the effects of tDCS may outlast the stimulation period. In a study by Nitsche and Paulus (2000), it was shown that a stimulus duration of at least 3 minutes at 1 mA (35 cm^2 surface electrode area, 0.29 A/m^2) or an intensity of 0.6 mA (35 cm^2 surface electrode area, 0.17 A/m^2) for 5 minutes could induce measurable after-effects in cortical excitability (Nitsche & Paulus, 2000). Using TMS-induced MEPs as a measure of cortical excitability, Nitsche and Paulus (2000) demonstrated a clear increase of MEP amplitude and endurance of the effect with rising stimulus duration and intensity. Indeed, the duration of stimulation plays a significant role in determining: (1) the occurrence and (2) the duration of after-effects in humans and animals (Bindman, Lippold, & Redfearn, 1964; Nitsche, Nitsche et al., 2003; Nitsche & Paulus, 2000; Nitsche & Paulus, 2001). For example, whereas 5- and 7-minute tDCS results in after-effects lasting for no longer than 5 minutes, 9- to 13-minute tDCS results in after-effects lasting from 30 to 90 minutes, respectively (Nitsche & Paulus, 2001). Therefore, when we discuss electrophysiological effects of tDCS it is important to distinguish between: (1) immediate effects (e.g., anodal tDCS as excitatory, cathodal tDCS as inhibitory); and (2) the after-effects of stimulation (e.g., facilitation vs. inhibition of activity) as they may be related to different mechanisms of action (e.g., membrane vs. synaptic mechanisms).

While the above neurophysiological studies only examined variation in duration of a single session of tDCS, behavioral evidence suggests that repeating sessions of tDCS over several consecutive days can enhance the effects of tDCS as well (Boggio, Nunes et al., 2007). Boggio et al. (2007) examined improvement of motor performance in stroke patients following four weekly sessions of tDCS and five consecutive daily sessions of tDCS. In both experimental paradigms, they found significant motor function improvement after either cathodal tDCS of the unaffected hemisphere or anodal tDCS of the affected hemisphere when compared to sham tDCS. Importantly, while they did not find a significant cumulative effect associated with weekly sessions of tDCS, consecutive daily sessions of tDCS were associated with significant improvement over time that was sustained for 2 weeks after treatment. Future neurophysiological studies should confirm whether the neuromodulatory effects of tDCS could indeed be enhanced by consecutive daily sessions.

Stimulation Polarity

Direct current appears to modulate spontaneous neuronal activity in a polarity-dependent fashion. For example, anodal tDCS applied over the motor cortex increases the excitability of the underlying motor cortex, while cathodal tDCS applied over the same area decreases it (Nitsche & Paulus, 2001; Wassermann & Grafman, 2005). Similarly, anodal tDCS applied over the occipital cortex produces short-lasting increases in visual cortex excitability (Antal, Kincses, Nitsche, & Paulus, 2003; Lang et al.,

2007). Purpura and McMurtry (1965) showed in an animal model that upon anodal stimulation membranes are depolarized at a subthreshold level, whereas upon cathodal stimulation they are hyperpolarized (Purpura & McMurtry, 1965). Hence, tDCS is believed to deliver its effects by polarizing brain tissue, and while anodal stimulation generally increases excitability and cathodal stimulation generally reduces excitability, the direction of polarization depends strictly on the orientation of axons and dendrites in the induced electric field.

In vitro experiments with slices of tissue from mammalian hippocampuses show that electric fields applied to brain tissue affect cellular properties in a predictable fashion (Jefferys et al., 2003). Specifically, the electric fields hyperpolarize the ends of cells closest to the negative part of the field (cathode), and depolarize the ends closest to the positive part (anode). In the case of neurons, this change in excitability results from alterations in the capacitance of the neuronal membrane. Indeed, changes to the capacitance are induced by an accumulation of charges along the conducting surface of the neuronal membrane due to the presence of the applied electric field. As charge builds on the outer surface of the neuronal membrane, charges of opposite polarity build up on the inner surface of the neuronal membrane, and the charges are separated by the insulating lipid bilayer. In this way, the neuronal membrane functions as an electric capacitor (by storing and separating charges) creating an electric field that in turn induces a directional capacitative current within the neuron. The polarity-dependent storage of charges along the neuronal membrane and the resulting current are at the heart of the depolarizing and hyperpolarizing differences between anodal and cathodal tDCS.

How these changes in transmembrane potential are distributed depends on the length, size, and geometry of the neuron, in addition to the pattern of dendritic arborization and relative orientation of axons, dendrites, and soma in the applied electric field. Although such properties of the neurons vary widely across the nervous system, a recent experiment by Radman et al. (2009) in rat cortical neurons suggests that the soma of layer V pyramidal cells are individually most sensitive to polarization by optimally oriented subthreshold fields. Moreover, Radman et al. (2009) also reveal that cortical layer V/VI neurons had the lowest absolute action potential thresholds. This suggests that while the electric field induced by tDCS likely has sensitizing effects at the dendrites of neurons in all six cortical layers (Radman, Datta, Ramos, Brumberg, & Bikson, 2009), it is the soma of the neurons in layers V and VI that are most susceptible to the polarizing and excitability modulating effects of tDCS (Radman, Ramos, Brumberg, & Bikson, 2009).

Importantly, anatomical changes due to pathology can significantly alter the current distribution induced by tDCS. For instance, in subjects with stroke, the affected cortical area is usually replaced by cerebrospinal fluid, which has a high conductance, and current can accumulate on the edges of cortical stroke lesions (Wagner, Fregni et al., 2007). Therefore, in cases of pathologies that affect neuroanatomy, such as stroke or traumatic brain injury, individual modeling might be recommended before tDCS application.

Stimulation Site

The location of the electrode placement in tDCS is critically important because placement of the electrodes in different areas will result in distribution of current density to those respective areas of the brain. Indeed, imaging studies confirm that the polarizing effects of tDCS are generally restricted to the area under the electrodes (Nitsche, Liebetanz et al., 2003; Nitsche, Niehaus et al., 2004). Stimulation of motor cortex (M1), occipital cortex (V1), somatosensory cortices, and dorsolateral prefrontal cortex all have been shown to deliver site-specific and differential effects on a gamut of cognitive, behavioral, psychosomatic, and electrophysiological tests (Zaghi et al., 2010). (It is worth noting that the position of the reference electrode is as important as the stimulating electrode for inducing the proper amount of current under the stimulating electrode.) Additionally, some evidence suggests that tDCS can have highly focal effects. In a study examining the combined effects of tDCS and peripheral nerve stimulation, Uy and Ridding (2003) optimized (using TMS) the site of tDCS for the first dorsal interosseous muscle and observed significant excitability changes for this muscle, but not the nearby abductor digiti minimi and flexor carpi ulnaris muscles (Uy & Ridding, 2003). A recent modeling study, however, has suggested that electric current might actually have its peak between the two electrodes (Datta et al., 2009).

While the polarizing effects of tDCS are generally confined to the areas under and surrounding the electrodes, the functional effects appear to perpetuate beyond the immediate site of stimulation. That is, tDCS induces distant effects that go beyond the direct application of current, likely via the influence of a stimulated region on other neural networks. For example, anodal tDCS of premotor cortex increases the excitability of the ipsilateral motor cortex (Boros, Poreisz, Munchau, Paulus, & Nitsche, 2008), and stimulation of the primary motor cortex has inhibitory effects on contralateral motor areas (Vines, Cerruti, & Schlaug, 2008). This supports the notion that tDCS has a functional effect not only on the underlying corticospinal excitability but also on distant neural networks (Nitsche et al., 2005). Indeed, fMRI studies reveal that although tDCS has the most activating effect on the underlying cortex (Kwon et al., 2008), the stimulation provokes sustained and widespread changes in other regions of the brain as well (Lang et al., 2005). EEG studies support these findings, showing that stimulation of a particular area (e.g., frontal cortex) induces changes to oscillatory activity that are synchronous throughout the brain (Ardolino, Bossi, Barbieri, & Priori, 2005; Marshall, Molle, Hallschmid, & Born, 2004).

Hence, this evidence suggests that the effects of DC stimulation are site-specific but not site-limited. That is, stimulation of one area will likely have effects on other areas, most probably via networks of interneuronal circuits (Lefaucheur, 2008). This phenomenon is not surprising given the neuroanatomic complexity of the brain, but it raises interesting questions as to: (1) how the effects are transmitted; and (2) whether the observed clinical effects (e.g., pain alleviation) are mediated primarily through the area of the cortex being stimulated or secondarily via activation or inhibition of other cortical or sub-cortical structures (Boggio, Zaghi, & Fregni, 2009; Boggio, Zaghi, Lopes et al., 2008). For instance, Roche et al. (2009) demonstrated that anodal tDCS of the motor cortex modifies excitability at the level of the spinal cord by showing that tDCS increases reflexive inhibition directed from the extensor carpi radialis to flexor carpi radialis, which is mediated by inhibitory interneurons located in the spinal cord (Roche, Lackmy, Achache, Bussel, & Katz, 2009). Therefore, observed clinical effects from tDCS might be explained by changes to several possible regions in the central nervous system (see Table 12.1 for a summary of the effects of varying parameters of tDCS).

Neurophysiological Effects of tDCS as Indexed by Cortical Excitability

Just as changes to motor evoked potentials and motor thresholds as measured by TMS provide insight into the excitability level of corticospinal neurons, so too changes to intracortical inhibition (ICI) and intracortical facilitation (ICF) as measured by TMS can provide helpful insight into the effects of tDCS on cortical interneurons. First we discuss the measurement of ICI and ICF, and then we describe the effect of tDCS on these

Table 12.1 Varying parameters of tDCS

Parameter	Standard range	Effect
Electrode size	20 cm^2–35 cm^2	Smaller electrode size results in greater final cortical current density, but also greater shunting to the scalp. Unipolar stimulation can be achieved through a small electrode by enlarging the area of the other electrode
Current intensity	1.0 mA–2.0 mA	A current intensity of 0.6 mA is necessary to observe after-effects. Larger current intensity results in greater amplitude of effect (as measured by MEPs) and longer-lasting effects
Current density on scalp surface	$24 \, \mu\text{A}/\text{cm}^2$–$29 \, \mu\text{A}/\text{cm}^2$	Larger current densities result in stronger effects of tDCS. Lower current densities (less than $24 \, \mu\text{A}/\text{cm}^2$) for a few minutes do not induce any significant effects. (This is the ratio of current intensity and electrode size)
Stimulation duration	5 min–30 min	Longer duration results in longer-lasting effects. Whereas 5- and 7-minute tDCS results in after-effects lasting for no longer than 5 minutes, tDCS from 9 to 13 minutes result in after-effects lasting from 30 to 90 minutes, respectively
Stimulation polarity	Anodal or cathodal (applied to cortical region of interest)	Effect depends strictly on the orientation of axons and dendrites in the induced electrical field. Generally, anodal tDCS increases the excitability of the underlying cortex by depolarizing neuronal membranes to subthreshold levels, while cathodal tDCS applied over the same area decreases it by hyperpolarizing neuronal membranes

(Continued)

Table 12.1 (Continued)

Parameter	Standard range	Effect
Stimulation site	M1, V1, somatosensory cortex, dorsolateral prefrontal cortex	Site-specific and differential effects on a gamut of cognitive, behavioral, psychosomatic, and electrophysiological tests. While the polarizing effects of tDCS are generally confined to the areas under the electrodes, the functional effects appear to perpetuate beyond the immediate site of stimulation. Anodal tDCS of the premotor cortex, for instance, increases the excitability of the ipsilateral motor cortex and inhibition of the contralateral motor areas

measures. We then discuss the effects of tDCS on transcallosal inhibition, cortical silent period, and paired-associative stimulation.

Intracortical Inhibition and Facilitation

Intracortical inhibition and facilitation are measured using a particular technique of TMS known as paired-pulse TMS. In this technique, the TMS device is used to produce two back-to-back stimuli separated by a range of inter-stimulus intervals (ISIs).

In the measurement of short interval intracortical inhibition (SICI), a sub-threshold conditioning stimulus precedes a supra-threshold stimulus by a short interval of 1 to 6 ms in time. Interestingly, the preceding conditioning pulse suppresses the amplitude of the MEP induced by the supra-threshold stimulus. In SICI, the subthreshold stimulus inhibits the effect of the supra-threshold pulse by activating low-threshold $GABA_A$-dependent inhibitory circuits (via inhibitory post-synaptic potentials, or IPSPs). In long interval intracortical inhibition (LICI), two TMS pulses are delivered at supra-threshold intensities at intervals of 50–200 ms. LICI is mediated by long-lasting $GABA_B$-dependent IPSPs and activation of pre-synaptic $GABA_B$ receptors on inhibitory interneurons, but this measurement is not frequently used. In intracortical facilitation, the amplitude of a test MEP can be enhanced if it is accompanied by a sub-threshold conditioning pulse applied 10–25 ms earlier. Glutamatergic interneurons at the level of M1 are likely to be involved in ICF since it is reduced by NMDA antagonists such as dextromethorphan. ICF is believed to result from the net facilitation of inhibitory and excitatory mechanisms mediated by $GABA_A$ and NMDA receptors, respectively.

Nitsche et al. (2005) used paired-pulse TMS techniques to examine the effects of tDCS on ICF, SICI, and LICI (Nitsche et al., 2005). They employed a protocol that included ISIs of 2, 3, and 4 ms to examine inhibitory effects and ISIs of 10 and 15 ms to examine facilitatory effects. Using TMS-induced MEPs as a measure, they tested for intra-tDCS excitability changes, short-lasting after-effects (5−10 minutes after stimulation) and long-lasting after-effects (up to 35 minutes after stimulation). With regard to intra-tDCS excitability changes, they found that anodal tDCS did not induce cortical inhibition or facilitation, while cathodal tDCS reduced facilitation. For the short-lasting after-effects, they found that anodal tDCS reduced inhibition and enhanced facilitation, while cathodal tDCS enhanced inhibition and reduced facilitation. Finally, for the long-lasting after-effects anodal tDCS decreased inhibition for ISIs of 3 ms, while cathodal tDCS increased inhibition at ISIs of 2 ms and 5 ms. Though for long-lasting effects the ISI of 15 ms condition did not show modified facilitation, anodal tDCS increased facilitation at ISI of 10 ms, while cathodal tDCS reduced facilitation.

These results suggest that intracortical inhibition and facilitation can be modified by tDCS. For the short-lasting and long-lasting effects, anodal tDCS can increase facilitation and decrease inhibition, while cathodal tDCS can produce the opposite effect. While intra-tDCS facilitatory effects are not observed for anodal stimulation, they are decreased for cathodal stimulation.

Transcallosal Inhibition

In transcallosal inhibition, the two motor cortices are stimulated with a delay of 10 ms. The first pulse (the conditioning pulse) is applied over the primary motor cortex and the second pulse (the test pulse) is applied after a delay of 10 ms in the contralateral primary motor cortex. It has been shown that the second pulse is associated with a significant inhibition in the MEP characteristics.

Transcallosal inhibition induced by tDCS has been explored for clinical use in rehabilitating motor function following stroke. Following stroke, the brain compensates for motor loss by increasing activity in the unaffected hemisphere and limb. Transcallosal inhibition from this cortical region can decrease activity in the affected hemisphere. Fregni et al. (2005) investigated whether reduction of activity in the unaffected hemisphere by cathodal tDCS would result in improved motor performance due to decreased transcallosal inhibition. Indeed, they found that cathodal stimulation of the unaffected hemisphere, as well as anodal stimulation of the affected hemisphere, significantly improved motor performance compared to sham tDCS (Fregni, Boggio, Mansur et al., 2005). In a recent study of healthy subjects, Williams, Pascual-Leone, and Fregni (2010) combined bilateral motor cortex tDCS with contralateral hand restraint of the dominant hand. When comparing active stimulation to sham stimulation, they found a decrease in cortical excitability in the dominant hemisphere and a decrease in transcallosal inhibition from the dominant hemisphere to the non-dominant hemisphere. The decrease in transcallosal inhibition correlated with motor performance enhancement in the non-dominant hand (Williams et al., 2010).

These findings therefore suggest that tDCS not only effects the proximal area of stimulation, but can have effects on more distal areas of the brain, which may have substantial implications for clinical treatments such as rehabilitation of motor function following stroke.

Cortical Silent Period

Another common phenomenon induced by transcranial stimulation that has been used as a measure of intra-cortical inhibition is known as cortical silent period (Hallett, 1995; Tergau et al., 1999). Similar to a refractory period, cortical silent period refers to an inhibitory response observed through electromyography following administration of TMS in which there is a period following the stimulation of the motor cortex during which a second stimulus would be ineffective. This period of depressed activity appears to be important for maintaining motor control as well as averting seizures. While cortical silent period has mainly been studied in TMS research, we expect that future investigation of this phenomenon following tDCS might yield comparable results due to the similar neuromodulatory effects tDCS can have when compared to TMS. Furthermore, evidence suggests that cortical silent period may also serve as a tool to index GABA activity, and may therefore be useful in confirming whether cathodal tDCS inhibits cortical excitability via a GABA-dependent pathway (McDonnell, Orekhov, & Ziemann, 2006; Ziemann, Lonnecker, Steinhoff, & Paulus, 1996).

Paired-Associative Stimulation

Classic theories of associative neuroplasticity predict that coactivation of two synaptic inputs modifies synaptic strength, having strong implications for learning processes. Paired-associative stimulation (PAS) has been proposed as a technique to explore the mechanisms by which this occurs (Classen et al., 2004). PAS refers to the administration of two stimuli at once or in close proximity so as to lead the subject to associate them. Wolters et al. (2003) showed that PAS increases or decreases motor cortical excitability (as measured by MEPs) when the interval between peripheral nerve stimulation and subsequent TMS pulse is 25 ms and 10 ms, respectively. This PAS-induced plasticity appears to be NMDA-receptor dependent and has been shown to influence motor learning (Stefan et al., 2006; Wolters et al., 2003; Ziemann, Ilic, Pauli, Meintzschel, & Ruge, 2004).

Nitsche et al. (2007) explored whether tDCS-induced background network activity changes effect PAS-induced plasticity. They hypothesized according to homeostatic plasticity theory that the effect of PAS would be enhanced with decreased background activity (Nitsche et al., 2007). Administering the PAS protocol to 12 healthy subjects, Nitsche et al. (2007) slowly stimulated the right ulnar nerve at the wrist at an intensity 300% above sensory threshold while a single TMS pulse was delivered over the contralateral motor cortical region representing the right abductor digiti minimi muscle. This protocol was performed alone, following anodal and cathodal tDCS, and simultaneously with anodal and cathodal tDCS. When administered simultaneously with PAS, excitability-enhancing (anodal) tDCS decreased the efficacy of PAS and excitability-diminishing (cathodal) tDCS increased the efficacy of PAS. This same effect was observed for prolonged administration of tDCS as well, but was not observed when tDCS was administered before PAS. This suggests, in accordance with theories of homeostatic plasticity, that tDCS has the potential to modify the efficacy of PAS by modulating background activity in the brain. For instance, decreased excitability of the cortex induced by cathodal tDCS, when applied in combination with PAS, has the potential to increase associative synaptic plasticity.

NEUROCHEMISTRY OF tDCS

As noted above, transcranial direct current results in polarity-specific changes during and after application of tDCS. Whereas anodal stimulation depolarizes membrane potentials to subthreshold levels leading to increased cortical excitability, cathodal stimulation hyperpolarizes membrane potentials leading to increases in cortical inhibition. Effects on cortical excitability can be immediate and short-lasting (up to 5 minutes following stimulation) and they can also be longer lasting (up to 1 hour following stimulation). These changes in cortical excitability are associated with changes of the underlying cortical neuronal activity. But what do we know from a neurochemistry standpoint about the effects of tDCS on neuronal activity?

Ion Channel Conductance and NMDA-Receptors

Several pharmacological studies have examined the roles of various ion channels and receptors in the modulation of cortical excitability by tDCS. Liebetanz, Nitsche, Tergau, & Paulus (2002) found that administration of the sodium channel blocker carbamazepine prior to tDCS eliminated the excitatory effects of anodal stimulation. Furthermore, the N-methyl-D-aspartate (NMDA)-receptor antagonist dextromethorphan eliminated the long-lasting after-effects of both anodal and cathodal stimulation (Liebetanz et al., 2002), suggesting that tDCS after-effects are associated with synaptic effects. In a later pharmacological study in healthy human subjects, Nitsche, Fricke et al. (2003) further examined the impact of carbamazepine, dextromethorphan, and the calcium channel blocker flunarizine on tDCS-elicited motor cortical excitability changes. They found similar effects resulting from blocking sodium channels and NMDA receptors, and further demonstrated that blocking calcium channels led to elimination of the excitatory effects of anodal stimulation (Nitsche, Fricke et al., 2003). Additionally, D-cylcoserine, a partial NMDA agonist shown to improve cognitive functions in humans, has also been found to prolong the cortical excitability induced by anodal tDCS (Nitsche, Jaussi et al., 2004). Extending these findings, a recent study using mouse M1 slices demonstrated that anodal tDCS combined with repetitive low-frequency synaptic activation induces long-term synaptic potentiation that is NMDA-receptor dependent and mediated by secretion of brain-derived neurotrophic factor (BDNF) (Fritsch et al., 2010). The combined results of these studies suggest that changes in cortical excitability during tDCS depend on membrane polarization, which is determined by the conductance of sodium and calcium channels. Moreover, they suggest that NMDA-dependent mechanisms are central to inducing the after-effects of tDCS. The above studies also suggest avenues for prolonging the effects of tDCS on cortical excitability and plasticity through the combination of tDCS with pharmacologic interventions.

Neurotransmitters Involved: GABA, Glutamate, and Dopamine

While the above studies suggest that sodium and calcium channels are central to the effects of tDCS, the evidence for the involvement of excitatory neurotransmitters such as glutamate or inhibitory neurotransmitters such as gamma-aminobutyric acid (GABA) is limited. In a magnetic resonance (MR) spectroscopy study, Stagg et al. (2009) found that anodal tDCS is related to decrease in GABA concentration and cathodal tDCS is related to decrease in both glutamate and GABA (Stagg et al., 2009). This suggests that tDCS affects activity of inhibitory interneurons, potentially explaining the mechanism by which cortical excitability increases and decreases upon stimulation. Nitsche et al. (2006) also found that dopaminergic mechanisms may be involved in NMDA-induced after-effects, as D2 receptor blocking by sulpiride eliminated the after-effects of cathodal tDCS, while enhancement of the receptors using pergolide consolidated tDCS-generated inhibition until the morning after stimulation (Nitsche et al., 2006).

Anodal tDCS has also been shown to manipulate cortical spreading depression (CSD), which is influenced by changes in the concentrations of ions and neurotransmitters that control cortical excitability like GABA and glutamate. CSD, which is thought to underlie migraine aura, is a wave of neuronal excitation followed by inhibition that spreads through the cortex (at a rate of $2-5$ mm/min) as a result of alterations in cortical ion homeostasis. Using a rat model, Liebetanz et al. demonstrated that the propagation velocity of CSD increases following the administration of anodal tDCS. Cathodal and sham tDCS did not influence the CSD propagation velocity (Liebetanz et al., 2006). Since anodal tDCS is known to increase cortical excitability, this study supports the theory that CSD propagation velocity reflects cortical excitability and suggests that anodal tDCS might increase the likelihood of migraine attacks in migraine patients.

Changes to Oxyhemoglobin Concentration

Studies of tDCS-induced cortical excitability have previously focused on the motor cortex and visual cortex since the effects of stimulation in these areas can be assessed by TMS motor evoked potentials and phosphene thresholds. To examine the effects of tDCS on other areas in the brain such as the prefrontal cortex, Merzagora et al. (2010) employed another technique called functional near-infrared spectroscopy (fNIRS), which allows for a non-invasive and portable measure of regional cerebral blood flow (rCBF) (Merzagora et al., 2010). fNIRS records cerebral concentrations of oxyhemoglobin and deoxyhemoglobin by observing the absorption of near-infrared light in particular regions of the brain and relating this to rCBF. In a sham-controlled study, Merzagora et al. (2010) stimulated two prefrontal locations for 10 minutes and found that oxyhemoglobin concentration was significantly increased following anodal stimulation compared to sham stimulation, suggesting that anodal stimulation increased rCBF in the stimulated regions. fNIRS data showed that this effect lasted for 8–10 minutes following stimulation, and that cathodal stimulation only induced a negligible effect on rCBF. This study potentially supports the use of changes to oxyhemoglobin concentration via fNIRS as an additional method for monitoring the neuromodulatory effects of tDCS.

Alterations to Membrane Phospholipids

Finally, one recent study suggests that tDCS may have some effects on membrane phospholipid metabolism. Myoinositol is an essential compound for the synthesis of inositol-containing phospholipids that has been found to be altered in many physiological and pathological conditions. Using proton magnetic resonance spectroscopy, Rango et al. (2008) showed that the concentration of myoinositol was increased with anodal tDCS of the right motor cortex compared to sham-tDCS (the effect was not observed in a control visual cortical region) (Rango et al., 2008). This study suggests that monitoring of the brain content of myoinositol may serve to further monitor the effects of tDCS.

While much remains to be explored regarding the neurochemistry of tDCS, studies to date have supported the understanding that tDCS exerts its effects primarily by depolarizing or hyperpolarizing neuronal membrane potentials, reinforcing these effects through NMDA-dependent mechanisms and increasing cerebral blood flow to the stimulated region.

SAFETY CONSIDERATIONS FOR tDCS

Numerous studies verify that low-intensity transcranial stimulation is safe for use in humans and that it is linked with only rare and relatively minor adverse effects (Poreisz, Boros, Antal, & Paulus, 2007). tDCS does not elevate the serum levels of molecular markers of neuronal injury such as neuron-specific enolase (Nitsche & Paulus, 2001) or N-acetyl-aspartate (Rango et al., 2008). Furthermore, both contrast-enhanced MRI and EEG studies have found no pathological changes associated with application of tDCS (Iyezr et al., 2005; Nitsche, Niehaus et al., 2004).

Additionally, no instances of epileptic seizures caused by tDCS have been observed in humans (Poreisz et al., 2007). In fact, pulsed transcranial stimulation has been correlated with an antiepileptic effect in rats (Liebetanz et al., 2006) and a previous tDCS study in patients with refractory epilepsy did not show an increase in seizures or EEG-epileptiform discharges (Fregni, Thome-Souza et al., 2006). The most common side effects observed with tDCS are mild tingling (70.6%), moderate fatigue (35.3%), sensations of light itching (30.4%), slight burning (21.6%), and mild pain (15.7%) under the electrodes (Poreisz et al., 2007).

Less commonly, some subjects report headache (11.8%), trouble concentrating (10.8%), nausea (2.9%), and sleep disturbances (1.0%) (Poreisz et al., 2007). Skin lesions in the form of burns following administration of tDCS have been reported (Palm, 2008). Visual sensations associated with turning the stimulation on or off have occurred in a small number of cases, but this can be avoided by slowly changing the current level at the start and end of stimulation. tDCS delivered at a level of 2 mA and administered according to current stimulation guidelines (Nitsche, 2008) has been shown to be safe for use in both healthy volunteers (Iyer et al., 2005) and patients with neurological injury (Boggio, Nunes et al., 2007). Using a rat model, researchers investigated the safety limits of extended cathodal tDCS and found the charge density threshold to be two orders of magnitude greater than the charge currently administered in humans (Liebetanz et al., 2009). The safety of tDCS use in pregnant women and children, however, has not yet been investigated.

CONCLUSIONS AND FUTURE DIRECTIONS

There is much left to be explored in understanding the neurophysiological effects of tDCS. Studies from electrophysiology and TMS have shown that tDCS can modulate cortical-excitability in a polarity-dependent fashion. Generally, anodal stimulation increases cortical excitability, while cathodal stimulation decreases it. Furthermore, these effects are dependent on current density and stimulation duration. tDCS has been shown to modulate activity in both the motor and visual cortices, and more recently has been shown to directly influence excitability of the spinal cord. Anodal tDCS has been shown to increase intracortical facilitation and diminish intracortical inhibition, while cathodal tDCS has been shown to have the reverse effect. Furthermore, tDCS appears to have substantial effects on transcallosal inhibition and may be a promising tool for enhancing the effects of PAS. While the neurochemical mechanisms underlying these effects are incompletely understood, neuropharmacology studies suggest that immediate effects are due to modulation of neuronal membrane potentials, thus increasing or decreasing the rate of action potential firing. Long-term effects, lasting for minutes to hours beyond the time of stimulation, likely involve NMDA-receptor dependent mechanisms. It is critical that we integrate the results from these studies as the neurophysiological effects and clinical applications of tDCS continue to be explored.

Future studies should combine other brain imaging methods such as functional magnetic resonance imaging (fMRI), positron emission tomography (PET), electroencephalography (EEG) before, during, and following the administration of tDCS. fMRI for instance has high spatial resolution that can assist in more precisely examining regions of the brain. PET can be utilized to monitor glucose or neurotransmitter uptake to observe the neurochemical effects of tDCS. Awake animal models combined with such imaging modalities might prove useful in probing the physiological effects of tDCS. Furthermore, additional research into the effects of tDCS on conditions such as chronic pain may shed light onto the neurophysiological mechanisms underlying these effects (see Zaghi et al., 2010, for recent review of the clinical applications of tDCS). Precise and stable positioning of the tDCS device remains one limitation of current tDCS research. Future engineering research should be targeted at improving the stability, focality, and depth of stimulation that can be administered by stimulation devices, as well as developing alternative stimulation parameters (e.g., alternating current, simultaneous administration of two tDCS devices), which would potentially enhance our ability to utilize tDCS in future research and clinical practice (Miranda et al., 2006). One interesting alternative that should be further explored is high-density tDCS (HD-tDCS) using ring electrodes to produce a more focal stimulation area (Datta et al., 2009). Finally, most research to date on the neurophysiological effects of tDCS has been conducted in healthy subjects, though we have reason to suspect such effects may be altered in patients with neuropsychiatric conditions who often exhibit differing baseline brain activity (Fregni, Boggio, Valle et al., 2006; Siebner et al., 2004). Future investigation should therefore examine whether the neurophysiological effects of tDCS vary in populations with neuropsychiatric conditions.

The key points from this chapter are summarized in Table 12.2.

Table 12.2 Transcranial direct current stimulation: summary of key points

Growing interest in the clinical applications of tDCS underscores the importance of elucidating the underlying neurophysiology of this brain stimulation technique

Transcranial magnetic stimulation is a method of neurostimulation and neuromodulation that has been central to the investigation of the neurophysiological effects of tDCS

Low amplitude current applied at the scalp can penetrate to the level of the cortex

Greater shunting to the scalp occurs with smaller electrode areas, although a greater final cortical current density can be achieved

Because of limitations in cortical current density, tDCS does not induce action potentials. The effects of tDCS on cortical neurons are transmitted as electrotonic potentials only, which spread along the neuron, altering the likelihood with which that neuron may reach an action potential

Larger current densities result in stronger effects of tDCS, while lower current densities for short periods of time do not induce any significant changes

Greater tDCS duration and intensity lead to greater endurance of its effects

Direct current modulates the spontaneous neuronal activity in a polarity-dependent fashion

Generally, anodal tDCS increases cortical excitability of the stimulated area, while cathodal tDCS decreases cortical excitability

Soma of the neurons in layers V and VI are most susceptible to the modulating effects of tDCS

Anodal tDCS of the motor cortex modifies excitability at the level of the spinal cord

Although tDCS has the most activating effect on the underlying cortex, the stimulation provokes sustained and widespread changes in other regions of the brain as well as through intracortical inhibition and facilitation

tDCS affects transcallosal inhibition. Cathodal stimulation of the unaffected hemisphere in stroke patients decreases transcallosal inhibition and significantly improves performance of motor tasks controlled by the affected hemisphere

Transcranial magnetic stimulation can induce a short cortical silent period, or refractory period, following stimulation. Future research should examine whether tDCS produces similar effects

tDCS has the potential to modify the efficacy of paired-associative stimulation by modulating background activity in the brain. For instance, decreased excitability of the cortex induced by cathodal tDCS, when applied in combination with paired-associative stimulation, has the potential to increase associative synaptic plasticity

Changes to cortical excitability during tDCS depend on membrane polarization, which is determined by the conductance of sodium and calcium channels. After-effects of tDCS may be additionally dependent on NMDA-receptors

(Continued)

Table 12.2 (Continued)

Anodal stimulation is associated with decrease in GABA concentration and cathodal tDCS is associated with decrease in both glutamate and GABA

Dopaminergic mechanisms may be involved in NMDA-induced after-effects

Oxyhemoglobin concentration significantly increases following anodal stimulation compared to sham stimulation, suggesting that anodal stimulation increases rCBF in the stimulated regions. The concentration of myoinositol increases with anodal tDCS as well

Neurochemistry studies to date have served to reinforce the understanding that tDCS exerts its effects primarily by depolarizing or hyperpolarizing neuronal membrane potential, reinforcing these effects through NMDA-dependent mechanisms and increasing cerebral blood flow to the stimulated region

Numerous studies verify that low-intensity transcranial stimulation is safe for use in humans (but not pregnant women and children) and that it is linked with only rare and relatively minor adverse effects

Future studies should examine the effects of tDCS using other imaging modalities. Research should also aim to understand the mechanisms underlying observed clinical effects, develop improved tDCS technologies and alternative parameters for enhanced use in research and clinical practice, and examine whether the neurophysiological effects of tDCS vary in populations with neuropsychiatric conditions

ACKNOWLEDGMENT

This publication was made possible with partial funding by grant number R21 7R21DK081773 from the National Institute of Diabetes and Digestive and Kidney Diseases (NIDDK) at the National Institutes of Health. Its contents are solely the responsibility of the authors and do not necessarily represent the official views of NIDDK.

REFERENCES

Antal, A., Kincses, T. Z., Nitsche, M. A., & Paulus, W. (2003). Manipulation of phosphene thresholds by transcranial direct current stimulation in man. *Experimental Brain Research, 150*(3), 375–378.

Ardolino, G., Bossi, B., Barbieri, S., & Priori, A. (2005). Non-synaptic mechanisms underlie the after-effects of cathodal transcutaneous direct current stimulation of the human brain. *Journal of Physiology, 568*(Pt 2), 653–663.

Barker, A. T., Jalinous, R., & Freeston, I. L. (1985). Non-invasive magnetic stimulation of human motor cortex. *Lancet, 1*(8437), 1106–1107.

Bindman, L. J., Lippold, O. C., & Redfearn, J. W. (1964). The action of brief polarizing currents on the cerebral cortex of the rat (1) during current flow and (2) in the production of long-lasting after-effects. *Journal of Physiology, 172*, 369–382.

Boggio, P. S., Bermpohl, F., Vergara, A. O., Muniz, A. L., Nahas, F. H., Leme, P. B., et al. (2007). Go-no-go task performance improvement after anodal transcranial DC stimulation of the left dorsolateral prefrontal cortex in major depression. *Journal of Affective Disorders, 101*(1–3), 91–98.

Boggio, P. S., Ferrucci, R., Rigonatti, S. P., Covre, P., Nitsche, M., Pascual-Leone, A., et al. (2006). Effects of transcranial direct current stimulation on working memory in patients with Parkinson's disease. *Journal of Neurological Sciences, 249*(1), 31–38.

Boggio, P. S., Nunes, A., Rigonatti, S. P., Nitsche, M. A., Pascual-Leone, A., & Fregni, F. (2007). Repeated sessions of noninvasive brain DC stimulation is associated with motor function improvement in stroke patients. *Restorative Neurology and Neuroscience, 25*(2), 123–129.

Boggio, P. S., Sultani, N., Fecteau, S., Merabet, L., Mecca, T., Pascual-Leone, A., et al. (2008). Prefrontal cortex modulation using transcranial DC stimulation reduces alcohol craving: a double-blind, sham-controlled study. *Drug and Alcohol Dependency, 92* (1–3), 55–60.

Boggio, P. S., Zaghi, S., & Fregni, F. (2009). Modulation of emotions associated with images of human pain using anodal transcranial direct current stimulation (tDCS). *Neuropsychologia, 47*(1), 212–217.

Boggio, P. S., Zaghi, S., Lopes, M., & Fregni, F. (2008). Modulatory effects of anodal transcranial direct current stimulation on perception and pain thresholds in healthy volunteers. *European Journal of Neurology, 15*(10), 1124–1130.

Boros, K., Poreisz, C., Munchau, A., Paulus, W., & Nitsche, M. A. (2008). Premotor transcranial direct current stimulation (tDCS) affects primary motor excitability in humans. *European Journal of Neuroscience, 27*(5), 1292–1300.

Classen, J., Wolters, A., Stefan, K., Wycislo, M., Sandbrink, F., Schmidt, A., et al. (2004). Paired associative stimulation. *Clinical Neurophysiology, 57*(Suppl.), 563–569.

Datta, A., Bansal, V., Diaz, J., Patel, J., Reato, D., & Bikson, M. (2009). Gyri-precise head model of transcranial DC stimulation: Improved spatial focality using a ring electrode versus conventional rectangular pad. *Brain Stimulation, 2*(4), 201–207.

Egner, T., & Sterman, M. B. (2006). Neurofeedback treatment of epilepsy: from basic rationale to practical application. *Expert Reviews in Neurotherapy, 6*(2), 247–257.

Fecteau, S., Pascual-Leone, A., Zald, D. H., Liguori, P., Theoret, H., Boggio, P. S., et al. (2007). Activation of prefrontal cortex by transcranial direct current stimulation reduces appetite for risk during ambiguous decision making. *Journal of Neuroscience, 27* (23), 6212–6218.

Floel, A., Rosser, N., Michka, O., Knecht, S., & Breitenstein, C. (2008). Noninvasive brain stimulation improves language learning. *Journal of Cognitive Neuroscience, 20*(8), 1415–1422.

Fregni, F., Boggio, P. S., Lima, M. C., Ferreira, M. J., Wagner, T., Rigonatti, S. P., et al. (2006). A sham-controlled, phase II trial of transcranial direct current stimulation for the treatment of central pain in traumatic spinal cord injury. *Pain, 122* (1-2), 197–209.

Fregni, F., Boggio, P. S., Mansur, C. G., Wagner, T., Ferreira, M. J., Lima, M. C., et al. (2005). Transcranial direct current stimulation of the unaffected hemisphere in stroke patients. *Neuroreport, 16*(14), 1551–1555.

Fregni, F., Boggio, P. S., Nitsche, M., Bermpohl, F., Antal, A., Feredoes, E., et al. (2005). Anodal transcranial direct current stimulation of prefrontal cortex enhances working memory. *Experimental Brain Research, 166*(1), 23–30.

Fregni, F., Boggio, P. S., Valle, A. C., Otachi, P., Thut, G., Rigonatti, S. P., et al. (2006). Homeostatic effects of plasma valproate levels on corticospinal excitability changes induced by 1Hz rTMS in patients with juvenile myoclonic epilepsy. *Clinical Neurophysiology, 117*(6), 1217–1227.

Fregni, F., Gimenes, R., Valle, A. C., Ferreira, M. J., Rocha, R. R., Natalle, L., et al. (2006). A randomized, sham-controlled, proof of principle study of transcranial direct current stimulation for the treatment of pain in fibromyalgia. *Arthritis and Rheumatism*, *54*(12), 3988–3998.

Fregni, F., Liguori, P., Fecteau, S., Nitsche, M. A., Pascual-Leone, A., & Boggio, P. S. (2008). Cortical stimulation of the prefrontal cortex with transcranial direct current stimulation reduces cue-provoked smoking craving: a randomized, sham-controlled study. *Journal of Clinical Psychiatry*, *69*(1), 32–40.

Fregni, F., Thome-Souza, S., Nitsche, M. A., Freedman, S. D., Valente, K. D., & Pascual-Leone, A. (2006). A controlled clinical trial of cathodal DC polarization in patients with refractory epilepsy. *Epilepsia*, *47*(2), 335–342.

Fritsch, B., Reis, J., Martinowich, K., Schambra, H. M., Ji, Y., Cohen, L. G., et al. (2010). Direct current stimulation promotes BDNF-dependent synaptic plasticity: potential implications for motor learning. *Neuron*, *66*(2), 198–204.

Gevensleben, H., Holl, B., Albrecht, B., Schlamp, D., Kratz, O., Studer, P., et al. (2010). Neurofeedback training in children with ADHD: 6-month follow-up of a randomised controlled trial. *European Child and Adolescent Psychiatry* (in press).

Goldensohn, E. S. (1998). Animal electricity from Bologna to Boston. *Electroencephalography and Clinical Neurophysiology*, *106*(2), 94–100.

Hallett, M. (1995). Transcranial magnetic stimulation. Negative effects. *Advances in Neurology*, *67*, 107–113.

Ilmoniemi, R. J., Virtanen, J., Ruohonen, J., Karhu, J., Aronen, H. J., Naatanen, R., et al. (1997). Neuronal responses to magnetic stimulation reveal cortical reactivity and connectivity. *Neuroreport*, *8*(16), 3537–3540.

Iyer, M. B., Mattu, U., Grafman, J., Lomarev, M., Sato, S., & Wassermann, E. M. (2005). Safety and cognitive effect of frontal DC brain polarization in healthy individuals. *Neurology*, *64*(5), 872–875.

Jefferys, J. G., Deans, J., Bikson, M., & Fox, J. (2003). Effects of weak electric fields on the activity of neurons and neuronal networks. *Radiation Protection Dosimetry*, *106*(4), 321–323.

Jo, J. M., Kim, Y. H., Ko, M. H., Ohn, S. H., Joen, B., & Lee, K. H. (2009). Enhancing the working memory of stroke patients using tDCS. *American Journal of Physical Medicine and Rehabilitation*, *88*(5), 404–409.

Kwon, Y. H., Ko, M. H., Ahn, S. H., Kim, Y. H., Song, J. C., Lee, C. H., et al. (2008). Primary motor cortex activation by transcranial direct current stimulation in the human brain. *Neuroscience Letters*, *435*(1), 56–59.

Lakhan, S. E., & Callaway, E. (2010). Deep brain stimulation for obsessive-compulsive disorder and treatment-resistant depression: systematic review. *BMC Research Notes*, *3*, 60.

Lang, N., Siebner, H. R., Chadaide, Z., Boros, K., Nitsche, M. A., Rothwell, J. C., et al. (2007). Bidirectional modulation of primary visual cortex excitability: a combined tDCS and rTMS study. *Investigative Ophthalmology and Visual Science*, *48*(12), 5782–5787.

Lang, N., Siebner, H. R., Ward, N. S., Lee, L., Nitsche, M. A., Paulus, W., et al. (2005). How does transcranial DC stimulation of the primary motor cortex alter regional neuronal activity in the human brain? *European Journal of Neuroscience*, *22*(2), 495–504.

Lefaucheur, J. P. (2008). Principles of therapeutic use of transcranial and epidural cortical stimulation. *Clinical Neurophysiology*, *119*(10), 2179–2184.

Liebetanz, D., Fregni, F., Monte-Silva, K. K., Oliveira, M. B., Amancio-dos-Santos, A., Nitsche, M. A., et al. (2006). After-effects of transcranial direct current stimulation (tDCS) on cortical spreading depression. *Neuroscience Letters*, *398*(1–2), 85–90.

Liebetanz, D., Koch, R., Mayenfels, S., Konig, F., Paulus, W., & Nitsche, M. A. (2009). Safety limits of cathodal transcranial direct current stimulation in rats. *Clinical Neurophysiology*, *120*(6), 1161–1167.

Liebetanz, D., Nitsche, M. A., Tergau, F., & Paulus, W. (2002). Pharmacological approach to the mechanisms of transcranial DC-stimulation-induced after-effects of human motor cortex excitability. *Brain, 125*(Pt 10), 2238−2247.

Lima, M. C., & Fregni, F. (2008). Motor cortex stimulation for chronic pain: systematic review and meta-analysis of the literature. *Neurology, 70*(24), 2329−2337.

Limousin, P., & Martinez-Torres, I. (2008). Deep brain stimulation for Parkinson's disease. *Neurotherapeutics, 5*(2), 309−319.

Marshall, L., Molle, M., Hallschmid, M., & Born, J. (2004). Transcranial direct current stimulation during sleep improves declarative memory. *Journal of Neuroscience, 24*(44), 9985−9992.

Mayberg, H. S., Lozano, A. M., Voon, V., McNeely, H. E., Seminowicz, D., Hamani, C., et al. (2005). Deep brain stimulation for treatment-resistant depression. *Neuron, 45*(5), 651−660.

McDonnell, M. N., Orekhov, Y., & Ziemann, U. (2006). The role of GABA(B) receptors in intracortical inhibition in the human motor cortex. *Experimental Brain Research, 173* (1), 86−93.

Merzagora, A. C., Foffani, G., Panyavin, I., Mordillo-Mateos, L., Aguilar, J., Onaral, B., et al. (2010). Prefrontal hemodynamic changes produced by anodal direct current stimulation. *Neuroimage, 49*(3), 2304−2310.

Miniussi, C., & Thut, G. (2010). Combining TMS and EEG offers new prospects in cognitive neuroscience. *Brain Topography, 22*(4), 249−256.

Miranda, P. C., Lomarev, M., & Hallett, M. (2006). Modeling the current distribution during transcranial direct current stimulation. *Clinical Neurophysiology, 117*(7), 1623−1629.

Murphy, D. N., Boggio, P., & Fregni, F. (2009). Transcranial direct current stimulation as a therapeutic tool for the treatment of major depression: insights from past and recent clinical studies. *Current Opinions in Psychiatry, 22*(3), 306−311.

Nitsche, M. (2008). Transcranial direct current stimulation: State of the art 2008. *Brain Stimulation, 1*(3), 206−223.

Nitsche, M. A., Fricke, K., Henschke, U., Schlitterlau, A., Liebetanz, D., Lang, N., et al. (2003). Pharmacological modulation of cortical excitability shifts induced by transcranial direct current stimulation in humans. *Journal of Physiology, 553*(Pt 1), 293−301.

Nitsche, M. A., Jaussi, W., Liebetanz, D., Lang, N., Tergau, F., & Paulus, W. (2004). Consolidation of human motor cortical neuroplasticity by D-cycloserine. *Neuropsychopharmacology, 29*(8), 1573−1578.

Nitsche, M. A., Lampe, C., Antal, A., Liebetanz, D., Lang, N., Tergau, F., et al. (2006). Dopaminergic modulation of long-lasting direct current-induced cortical excitability changes in the human motor cortex. *European Journal of Neuroscience, 23*(6), 1651−1657.

Nitsche, M. A., Liebetanz, D., Lang, N., Antal, A., Tergau, F., & Paulus, W. (2003). Safety criteria for transcranial direct current stimulation (tDCS) in humans. *Clinical Neurophysiology, 114*(11), 2220−2222, author reply 2222-2223.

Nitsche, M. A., Niehaus, L., Hoffmann, K. T., Hengst, S., Liebetanz, D., Paulus, W., et al. (2004). MRI study of human brain exposed to weak direct current stimulation of the frontal cortex. *Clinical Neurophysiology, 115*(10), 2419−2423.

Nitsche, M. A., Nitsche, M. S., Klein, C. C., Tergau, F., Rothwell, J. C., & Paulus, W. (2003). Level of action of cathodal DC polarisation induced inhibition of the human motor cortex. *Clinical Neurophysiology, 114*(4), 600−604.

Nitsche, M. A., & Paulus, W. (2000). Excitability changes induced in the human motor cortex by weak transcranial direct current stimulation. *Journal of Physiology, 527*(Pt 3), 633−639.

Nitsche, M. A., & Paulus, W. (2001). Sustained excitability elevations induced by transcranial DC motor cortex stimulation in humans. *Neurology, 57*(10), 1899−1901.

Nitsche, M. A., Roth, A., Kuo, M. F., Fischer, A. K., Liebetanz, D., Lang, N., et al. (2007). Timing-dependent modulation of associative plasticity by general network excitability in the human motor cortex. *Journal of Neuroscience, 27*(14), 3807−3812.

Nitsche, M. A., Seeber, A., Frommann, K., Klein, C. C., Rochford, C., Nitsche, M. S., et al. (2005). Modulating parameters of excitability during and after transcranial direct current stimulation of the human motor cortex. *Journal of Physiology, 568*(Pt 1), 291−303.

Nowak, D. A., Grefkes, C., Ameli, M., & Fink, G. R. (2009). Interhemispheric competition after stroke: brain stimulation to enhance recovery of function of the affected hand. *Neurorehabilitation and Neural Repair, 23*(7), 641−656.

Palm, U., Keeser, D., Schiller, C., Fintescu, Z., Reisinger, E., Padberg, F., & Nitsche, M. (2008). Skin lesions after treatment with transcranial direct current stimulation (tDCS). *Brain Stimulation, 1*, 386−387.

Paulus, W. (2004). Outlasting excitability shifts induced by direct current stimulation of the human brain. *Clinical Neurophysiology, 57*(Suppl), 708−714.

Petersen, N. T., Pyndt, H. S., & Nielsen, J. B. (2003). Investigating human motor control by transcranial magnetic stimulation. *Experimental Brain Research, 152*(1), 1−16.

Poreisz, C., Boros, K., Antal, A., & Paulus, W. (2007). Safety aspects of transcranial direct current stimulation concerning healthy subjects and patients. *Brain Research Bulletin, 72*(4−6), 208−214.

Priori, A. (2003). Brain polarization in humans: a reappraisal of an old tool for prolonged non-invasive modulation of brain excitability. *Clinical Neurophysiology, 114*(4), 589−595.

Priori, A., Hallett, M., & Rothwell, J. C. (2009). Repetitive transcranial magnetic stimulation or transcranial direct current stimulation? *Brain Stimulation, 2*(4), 241−245.

Purpura, D. P., & McMurtry, J. G. (1965). Intracellular activities and evoked potential changes during polarization of motor cortex. *Journal of Neurophysiology, 28*, 166−185.

Radman, T., Datta, A., Ramos, R. L., Brumberg, J. C., & Bikson, M. (2009). One-dimensional representation of a neuron in a uniform electric field. *Conference Proceedings IEEE Engineering in Medicine and Biology Society, 2009*, 6481−6484.

Radman, T., Ramos, R. L., Brumberg, J. C., & Bikson, M. (2009). Role of cortical cell type and morphology in sub- and suprathreshold uniform electric field stimulation. *Brain Stimulation, 2*(4), 215−228.

Rango, M., Cogiamanian, F., Marceglia, S., Barberis, B., Arighi, A., Biondetti, P., et al. (2008). Myoinositol content in the human brain is modified by transcranial direct current stimulation in a matter of minutes: A (1)H-MRS study. *Magnetic Resonance in Medicine, 60*(4), 782−789.

Roche, N., Lackmy, A., Achache, V., Bussel, B., & Katz, R. (2009). Impact of transcranial direct current stimulation on spinal network excitability in humans. *Journal of Physiology, 587*(Pt, 23), 5653−5664.

Siebner, H. R., Lang, N., Rizzo, V., Nitsche, M. A., Paulus, W., Lemon, R. N., et al. (2004). Preconditioning of low-frequency repetitive transcranial magnetic stimulation with transcranial direct current stimulation: evidence for homeostatic plasticity in the human motor cortex. *Journal of Neuroscience, 24*(13), 3379−3385.

Silva, G., Miksad, R., Freedman, S. D., Pascual-Leone, A., Jain, S., Gomes, D. L., et al. (2007). Treatment of cancer pain with noninvasive brain stimulation. *Journal of Pain Symptom Management, 34*(4), 342−345.

Stagg, C. J., Best, J. G., Stephenson, M. C., O'Shea, J., Wylezinska, M., Kincses, Z. T., et al. (2009). Polarity-sensitive modulation of cortical neurotransmitters by transcranial stimulation. *Journal of Neuroscience, 29*(16), 5202−5206.

Stefan, K., Wycislo, M., Gentner, R., Schramm, A., Naumann, M., Reiners, K., et al. (2006). Temporary occlusion of associative motor cortical plasticity by prior dynamic motor training. *Cerebral Cortex, 16*(3), 376–385.

Tehovnik, E. J. (1996). Electrical stimulation of neural tissue to evoke behavioral responses. *Journal of Neuroscience Methods, 65*(1), 1–17.

Tergau, F., Wanschura, V., Canelo, M., Wischer, S., Wassermann, E. M., Ziemann, U., et al. (1999). Complete suppression of voluntary motor drive during the silent period after transcranial magnetic stimulation. *Experimental Brain Research, 124*(4), 447–454.

Thut, G., Ives, J. R., Kampmann, F., Pastor, M. A., & Pascual-Leone, A. (2005). A new device and protocol for combining TMS and online recordings of EEG and evoked potentials. *Journal of Neuroscience Methods, 141*(2), 207–217.

Uy, J., & Ridding, M. C. (2003). Increased cortical excitability induced by transcranial DC and peripheral nerve stimulation. *Journal of Neuroscience Methods, 127*(2), 193–197.

Vines, B. W., Cerruti, C., & Schlaug, G. (2008). Dual-hemisphere tDCS facilitates greater improvements for healthy subjects' non-dominant hand compared to uni-hemisphere stimulation. *BMC Neuroscience, 9*(1), 103.

Wagner, T., Fregni, F., Fecteau, S., Grodzinsky, A., Zahn, M., & Pascual-Leone, A. (2007). Transcranial direct current stimulation: a computer-based human model study. *Neuroimage, 35*(3), 1113–1124.

Wagner, T., Valero-Cabre, A., & Pascual-Leone, A. (2007). Noninvasive human brain stimulation. *Annual Review of Biomedical Engineering, 9*, 527–565.

Wassermann, E. M., & Grafman, J. (2005). Recharging cognition with DC brain polarization. *Trends in Cognitive Science, 9*(11), 503–505.

Williams, J. A., Pascual-Leone, A., & Fregni, F. (2010). Interhemispheric modulation induced by cortical stimulation and motor training. *Physical Therapy, 90*(3), 398–410.

Wolters, A., Sandbrink, F., Schlottmann, A., Kunesch, E., Stefan, K., Cohen, L. G., et al. (2003). A temporally asymmetric Hebbian rule governing plasticity in the human motor cortex. *Journal of Neurophysiology, 89*(5), 2339–2345.

Zaghi, S., Acar, M., Hultgren, B., Boggio, P. S., & Fregni, F. (2010). Noninvasive brain stimulation with low-intensity electrical currents: putative mechanisms of action for direct and alternating current stimulation. *Neuroscientist, 16*(3), 285–307.

Zaghi, S., Heine, N., & Fregni, F. (2009). Brain stimulation for the treatment of pain: A review of costs, clinical effects, and mechanisms of treatment for three different central neuromodulatory approaches. *Journal of Pain Management, 2*(3), 339–352.

Ziemann, U., Ilic, T. V., Pauli, C., Meintzschel, F., & Ruge, D. (2004). Learning modifies subsequent induction of long-term potentiation-like and long-term depression-like plasticity in human motor cortex. *Journal of Neuroscience, 24*(7), 1666–1672.

Ziemann, U., Lonnecker, S., Steinhoff, B. J., & Paulus, W. (1996). Effects of antiepileptic drugs on motor cortex excitability in humans: a transcranial magnetic stimulation study. *Annals of Neurology, 40*(3), 367–378.

PART Four

Mechanism of Change and Long-Term Consolidation: Beginning Evidence

CHAPTER 13

Functional Neuroimaging Evidence Supporting Neurofeedback in ADHD

Johanne Lévesque[1] and Mario Beauregard[2]

[1]Institut PsychoNeuro, Laval, Canada
[2]Centre de Recherche en Neuropsychologie et Cognition (CERNEC), Département de Psychologie, Université de Montréal; Département de Radiologie, Université de Montréal; Centre de Recherche en Sciences Neurologiques (CRSN), Université de Montréal, and Centre de Recherche du Centre Hospitalier de l'Université de Montréal (CRCHUM), Canada

Contents

INTRODUCTION

Attention deficit hyperactivity disorder (ADHD) was first described more than a century ago under the name "hyperkinesis disorder in childhood" (Still, 1902). In the 1960s the National Institutes of Health adopted the term "minimal brain dysfunction" to describe this disorder. Following this renaming, the focus on "attention" led to the analysis of the brain localization of attention deficits (Barkley, 1997; Mattes, 1980). This effort was supported by new conceptualizations in the neurobiological bases of attentional processes (Heilman, Pandya, & Geschwind, 1970; Heilman, Watson, Bower, & Valenstein, 1983; Mesulam, 1990; Posner & Petersen, 1990). Based on these new insights, a large number of studies were performed over the last decades to circumscribe the brain basis of ADHD.

Neurofeedback and Neuromodulation Techniques and Applications
DOI: 10.1016/B978-0-12-382235-2.00013-5

ADHD is a frequent neurodevelopmental disorder of childhood, which affects 3—7% of children worldwide, and frequently continues into adulthood (Barkley, 1996). This disorder negatively affects academic performance in childhood and leads to increased risk for antisocial disorders and drug abuse in adulthood (Mannuzza, Klein, Bessler, Malloy, & Hynes, 1997). The ADHD syndrome is mainly characterized by deficits in selective attention and response inhibition (Barkley, 1997). These symptoms reflect impairments in executive functions. The latter functions refer to the dynamic regulatory capacities for the initiation and maintenance of efficient attainment of goals (Lezak, 1990), as well as the inhibition of behavioral responses that are inappropriate in the current context (Shallice, 1988). This type of behavioral regulation is essential to successfully adapt one's behavior to changing environmental demands. Executive functions are closely related to prefrontal and striatal brain systems (Godefroy, Lhullier, & Rousseaux, 1996; Leimkuhler & Mesulam, 1985; Smith & Jonides, 1999). Of special importance and relevance to this chapter, there is mounting evidence indicating that neurofeedback may be efficacious in treating individuals with ADHD.

Aetiologically and clinically, ADHD is more a heterogeneous than a homogenous syndrome. This has led to the idea that this disorder can be caused by a multitude of factors (Steinhausen, 2009). In keeping with this idea, a variety of factors have been proposed to explain the different aspects of this neurobiological disorder. In the second section of this chapter we cover these factors, which include genes and brain abnormalities (measured with various neuroimaging techniques). In the following section we review the functional neuroimaging findings supporting the view that neurofeedback can significantly improve cognitive and executive functions in ADHD individuals. In the fourth section we discuss putative neural mechanisms underlying the effects of neurofeedback in ADHD. Finally, in the last section, we provide a few concluding remarks and propose new opportunities for expanding the neuroscientific study of the effects of neurofeedback in individuals with ADHD.

BIOLOGICAL BASIS OF ADHD

Neurogenetics

Over the past decades considerable progress has been made in understanding the aetiology of ADHD because of the publication of several twin studies. These twin studies are consistent in advocating large genetic influences (i.e., heritability ranging from 60% to 90%), non-shared environmental influences that are small-to-moderate in magnitude (i.e., ranging from 10% to 40%), and little-to-no shared environmental influences (Waldman & Gizer, 2006). A polygenic transmission model seems likely (Faraone & Doyle 2001; Morrison & Stewart 1974). Still, the genetic architecture of ADHD is not currently clear. Indeed, it has proven difficult to identify the individual genes contributing to the genetic variance of ADHD. Three approaches have been used in attempts to circumscribe the genetic influences: hypothesis-driven candidate gene association studies, hypothesis-free genome-wide linkage analysis, and the genome-wide association study methodology.

Candidate Gene Association Methodology

The candidate gene association methodology is limited to hypothesis-driven studies on candidate genes. Such an approach is largely conditioned by the amount of existing knowledge regarding disease aetiology. Since this knowledge is still limited for ADHD, candidate gene-based studies are likely to miss at least part of the genetic variance. To date, such studies cannot explain more than 3–5% of the total genetic components of ADHD (Li, Sham, Owen, & He, 2006). These studies have mainly concentrated on genes involved in catecholaminergic neurotransmission.

Genes associated with the dopaminergic system – in particular the D4 dopamine receptor gene (DRD4) and the human dopamine transporter gene (DAT1/SLC6A3) – have been frequently investigated. The particular interest in this neurotransmission system comes from the effectiveness of methylphenidate in treating ADHD symptoms (this psychostimulant drug acts by blocking the dopamine transporter). The dopaminergic system has also been investigated because of the association between ADHD, executive functions, and fronto-striatal pathways (Swanson et al., 2007). The DRD4 gene – encoding a receptor expressed primarily in the prefrontal cortex – is the strongest and most consistently replicated molecular genetics finding in ADHD. A meta-analysis of more than 30 studies found that the DRD4 7-repeat (DRD4-7r) allele increases the risk for ADHD, although this increase is only moderate with a pooled odds ratio of 1.34 (Faraone, Doyle, Mick, & Biederman, 2001; Li et al., 2006). According to Asghari and colleagues (1995), this allele seems to alter the function of the encoded receptor by making it less sensitive to dopamine than the alternative alleles. Despite mixed results across studies (for a review, see Banaschewski, Becker, Scherag, Franke, & Coghill 2010), the

7-repeat allele might be associated with behavioral features rather than cognitive deficits (Asghari et al., 1995). In fact, association of high reaction time variability with the 7-repeat allele absence appears to be the most consistent result and seems to be specific to ADHD (Kebir, Grizenk, Sengupta, & Joober 2009). Regarding structural anatomical correlates, Durston and colleagues (2005) suggested that variations in DRD4 influence prefrontal gray matter volume in a sample of subjects that included individuals with ADHD as well as their unaffected siblings, and healthy controls. Monuteaux and collaborators (2009) also reported findings in adults with ADHD showing that 7-repeat allele carriers have a significantly smaller mean volume in the superior frontal cortex and cerebellum cortex when compared to subjects without this particular allele.

The dopamine transporter DAT1 is expressed primarily in the striatum and the nucleus accumbens, and is a site of action of methylphenidate. Consequently, the relationship between ADHD and variations in the DAT1 gene has been largely investigated. A recent meta-analysis has shown positive and negative associations between DAT1 and ADHD (Li et al., 2006). Based on these contradictory findings, further studies of the association of the DAT1 alleles and ADHD in large datasets are needed before drawing any conclusion. Durston et al. (2005) reported that DAT1 variability seems to influence caudate nucleus volume. At the functional level, the results of a neuroimaging study suggested that the DAT1 genotype affects activation in the striatum, and that the familial risk of ADHD is related to this cerebral structure (Durston, Fossella, Mulder, Casey, Ziermans et al., 2008).

Adrenergic neurotransmitter systems are hypothesized to mediate attentional processes and certain dimensions of executive control (Arnsten, 2006). In this regard, there is growing evidence for involvement of genetic variants of the adrenergic receptor alpha-2A gene (ADRA2A) in ADHD (Anney et al., 2008; Cho et al., 2008; Deupree et al., 2006; Schmitz et al., 2006; Wang et al., 2006). These variants seem to be more relevant for inattentive than hyperactive/impulsive symptoms (Roman et al., 2002; Schmitz et al., 2006). Cho et al. (2008) reported associations between variants of the alpha-2C adrenergic receptor gene (ADRA2C) and ADHD in their sample of Korean subjects while Guan and colleagues (2009) reported an association of ADRA2C variants with ADHD combined type.

As for the serotoninergic system, serotonin dysregulation has been related to impulsive behavior in children (Halperin et al., 1997). Consequently, this neurotransmitter/neuromodulator has been hypothesized to be causally involved in ADHD (Oades et al. 2008) "knockout" gene studies in mice, in which the behavioral effects of the deactivation of specific genes are examined, have further evidenced the potential implication of serotoninergic genes (Gainetdinov et al., 1999). The main candidate genes studied within the serotoninergic system are those coding for the serotonin transporter (5-HTT/SLC6A4), the 1B and 2A serotonin receptors (HTR1B) and (HTR2A), and the tryptophan hydroxylase (TPH2) genes. There are contradictory findings for the potential association of the serotonin receptors with ADHD. A meta-analysis supported an association between the HTR1B gene and ADHD (Faraone et al., 2005). However, such an association was not found in subsequent investigations (Brookes et al., 2006; Ickowicz et al., 2007). Similarly, several groups have reported positive findings for HTR2A (Guimaraes et al., 2007, Ribases et al., 2009), whilst others have failed to find an association (Dorval et al., 2007; Romanos et al., 2008). In addition, a meta-analysis has supported an association between ADHD and a 44-base-pair insertion/deletion (5-HTTLPR) in the promoter region of the serotonin transporter gene (5-HTT/SLC6A4). However, although there have been further replications since this meta-analysis (Li, Kang, Zhang, Wang, Zhou, et al., 2007; Kopeckova et al., 2008; Retz et al., 2008), several studies have failed to replicate this finding (Brookes et al., 2006; Grevet et al., 2007; Mick & Faraone, 2008; Wigg et al., 2006; Xu et al., 2008). Finally, Li and colleagues (2003, 2006) have reported on ADHD associations for the tryptophan hydroxylase 2 gene (TPH2), which mediates the transformation of tryptophan to 5-hydroxytryptophan, and these findings have been replicated (Lasky-Su et al., 2008; Sheehan et al., 2005; Walitza et al., 2005).

Genome-Wide Linkage Analysis

Genome-wide, hypothesis-free linkage analysis has been performed in ADHD using qualitative and quantitative definitions of the disease phenotype (Arcos-Burgos et al., 2004; Asherson et al., 2008; Bakker et al., 2003; Hebebrand et al., 2006; Ogdie et al., 2006; Romanos et al., 2008; Zhou, Dempfle et al., 2008), and recently also using ADHD endophenotypes at the level of neuropsychological functioning (Doyle et al., 2008; Rommelse et al., 2008). The linkage studies in ADHD have identified a number of genetic loci potentially harbouring genes for ADHD, but very little overlap was observed between studies, so far. However, a recent meta-analysis of ADHD linkage studies confirmed one locus, on chromosome 16 (Zhou, Chen et al., 2008).

Genome-Wide Association Study Methodology

Using the genome-wide association study methodology, it is now possible to perform hypothesis-free analyses of the entire genome. Taken together, results from the genome-wide association study performed in ADHD have failed to show genome-wide significant association with ADHD according to the thresholds currently used (Dudbridge & Gusnanto, 2008; Peter, Yelensky, Altshuler, & Daly, 2008; van Steen & Lange, 2005). Indeed, little overlap is observed between studies, except for the CDH13 gene (Lasky-Su et al., 2008; Lesch, Timmesfeld, Renner, Halperin, Roser et al., 2008; Neale et al., 2008). Interestingly, this gene is thought to participate in neuronal cell−cell communication during development and maturation of the brain.

Brain Abnormalities

Structural Anomalies

Consistent with the clinical picture of ADHD, anatomical magnetic resonance imaging (MRI) has identified abnormalities in brain regions playing a key role in attention, behavioral inhibition or motor control (Seidman, Valera & Makris, 2005; Valera, Faraone, Murray, & Seidman, 2007).

MRI investigations have reported that children with ADHD, compared with non-ADHD children, show a slight reduction in total brain volume (Castellanos et al., 2002), and that individuals with ADHD show smaller prefrontal volumes (Aylward et al., 1996; Castellanos et al., 1994, 1996, 2001; Durston et al., 2004; Filipek et al., 1997; Garavan, Ross, Murphy, Roche, & Stein, 2002; Hill et al., 2003; Kates et al., 2002; Mataro, Garcia-Sanchez, Junque, Estevez-Gonzalez, & Pujol, 1997; Mostofsky, Cooper, Kates, Denckla, & Kaufmann, 2002; Overmeyer et al., 2001; Shaw et al., 2006; Sowell et al., 2003). Additionally, adults with ADHD have a smaller anterior cingulate cortex (ACC) volume than healthy controls (Duncan & Owen, 2000). About this cerebral structure, two studies revealed volumetric decreases on the right ACC in treatment-naïve children with ADHD relative to treated children with ADHD and normal children (Pliszka et al., 2006; Semrud-Clikeman, Pliszka, Lancaster, & Liotti, 2006). The ACC is thought to be centrally important in cognition and motor control, and to be involved in processes underlying the arousal/drive state of the organism (Dum & Strick, 1993; Paus, 2001). The dorsal part of the ACC (dACC) is known to play a role in complex cognitive operations (Bush, Luu, & Posner, 2000) such as target detection, response selection, error detection, action monitoring and reward-based decision-making (Bush et al., 2002; Carter et al., 1998, 2000; Gehring & Knight, 2000), all important aspects of executive functions known to be impaired in children diagnosed with ADHD (Makris, Biederman, Monuteaux, & Seidman, 2009).

A growing body of neuroimaging studies supports a role for the basal ganglia in ADHD. Most investigations have demonstrated significantly smaller total caudate or smaller caudate head, either on the left or right side (Castellanos et al., 1994, 2002; Semrud-Clikeman et al., 1994). Studies of children with ADHD have revealed that the globus pallidus is smaller on the right (Castellanos et al., 1996; Overmeyer et al., 2001) or the left (Aylward et al., 1996; Castellanos et al., 2001, 2002). Furthermore, Castellanos et al. (2002) demonstrated that significant differences between children with ADHD and controls in caudate volume attenuated by the oldest age studied (19 years), thus showing a normalization of brain volume over time. Bilateral caudate volumetric decrease has been shown in treatment-naïve children with ADHD compared to treated children with ADHD and controls (Semrud-Clikeman, Pliszka, Lancaster, & Liotti, 2006). Additionally, Seidman et al. (2006) demonstrated that the nucleus accumbens is larger in adults with ADHD.

The cerebellum also has been demonstrated to be structurally altered in ADHD. Cerebellar structural abnormalities can manifest with impairments in executive functions since the cerebellum innervates frontal and parietal association areas involved in higher cognitive processes (Timmann & Daum, 2007). Interestingly, volumetric reductions in lobules VIII, IX, and X of the vermis have been noted in both ADHD boys (Berquin et al., 1998; Castellanos et al., 1996; Mostofsky, Reiss, Lokhart, & Denck-La, 1998) and girls (Castellanos et al., 2001; Hill et al., 2003). Bussing and colleagues (2002) also found reductions in vermal lobules VI and VII. Furthermore, Castellanos and collaborators (2002) found that once they adjusted for total cerebral volume, only the cerebellar volume was smaller in 152 ADHD adolescents compared to 139 matched control subjects. This measure also correlated significantly and negatively with measures of attentional difficulties. Durston et al. (2004) corroborated the finding of a smaller cerebellum in a group of 30 ADHD children.

Volumetric differences have also been observed in the inferior parietal lobule, a cortical region known to be associated with attentional processes. Sowell and colleagues (2003) reported an increased size of cortex in the inferior parietal lobule of children and adolescents with ADHD. On the other hand, another study reported a decrease in cortical thickness of that region in adults with ADHD (Makris et al., 2007). These results may appear contradictory, but volume and cortical thickness are distinct measures and may not correlate with one another.

In other respects, there is some evidence from MRI structural investigations that white matter abnormalities are present in children, adolescents and adults with ADHD (Castellanos et al., 2002; Filipek et al., 1997; Hynd, Semrud-Clikeman, Lorys, Novey & Eliopulos, 1990; Overmeyer et al., 2001; Seidman et al., 2006). The studies involving ADHD children and adolescents indicate a decrease in overall white matter volume (Castellanos et al., 2002) whereas the studies conducted in adults with ADHD reveal a tendency toward an overall increase in white matter volume (Seidman et al., 2006). It is noteworthy that these investigations, instead of examining specific fiber pathways, considered the cerebral white matter in its entirety.

To date there are only a few published MR studies that used diffusion tensor imaging (DTI) in individuals with ADHD. In the first of these studies, Ashtari et al. (2005) demonstrated that ADHD children had decreased fractional anisotropy (FA, an index of white matter integrity) in regions that have been implicated in the pathophysiology of ADHD, such as the premotor cortex, striatum, cerebellum, and parieto-occipital areas. These findings support the hypothesis that alterations in brain white matter integrity occur in ADHD. Decreased FA has also been reported in ADHD children and adolescents in the anterior corona radiata, anterior limb of the internal capsule, and superior region of the internal capsule (Pavuluri et al., 2009). Reduced FA implies an impaired fiber density or reduced myelination in these pathways. In adults with ADHD, decreased FA has been found in fiber pathways such as the superior longitudinal fascicle II and the cingulum bundle, both known to be affiliated with attention and executive functions (Makris et al., 2008).

Regional Brain Dysfunction

During resting state, single photon emission computed tomography (SPECT) and positron emission tomography (PET) studies carried out in ADHD children, adolescents, or adults have shown decreased metabolism in the striatum and various prefrontal areas involved in the control of attentional processes (Amen & Carmichael, 1997; Kim, Lee, Shin, Cho, & Lee, 2002; Lou, Henriksen, Bruhn, Borner, & Nielsen, 1989; Sieg, Gaffney, Preston, & Hellings, 1995; Zametkin et al., 1990).

Functional neuroimaging studies have demonstrated that differences in cognitive control between individuals with and without ADHD are related to differences in brain activation patterns (e.g., Bush et al., 1999; Durston & Casey, 2006; Durston et al., 2003; Konrad et al., 2006; Rubia, Overmeyer, Taylor, Brammer, Williams, et al., 1999; Vaidya et al., 1998). These studies have shown reduced activation in prefrontal and striatal regions during tasks that require subjects to inhibit prepotent tendencies such as GO/NO-GO or Stroop paradigms (Booth et al., 2005; Bush et al., 1999; Durston et al., 2003; Durston, Mulder, Casey, Ziermans, & van Engeland, 2006; Konrad et al., 2006; Pliszka et al., 2006; Rubia et al., 1999; Rubia, Smith, Brammer, Toone, & Tayler, 2005; Shafritz, Marchione, Gore, Shaywitz, & Shaywitz, 2004; Schulz, Newcorn, Fan, Tang, & Halperin 2005; Suskauer et al., 2008; Tamm, Menon, Ringel, & Reiss, 2004; Vaidya et al., 1998). Other studies have used paradigms that investigate other aspects of behavior, such as aspects of attention (Bush et al., 2008; Konrad et al., 2006; Konrad, Neufang, Fink, & Herpertz-Dahlmann, 2007; Stevens, Pearlson, & Kiehl, 2007; Tamm, Menon, & Reiss, 2006), mental rotation paradigms (Silk et al., 2005) and motivated behavior (Scheres, Miham, Knutson, & Castellanos, 2007; Ströhle et al., 2008). Again, deficits in striatal (Konrad et al., 2006; Scheres et al., 2007; Shafritz et al., 2004; Silk et al., 2005; Ströhle et al., 2008) and prefrontal (Konrad et al., 2006; Silk et al., 2005) activation have been found, as well as changes in activation in parietal areas (Konrad et al., 2006; Shafritz et al., 2004; Silk et al., 2005; Stevens et al., 2007). These findings underscore the importance of fronto-striatal networks in ADHD, as deficits in these networks have been associated with various cognitive functions.

Additionally, a recent study using DTI has shown that reduced fronto-striatal activation during a GO/NO-GO task was associated with reduced white matter integrity in both children with ADHD and their affected parents (Casey, Epstein, Buhle, Liston, Davidson, et al., 2007). These findings suggest that disruption of fronto-striatal white matter tracts may contribute to a familial form of the disorder.

IMPACT OF NEUROFEEDBACK TRAINING ON THE NEURAL SUBSTRATES OF SELECTIVE ATTENTION AND RESPONSE INHIBITION IN CHILDREN WITH ADHD

The results of several clinical studies performed during the last three decades suggest that neurofeedback may be efficacious in treating individuals with ADHD (Fuchs, Birbaumer, Lutzenberger, Gruzelier, & Kaiser, 2003; Gevensleben et al., 2009; Kropotov et al., 2005; Linden, Habib, & Radojevic, 1996; Lubar & Lubar, 1984; Lubar & Shouse, 1976; Lubar, Swartwood, Swartwood, & O"Donnell, 1995; Monastra, Monastra, & George, 2002; Rossiter, 2004; Rossiter & LaVaque, 1995; Shouse & Lubar, 1979; Strehl, Leins, Goth, Klinger, Hinterberger, et al., 2006; Tansey, 1984, 1985; Thompson & Thompson, 1998). In many of these studies, the operant enhancement of sensorimotor rhythm (SMR) (12–15 Hz) and/or beta 1 (15–20 Hz) EEG activity from the regions overlying the Rolandic area, was trained concomitantly with suppression of theta (4–7 Hz) activity. The basic assumption guiding this approach is that SMR enhancement reduces problems of hyperactivity, whereas increasing beta 1 activity and suppressing theta activity diminishes attention deficits (Lubar & Shouse, 1976). In line with this assumption, these studies demonstrated that neurofeedback training (NFT) can significantly reduce attention deficits and hyperactivity in children with ADHD.

Recently, we used fMRI to measure the effects of NFT — in ADHD children — on the neural substrates of selective attention and response inhibition (Beauregard & Lévesque, 2006; Lévesque, Beauregard, & Mensour, et al., 2006). Brain activity was measured during a Counting Stroop task (Experiment 1) and a GO/NO-GO task (Experiment 2). The Counting Stroop task, which implicates selective attention and response inhibition, exploits the conflict between a well-learned behavior (i.e., reading) and a decision rule that requires this behavior to be inhibited. Converging evidence from PET and fMRI indicate that the dorsal division of the ACC (or ACcd, Brodmann area-BA-24b'-c' and 32') plays an important role in the various cognitive processes involved in the Stroop task (e.g., interference, allocation of attentional resources, response selection) (Bush et al., 1998, 2000). In GO/NO-GO tasks, subjects are required to refrain from responding to designated items within a series of stimuli. FMRI studies have shown that several prefrontal areas (ACC, dorsolateral prefrontal cortex, orbitofrontal cortex, ventrolateral prefrontal cortex) (Casey, Durston, & Fossella, 2001; Garavan et al., 1999, 2002; Kiehl, Liddle, & Hopfinger, 2000; Liddle, Kiehl & Smith, 2001 Konishi, Nakajima, Uchida, Sekihara, & Miyashita, 1998; Menon, Adleman, White, Glover, & Reiss, 2001; Rubia, Smith, Brammer, & Taylor, 2003) and the striatum (Menon et al., 2001) are crucially involved in response inhibition.

The study sample was composed of 20 ADHD children. These ADHD children were randomly assigned to either an Experimental (EXP) group or a control (CON) group. Fifteen children diagnosed as ADHD comprised the EXP group (4 girls and 11 boys, mean age: 10.2, range: 8–12) and five children also diagnosed as ADHD comprised the CON group (5 boys, mean age: 10.2, range: 9–11). The EXP group received NFT whereas the CON group received no treatment (the CON group served specifically to measure the effect of passage of time). Subjects were not taking any psychostimulant drug during the study (subjects in both EXP and CON groups had been treated with methylphenidate before the beginning of the study). Clinical assessment of the subjects included: (1) psychiatric, medical, and neurologic evaluations by a board certified child psychiatrist; (2) structured diagnostic interview with the Structured Clinical Interview (Spitzer, Williams, Gibbon, & First, 1992) and an ADHD symptom checklist from DSM-IV (1994). Neuropsychological testing included the Digit Span subtest of the Wechsler Intelligence Scale for Children–Revised (WISC–R) (Wechsler, 1981) to assess attention span, and the Integrated Visual and Auditory Continuous Performance Test (IVA) (Full Scale Attention Quotient and Full Scale Response Control Quotient) to evaluate visual and auditory attention (Sandford & Turner, 1995). The Conners Parent Rating Scale–Revised (CPRS–R), was also used to obtain parental reports of subjects' behavioral problems regarding specifically inattention and hyperactivity (Conners et al., 1997).

The Digit Span, the IVA, and the CPRS-R were administered at Time 1 (1 week before the beginning of the NFT) and Time 2 (1 week after the end of the NFT). Before treatment the EXP and CON groups did not differ cognitively or behaviourally in regard to these measures.

NFT was based on a protocol previously developed by Lubar and Lubar (1984). It was conducted over a period of 13½ weeks (40 sessions, three training sessions per week). The training was divided into two phases (20 sessions in each phase): in the first phase, subjects in the EXP group were trained to enhance the amplitude of the SMR (12–15 Hz) and decrease the amplitude of theta activity (4–7 Hz); in the second phase, EXP subjects learned to inhibit the amplitude of their theta waves (4–7 Hz) and increase the amplitude of their beta 1 waves (15–18 Hz). EEG was recorded from CZ, with reference placed on the left earlobe and ground electrode on the right earlobe. The pertinent frequencies were extracted from EEG recordings and fed back using an audio-visual online feedback loop in the form of a video game. Each session was subdivided into 2 min periods (that were gradually increased up to 10 min). During the training sessions, subjects were either attempting to maintain a state of relaxation, solve mathematical problems or read texts.

The scores of the CON subjects on the three neuropsychological tests were not significantly different at Time 2 than those at Time 1. For the EXP group, however, the scores on the Digit Span ($p < 0.05$) and the IVA ($p < 0.005$) significantly increased at Time 2, compared to Time 1. Moreover, at Time 2 the scores on the Inattention ($p < 0.0001$) and Hyperactivity ($p < 0.05$) components of the CPRS-R significantly decreased relative to Time 1.

As for the Counting Stroop task (Experiment 1), at Time 1 the average accuracy scores (percentage of correct responses) were not statistically different between the CON and EXP groups. At Time 2, the average accuracy score of the CON subjects was comparable to that of Time 1. For the EXP group, this score was significantly higher at Time 2 than Time 1 ($p < 0.05$).

With respect to brain activation patterns in the CON group, at Time 1 the Counting Stroop task (Interference minus Neutral contrast) generated a significant locus of activation in the left superior parietal lobule (Brodmann area [BA] 7) ($p < 0.001$). At Time 2, this contrast was associated with another locus of blood oxygenation level-dependent (BOLD) activation in the left superior parietal lobule (BA 7) ($p < 0.001$). For the EXP group, at Time 1 a significant locus of activation was noted in the left superior parietal lobule (BA 7) ($p < 0.001$). At Time 2, significant loci of activation were detected in the left superior parietal lobule (BA 7), right ACcd (BA 32), left caudate nucleus, and left substantia nigra ($p < 0.001$) (Figure 13.1).

In Experiment 2 (GO/NO-GO task), the average accuracy scores for GO and NO-GO trials were not statistically different between both groups of subjects at Time 1. For CON subjects, these scores were comparable at Time 1 and Time 2. For EXP subjects, however, the average accuracy scores for GO ($p < 0.05$) and NO-GO trials ($p < 0.0005$) were significantly higher at Time 2 than Time 1.

In regard to brain responses, at both Time 1 and Time 2 the GO/NO-GO task (NO-GO minus GO contrast) did not produce any significant locus of activation in CON subjects. As for the members of the EXP group, the NO-GO minus GO contrast did not reveal any significant locus of activation at Time 1. Nevertheless, at Time 2 significant loci of activation were noted in these subjects in the right ACcd (BA 24/32), right ventrolateral prefrontal cortex (BA 47), left

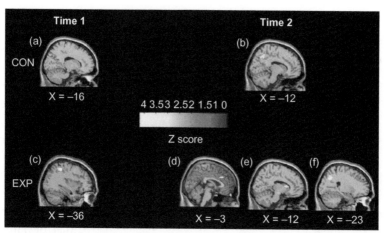

Figure 13.1 *(See Color Plate section)* Statistical activation maps at Time 1 and Time 2 produced by the Interference minus Neutral contrast. Images are sagittal sections for the data averaged across subjects. At Time 1, significant loci of activation were detected in the left superior parietal lobule for both the CON (a) and EXP (c) groups. At Time 2, activations were also noted in this cortical region for the CON (b) and EXP (f) groups. In addition, for the EXP group only, significant loci of activation were measured in the right ACcd (d), as well as the left caudate nucleus and left substantia nigra (e). *(Reproduced from Beauregard & Lévesque (2006) by permission of Springer Science + Business Media.)*

thalamus, left caudate nucleus, and left substantia nigra (p < 0.001) (Figure 13.2).

The post- vs. pre-treatment comparison of the average scores on the Digit Span, the IVA, and the CPRS-R suggests that NFT led to a significant decrease of inattention and hyperactivity in the EXP group. Furthermore, this improvement was associated with better performance on the Counting Stroop task and on the GO/NO-GO task. These findings accord with those of previous studies showing that NFT can significantly improve attention and response inhibition in ADHD children (Fuchs et al., 2003; Kropotov et al., 2005; Linden et al., 1996; Lubar & Lubar, 1984; Lubar & Shouse, 1976; Lubar et al., 1995; Monastra et al., 2002; Rossiter, 2004; Rossiter & LaVaque, 1995; Shouse & Lubar, 1979; Tansey, 1984, 1985; Thompson & Thompson, 1998). We posited that these improvements were related to an enhancement, following NFT, of neural activity in brain regions and networks involved in diverse attentional processes (e.g., ACcd) and in suppression of inappropriate

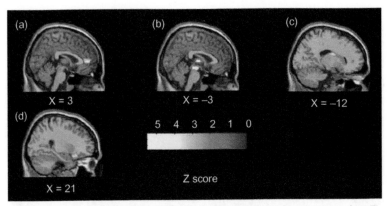

Figure 13.2 *(See Color Plate Section)* Statistical activation maps measured at Time 2 in the EXP group (NO-GO minus GO contrast). Significant loci of activation were measured in the right ACcd (a), left thalamus and left substantia nigra (b), left caudate nucleus (c), and right ventrolateral prefrontal cortex (d). *(Reproduced from Beauregard & Lévesque (2006) by permission of Springer Science + Business Media.)*

behavioral responses (e.g., caudate nucleus, thalamus, ventrolateral prefrontal cortex) (Beauregard & Lévesque, 2006; Lévesque et al., 2006).

PUTATIVE NEURAL MECHANISMS UNDERLYING THE EFFECTS OF NEUROFEEDBACK IN ADHD

ADHD is currently hypothesized to originate from genetic and perinatal environmental factors whose effects unfold across development. The resulting pathophysiology is characterized by structural and functional abnormalities in cortico-cortical and fronto-subcortical neural networks presumably mediating attention, executive functions, and motor regulation. Regarding this issue, Makris and colleagues (2009) proposed that the attention network includes the cingulate gyrus, the lateral and medial prefrontal cortices (middle and superior lateral frontal gyri), the lateral-inferior parietal and temporo-occipito-parietal cortices (the inferior parietal lobule including the angular and supramarginal gyri) and a few thalamic nuclei (medial dorsal, reticular, and pulvinar). The main connecting fiber pathways are three subcomponents of the superior longitudinal fascicle (I, II, and III), the cingulum bundle, and the inferior longitudinal fascicle. According to Makris et al. (2009), the executive functions network involves prefrontal cortical and striatal areas, as well as cortical limbic structures such as the ACC. The principal fiber tracts mediating the connections between these brain regions are the cingulum bundle and the corticostriatal projections. As for motor regulation, Makris and colleagues (2009) postulate that the network consists of parallel networks (cortico-striatal, cortico-pallidal, fronto-cerebellar) mediating motor and cognitive functions. In the cortico-striatal circuit, the caudate nucleus receives projections from the extrastriate, lateral parietal and lateral frontal areas, and the temporal cortices. The cortico-pallidal projections are from premotor cortex and from primary somatosensory and motor cortices. The fronto-cerebellar circuit connects frontal cortical areas with the cerebellum. The latter structure is topologically connected to distinct sensorimotor and association regions by way of the pons via the feed-forward pathway, and through the thalamus via the feedback pathway.

It is conceivable that the NFT administered in our study (Beauregard & Lévesque, 2006; Lévesque et al., 2006) significantly improved activity in the neural networks supporting attention, executive functions, and motor regulation. In this study, subjects were trained to enhance the amplitude of the SMR and Beta 1 activity. Lubar (1997) submitted that although thalamic pacemakers generate different brain rhythms depending on which cortical loops they activate, changes in cortical loops can modify the firing rate of thalamic pacemakers and, hence, alter their intrinsic firing pattern. In this view, the neurofeedback protocol used in our investigation might have influenced central and frontal loops which, in turn, might have linked dynamically through regional resonances to other brain regions including the thalamus. Furthermore, it is likely that dopamine is critically affected by this neurofeedback protocol.

Dopamine is known to exert a pivotal neuromodulatory effect in the brain (Seamans & Yang, 2004). A wealth of evidence suggests that a dysfunction in dopaminergic transmission in fronto-striatal networks is implicated in the pathophysiology of ADHD. First, ADHD symptoms can be successfully treated with methylphenidate, a potent blocker of the reuptake of dopamine which augments the availability of this neuromodulator/neurotransmitter in the extraneuronal space (Dresel et al., 2000). Second, molecular genetic data suggests an association between ADHD and polymorphism of the dopamine transporter gene, as well as the dopamine D4 receptor gene. Third, structural MRI studies of individuals with ADHD have reported volumetric reductions in brain regions heavily innervated by dopaminergic neurons (e.g., frontal lobes and striatum). Fourth, SPECT and PET studies carried out in ADHD children, adolescents or adults have found decreased metabolism in the same regions.

Fifth, as the nigrostriatal dopaminergic system is implicated in motor control whereas the mesocortical dopaminergic is involved in attention processes (Nieoullon & Coquerel, 2003), it is probable that a hypofunction of the dopaminergic pathways results in deficient attention, poor executive function, and impaired modulation of motor activity. Last, there are also some data indicating that dopamine supports synaptic plasticity processes such as long-term potentiation (Calabresi, Pisani, Mercuri, & Bernardi, 1996). On this basis, we postulate that the neurofeedback protocol used in our study led to the neuromodulation by dopamine of neural activity in fronto-striatal networks. Furthermore, given the association between ADHD and polymorphism of the D4 receptor gene, we hypothesize that this neuroplastic phenomenon implicated long-term potentiation and D4 receptors.

CONCLUSION

The cognitive deficits that are the hallmarks of the ADHD syndrome appear to result from dopaminergic dysregulation, as well as structural and functional abnormalities in cortico-cortical and fronto-subcortical neural networks mediating attention, executive functions, and motor regulation. Our neuroimaging work in ADHD children suggests that NFT can significantly improve cognitive function and neural activity in these networks. We propose that a neuromodulatory action of dopamine is centrally implicated in these improvements. SPECT and/or PET could be used to test this hypothesis.

In recent years, a few structural MRI studies using morphometry have shown that short periods of intensive learning (ranging from a few weeks to a few months) can be associated with regional volume increases in the gray matter (Ceccarelli et al., 2009; Draganski et al., 2006). The gray matter volume increases noted in these studies may be related to cellular events such as sprouting of new synaptic connections and dendritic spine growth. Other MRI studies using DTI demonstrated that learning can also lead rapidly to microstructural white matter changes (i.e., increased FA) (Johansen-Berg, 2007). These changes may reflect increased axon caliber and myelination. In this context, morphometry and DTI could be utilized to verify if a few months of neurofeedback training can lead to grey matter and white matter changes in ADHD individuals. PET could also be used to measure the impact of neurofeedback on various neurotransmitters, including dopamine.

REFERENCES

Amen, D. G., & Carmichael, B. D. (1997). High-resolution brain SPECT imaging in ADHD. *Annals of Clinical Psychiatry, 9*, 81−86.

Anney, R. J., Hawi, Z., Sheehan, K., Mulligan, A., Pinto, C., Brookes, K. J., et al. (2008). Parent of origin effects in attention/deficit hyperactivity disorder (ADHD): Analysis of data from the international multicenter ADHD genetics (IMAGE) program. *American Journal of Medical Genetics B Neuropsychiatry and Genetics, 147B,* 1495−1500.

Arcos-Burgos, M., Castellanos, F. X., Pineda, D., Lopera, F., Palacio, J. D., Palacio, L. G., et al. (2004). Attention-deficit/hyperactivity disorder in a population isolate: Linkage to loci at 4q13.2, 5q33.3, 11q22, and 17p11. *American Journal of Human Genetics, 75,* 998−1014.

Arnsten, A. F. (2006). Fundamentals of attention-deficit/hyperactivity disorder: Circuits and pathways. *Journal of Clinical Psychiatry, 67*(Suppl 8), 7−12.

Asghari, V., Sanyal, S., Buchwaldt, S., Paterson, A., Jovanovic, V., & Van Tol, H. H. (1995). Modulation of intracellular cyclic AMP levels by different human dopamine D4 receptor variants. *Journal of Neurochemistry, 65,* 1157−1165.

Asherson, P., Zhou, K., Anney, R. J., Franke, B., Buitelaar, J., Ebstein, R., et al. (2008). A high-density SNP linkage scan with 142 combined subtype ADHD sib pairs identifies linkage regions on chromosomes 9 and 16. *Molecular Psychiatry, 13,* 514−521.

Ashtari, M., Kumra, S., Bhaskar, S. L., Clarke, T., Thaden, E., Cervellione, K. L., et al. (2005). Attention-deficit/hyperactivity disorder: a preliminary diffusion tensor imaging study. *Biological Psychiatry, 57,* 448−455.

Aylward, E. H., Reiss, A. L., Reader, M. J., Singer, H. S., Brown, J. E., & Denckla, M. B. (1996). Basal ganglia volumes in children with attention-deficit hyperactivity disorder. *Journal of Child Neurology, 11,* 112−115.

Bakker, S. C., van der Meulen, E. M., Buitelaar, J. K., Sandkuijl, L. A., Pauls, D. L., Monsuur, A. J., et al. (2003). A whole-genome scan in 164 Dutch sib pairs with attention-deficit/hyperactivity disorder: Suggestive evidence for linkage on chromosomes 7p and 15q. *American Journal of Human Genetics, 72,* 1251−1260.

Banaschewski, T., Becker, K., Scherag, S., Franke, B., & Coghill., D. (2010). Molecular genetics of attention-deficit/hyperactivity disorder: An overview. *European Child and Adolescent Psychiatry, 19*(3), 237−257.

Barkley, R. A. (1996). *Attention Deficit Hyperactivity Disorder: A handbook for diagnosis and treatment.* New York: Guilford Press.

Barkley, R. A. (1997). Behavioral inhibition, sustained attention, and executive functions: Constructing a unifying theory of ADHD. *Psychology Bulletin, 121,* 65−94.

Beauregard, M., & Lévesque, J. (2006). Functional magnetic resonance imaging investigation of the effects of neurofeedback training on the neural bases of selective attention and response inhibition in children with attention-deficit/hyperactivity disorder. Putative neural mechanisms underlying the effects of neurofeedback in ADHD. *Applied Psychophysiology and Biofeedback, 31*(1), 3−20.

Berquin, P. C., Giedd, J. N., Jacobsen, L. K., Hamburger, S. D., Krain, A. L., Rapoport, J. L., et al. (1998). Cerebellum in attention-deficit hyperactivity disorder: A morphometric MRI study. *Neurology, 50,* 1087−1093.

Booth, J. R., Burman, D. D., Meyer, J. R., Lei, Z., Trommer, B. L., Davenport, N. D., et al. (2005). Larger deficits in brain networks for response inhibition than for visual selective attention in attention deficit hyperactivity disorder (ADHD). *Journal of Child Psychology and Psychiatry, 46,* 94−111.

Brookes, K. J., Mill, J., Guindalini, C., Curran, S., Xu, X., Knight, J., et al. (2006). A common haplotype of the dopamine transporter gene associated with attention-deficit/hyperactivity disorder and interacting with maternal use of alcohol during pregnancy. *Archives of General Psychiatry, 63*, 74—81.

Bush, B., Biederman, J., Cohen, L. G., Sayer, J. M., Monuteaux, M. C., Mick, E., et al. (2002). Correlates of ADHD among children in pediatric and psychiatric clinics. *Psychiatric Services, 53*(9), 1103—1111.

Bush, G., Frazier, J. A., Rauch, S. L., Seidman, L. J., Whalen, P. J., Jenike, M. A., et al. (1999). Anterior cingulated cortex dysfunction in attention-deficit hyperactivity disorder revealed by fMRI and the Counting Stroop. *Biological Psychiatry, 45*, 1542—1552.

Bush, G., Luu, P., & Posner, M. I. (2000). Cognitive and emotional influences in anterior cingulate cortex. *Trends in Cognitive Sciences, 4*, 215—222.

Bush, G., Spencer, T. J., Holmes, J., Shin, L. M., Valera, E. M., Seidman, L. J., et al. (2008). Functional magnetic resonance imaging of methylphenidate and placebo in attention-deficit/hyperactivity disorder during the multi-source interference task. *Archives of General Psychiatry, 65*(1), 102—114.

Bush, G., Whalen, P. J., Rosen, B. R., Jenike, M. A., McInerney, S. C., & Rauch, S. L. (1998). The counting Stroop: An interference task specialized for functional neuroimaging—validation study with functional MRI. *Human Brain Mapping, 6*, 270—282.

Bussing, R., Grudnik, J., Mason, D., Wasiak, M., & Leonard, C. (2002). ADHD and conduct disorder: An MRI study in a community sample. *World Journal of Biological Psychiatry, 3*, 216—220.

Calabresi, P., Pisani, A., Mercuri, N. B., & Bernardi, G. (1996). The corticostriatal projection: From synaptic plasticity to dysfunctions of the basal ganglia. *Trends in Neurosciences, 19*, 19—24.

Carter, A. S., O'Donnell, D. A., Schultz, R. T., Scahill, L., Leckman, J. F., & Pauls, D. L. (2000). Social and emotional adjustment in children affected with Gilles de la Tourette's syndrome: Associations with ADHD and family functioning. Attention deficit hyperactivity disorder. *Journal of Child Psychology and Psychiatry, 41*(2), 215—223.

Carter, C. S., Braver, T. S., Barch, D. M., Botvinick, M. M., Noll, D., & Cohen, J. D. (1998). Anterior cingulate cortex, error detection, and the online monitoring of performance. *Science, 280*, 747—749.

Casey, B. J., Durston, S., & Fossella, J. A. (2001). Evidence for a mechanistic model of cognitive control. *Clinical Neuroscience Research, 1*, 267—282.

Casey, B. J., Epstein, J. N., Buhle, J., Liston, C., Davidson, M. C., Tonev, S. T., et al. (2007). Frontostriatal connectivity and its role in cognitive control in parent-child dyads with ADHD. *American Journal of Psychiatry, 164*(11), 1729—1736.

Castellanos, F. X., Giedd, J. N., Berquin, P. C., Walter, J. M., Sharp, W., Tran, T., et al. (2001). Quantitative brain magnetic resonance imaging in girls with attention-deficit/hyperactivity disorder. *Archives of General Psychiatry, 58*, 289—295.

Castellanos, F., Giedd, J., Eckburg, P., Marsh, W., Vaituzis, C., Kaysen, D., et al. (1994). Quantitative morphology of the caudate nucleus in attention deficit hyperactivity disorder. *American Journal of Psychiatry, 151*, 1791—1796.

Castellanos, F., Giedd, J., Marsh, W., Hamburger, S., Vaituzis, A., Dickstein, D., et al. (1996). Quantitative brain magnetic resonance imaging in attention deficit hyperactivity disorder. *Archives of General Psychiatry, 53*, 607—616.

Castellanos, F. X., Lee, P. P., Sharp, W., Jeffries, N. O., Greenstein, D. K., Clasen, L. S., et al. (2002). Developmental trajectories of brain volume abnormalities in children and adolescents with attention-deficit/hyperactivity disorder. *JAMA, 288*, 1740—1748.

Ceccarelli, A., Rocca, M. A., Pagani, E., Falini, A., Comi, G., & Filippi, M. (2009). Cognitive learning is associated with gray matter changes in healthy human individuals: A tensor-based morphometry study. *Neuroimage, 48*(3), 585—589.

Cho, S. C., Kim, J. W., Kim, B. N., Hwang, J. W., Shin, M. S., Park, M., et al. (2008). Association between the alpha-2C-adrenergic receptor gene and attention deficit hyperactivity disorder in a Korean sample. *Neuroscience Letters, 446*, 108−111.

Conners, C. K., Wells, K. C., Parker, J. D. A., Sitarenios, G., Diamond, J. M., & Powell, J. W. (1997). A new self-report scale for the assessment of adolescent psychopathology: Factor structure, reliability, validity and diagnostic sensitivity. *Journal of Abnormal Child Psychology, 25*, 487−497.

Deupree, J. D., Smith, S. D., Kratochvil, C. J., Bohac, D., Ellis, C. R., Polaha, J., et al. (2006). Possible involvement of alpha-2A adrenergic receptors in attention deficit hyperactivity disorder:radioligand binding and polymorphism studies. *American Journal of Medical Genetics B Neuropsychiatric Genetics, 141B*, 877−884.

Dorval, K. M., Wigg, K. G., Crosbie, J., Tannock, R., Kennedy, J. L., Ickowicz, A., et al. (2007). Association of the glutamate receptor subunit gene GRIN2B with attention-deficit/hyperactivity disorder. *Genes Brain and Behavior, 6*, 444−452.

Doyle, A. E., Ferreira, M. A., Sklar, P. B., Lasky-Su, J., Petty, C., Fusillo, S. J., et al. (2008). Multivariate genomewide linkage scan of neurocognitive traits and ADHD symptoms: Suggestive linkage to 3q13. *American Journal of Medical Genetics B Neuropsychiatric Genetics, 147B*, 1399−1411.

Draganski, B., Gaser, C., Kempermann, G., Kuhn, H. G., Winkler, J., Büchel, C., et al. (2006). Temporal and spatial dynamics of brain structure changes during extensive learning. *Journal of Neuroscience, 26*(23), 6314−6317.

Dresel, S., Krause, J., Krause, K. H., LaFougere, C., Brinkbaumer, K., Kung, H. F., et al. (2000). Attention deficit hyperactivity disorder: Binding of [99mTc]TRODAT-1 to the dopamine transporter before and after methylphenidate treatment. *European Journal of Nuclear Medicine, 27*, 1518−1524.

Dudbridge, F., & Gusnanto, A. (2008). Estimation of significance thresholds for genome-wide association scans. *Genetic Epidemiology, 32*(3), 227−234.

Dum, R., & Strick, P. (1993). Cingulate motor areas. In B. A. Vogt & M. Gabriel (Eds.), *Neurobiology of cingulate cortex and limbic thalamus: A comprehensive handbook*. Boston, MA: Birkhauser.

Duncan, J., & Owen, A. M. (2000). Common regions of the human frontal lobe recruited by diverse cognitive demands. *Trends in Neuroscience, 23*, 475−483.

Durston, S., & Casey, B. J. (2006). What have we learned about cognitive development from neuroimaging? *Neuropsychologia, 44*(11), 2149−2157.

Durston, S., Fossella, J. A., Casey, B. J., Hulshoff Pol, H. E., Galvan, A., Schnack, H. G., et al. (2005). Differential effects of DRD4 and DAT1genotype on fronto-striatal gray matter volumes in a sample of subjects with attention deficit hyperactivity disorder, their unaffected siblings, and controls. *Molecular Psychiatry, 10*, 678−685.

Durston, S., Fossella, J. A., Mulder, M. J., Casey, B. J., Ziermans, T. B., Vessaz, M. N., et al. (2008). Dopamine transporter genotype conveys familial risk of attention-deficit/hyperactivity disorder through striatal activation. *Journal of the American Academy of Child and Adolescent Psychiatry, 47*, 61−67.

Durston, S., Hulshoff Pol, H. E., Schnack, H. G., Buitelaar, J. K., Steenhuis, M. P., Minderaa, R. B., et al. (2004). Magnetic resonance imaging of boys with attention-deficit/hyperactivity disorder and their unaffected siblings. *Journal of the American Academy of Child and Adolescent Psychiatry, 43*, 332−340.

Durston, S., Mulder, M., Casey, B. J., Ziermans, T., & van Engeland, H. (2006). Activation in ventral prefrontal cortex is sensitive to genetic vulnerability for attention-deficit hyperactivity disorder. *Biological Psychiatry, 60*(10), 1062−1070.

Durston, S., Tottenham, N. T., Thomas, K. M., Davidson, M. C., Eigsti, I. M., Yang, Y., et al. (2003). Differential patterns of striatal activation in young children with and without ADHD. *Biological Psychiatry, 53*, 871−878.

Faraone, S. V., & Doyle, A. E. (2001). The nature and heritability of attention-deficit/ hyperactivity disorder. *Child and Adolescent Psychiatry Clinics of North America, 10*(2), 299–316, viii–ix.

Faraone, S. V., Doyle, A. E., Mick, E., & Biederman, J. (2001). Metaanalysis of the association between the 7-repeat allele of the dopamine D(4) receptor gene and attention deficit hyperactivity disorder. *American Journal of Psychiatry, 158,* 1052–1057.

Faraone, S. V., Perlis, R. H., Doyle, A. E., Smoller, J. W., Goralnick, J. J., Holmgren, M. A., et al. (2005). Molecular genetics of attention deficit/hyperactivity disorder. *Biological Psychiatry, 57,* 1313–1323.

Filipek, P. A., Semrud-Clikeman, M., Steingard, R. J., Renshaw, P. F., Kennedy, D. N., & Biederman, J. (1997). Volumetric MRI analysis comparing subjects having attention-deficit hyperactivity disorder with normal controls. *Neurology, 48,* 589–601.

Fuchs, T., Birbaumer, N., Lutzenberger, W., Gruzelier, J. H., & Kaiser, J. (2003). Neurofeedback treatment for attention-deficit/hyperactivity disorder in children: A comparison with methylphenidate. *Applied Psychophysiology and Biofeedback, 28,* 1–12.

Gainetdinov, R. R., Wetsel, W. C., Jones, S. R., Levin, E. D., Jaber, M., & Caron, M. G. (1999). Role of serotonin in the paradoxical calming effect of psychostimulants on hyperactivity. *Science, 283,* 397–401.

Garavan, H., Ross, T. J., Murphy, K., Roche, R. A., & Stein, E. A. (2002). Dissociable executive functions in the dynamic control of behavior: Inhibition, error detection, and correction. *Neuroimage, 17*(4), 1820–1829.

Garavan, H., Ross, T. J., & Stein, E. A. (1999). Right hemispheric dominance of inhibitory control: An event-related functional MRI study. *Proceedings of the National Academy of Sciences of the U S A, 96,* 8301–8306.

Gehring, W. J., & Knight, R. T. (2000). Prefrontal-cingulate interactions in action monitoring. *Nature Neuroscience, 3,* 516–520.

Gevensleben, H., Holl, B., Albrecht, B., Vogel, C., Schlamp, D., Kratz, O., et al. (2009). Is neurofeedback an efficacious treatment for ADHD? A randomised controlled clinical trial. *Journal of Child Psychology and Psychiatry, 50*(7), 780–789.

Godefroy, O., Lhullier, C., & Rousseaux, M. (1996). Non-spatial attention disorders in patients with frontal or posterior brain damage. *Brain, 119,* 191–202.

Grevet, E. H., Marques, F. Z., Salgado, C. A., Fischer, A. G., Kalil, K. L., Victor, M. M., et al. (2007). Serotonin transporter gene polymorphism and the phenotypic heterogeneity of adult ADHD. *Journal of Neural Transmission, 114,* 1631–1636.

Guan, L., Wang, B., Chen, Y., Yang, L., Li, J., Qian, Q., et al. (2009). A high-density single-nucleotide polymorphism screen of 23 candidate genes in attention deficit hyperactivity disorder: Suggesting multiple susceptibility genes among Chinese Han population. *Molecular Psychiatry, 14,* 546–554.

Guimaraes, A. P., Zeni, C., Polanczyk, G. V., Genro, J. P., Roman, T., Rohde, L. A., et al. (2007). Serotonin genes and attention deficit/hyperactivity disorder in a Brazilian sample: Preferential transmission of the HTR2A 452His allele to affected boys. *American Journal of Medical Genetics B Neuropsychiatric Genetics, 144B,* 69–73.

Halperin, J. M., Newcorn, J. H., Schwartz, S. T., Sharma, V., Siever, L. J., Koda, V. H., et al. (1997). Age-related changes in the association between serotonergic function and aggression in boys with ADHD. *Biological Psychiatry, 41,* 682–689.

Hebebrand, J., Dempfle, A., Saar, K., Thiele, H., Herpertz-Dahlmann, B., Linder, M., et al. (2006). A genome-wide scan for attention-deficit/hyperactivity disorder in 155 German sib-pairs. *Molecular Psychiatry, 11,* 196–205.

Heilman, K. M., Pandya, D. N., & Geschwind, N. (1970). Trimodal inattention following parietal lobe ablations. *Transactions of the American Neurological Association, 95,* 259–261.

Heilman, K. M., Watson, R. T., Bower, D., & Valenstein, E. (1983). Right hemisphere dominance for attention (in French). *Revue Neurologie (Paris)*, *139*, 15–17.

Hill, D. E., Yeo, R. A., Campbell, R. A., Hart, B., Vigil, J., & Brooks, W. (2003). Magnetic resonance imaging correlates of attention-deficit/hyperactivity disorder in children. *Neuropsychology*, *17*, 496–506.

Hynd, G. W., Semrud-Clikeman, M. S., Lorys, A. R., Novey, E. S., & Eliopulos, D. (1990). Brain morphology in developmental dyslexia and attention deficit/hyperactivity. *Archives of Neurology*, *47*, 919–926.

Ickowicz, A., Feng, Y., Wigg, K., Quist, J., Pathare, T., Roberts, W., et al. (2007). The serotonin receptor HTR1B: Gene polymorphisms in attention deficit hyperactivity disorder. *American Journal of Medical Genetics B Neuropsychiatric Genetics*, *144B*, 121–125.

Johansen-Berg, H. (2007). Structural plasticity: Rewiring the brain. *Current Biology*, *17*(4), R141–R144.

Kates, W. R., Frederikse, M., Mostofsky, S. H., Folley, B. S., Cooper, K., Mazur-Hopkins, P., et al. (2002). MRI parcellation of the frontal lobe in boys with attention deficit hyperactivity disorder or Tourette syndrome. *Psychiatry Research*, *116*, 63–81.

Kebir, O., Grizenko., N., Sengupta, S., & Joober, R. (2009). Verbal but not performance IQ is highly correlated to externalizing behavior in boys with ADHD carrying both DRD4 and DAT1 risk genotypes. *Progress in Neuro-Psychopharmacology and Biological Psychiatry*, *33*, 939–944.

Kiehl, K. A., Liddle, P. F., & Hopfinger, J. B. (2000). Error processing and the rostral anterior cingulate: An event-related fMRI study. *Psychophysiology*, *37*, 216–223.

Kim, B. N., Lee, J. S., Shin, M. S., Cho, S. C., & Lee, D. S. (2002). Regional cerebral perfusion abnormalities in attention deficit/hyperactivity disorder. Statistical parametric mapping analysis. *European Archives of Psychiatry and Clinical Neuroscience*, *252*, 219–225.

Konishi, S., Nakajima, K., Uchida, I., Sekihara, K., & Miyashita, Y. (1998). No-Go dominant brain activity in human inferior prefrontal cortex revealed by functional magnetic resonance imaging. *European Journal of Neuroscience*, *10*, 1209–1213.

Konrad, K., Neufang, S., Fink, G. R., & Herpertz-Dahlmann, B. (2007). Long-term effects of methylphenidate on neural networks associated with executive attention in children with ADHD: Results from a longitudinal functional MRI study. *Journal of the American Academy of Child and Adolescent Psychiatry*, *46*(12), 1633–1641.

Konrad, K., Neufang, S., Hanisch, C., Fink, G. R., & Herpertz-Dahlmann, B. (2006). Dysfunctional attentional networks in children with attention deficit/hyperactivity disorder: Evidence from an event-related functional magnetic resonance imaging study. *Biological Psychiatry*, *59*(7), 643–651.

Kopeckova, M., Paclt, I., Petrasek, J., Pacltova, D., Malikova, M., & Zagatova, V. (2008). Some ADHD polymorphisms (in genes DAT1, DRD2, DRD3, DBH, 5-HTT) in case–control study of 100 subjects 6–10 age. *Neuroendocrinology Letters*, *29*, 246–251.

Kropotov, J. D., Grin-Yatsenko, V. A., Ponomarev, V. A., Chutko, L. S., Yakovenko, E., & Nikishena, I. S. (2005). ERPs correlates of EEG relative beta training in ADHD children. *International Journal of Psychophysiology*, *55*, 23–34.

Lasky-Su, J., Neale, B. M., Franke, B., Anney, R. J., Zhou, K., Maller, J. B., et al. (2008). Genome-wide association scan of quantitative traits for attention deficit hyperactivity disorder identifies novel associations and confirms candidate gene associations. *American Journal of Medical Genetics B Neuropsychiatric Genetics*, *147B*, 1345–1354.

Leimkuhler, M. E., & Mesulam, M. M. (1985). Reversible go-no go deficits in a case of frontal lobe tumor. *Annals of Neurology*, *18*, 617–619.

Lesch, K. P., Timmesfeld, N., Renner, T. J., Halperin, R., Roser, C., Nguyen, T. T., et al. (2008). Molecular genetics of adult ADHD: Converging evidence from genome-wide association and extended pedigree linkage studies. *Journal of Neural Transmission, 115*, 1573—1585.

Lévesque, J., Beauregard, M., & Mensour, B. (2006). Effect of neurofeedback training on the neural substrates of selective attention in children with attention-deficit/hyperactivity disorder: A functional magnetic resonance imaging study. *Neuroscience Letters, 394*(3), 216—221.

Lezak, M. D. (1990). Neuropsychological assessment. In J. Frederiks (Ed.), *Handbook of clinical neurology: Vol. 1. Clinical neuropsychology* (pp. 515—530). New York: Elsevier.

Li, D., Sham, P. C., Owen, M. J., & He, L. (2006). Meta-analysis shows significant association between dopamine system genes and attention deficit hyperactivity disorder (ADHD). *Human Molecular Genetics, 15*, 2276—2284.

Li, J., Kang, C., Zhang, H., Wang, Y., Zhou, R., Wang, B., et al. (2007). Monoamine oxidase A gene polymorphism predicts adolescent outcome of attention-deficit/hyperactivity disorder. *American Journal of Medical Genetics B Neuropsychiatric Genetics, 144B*, 430—433.

Li, J., Wang, Y. F., Zhou, R. L., Yang, L., Zhang, H. B., & Wang, B. (2003). Association between tryptophan hydroxylase gene polymorphisms and attention deficit hyperactivity disorder with or without learning disorder. *Zhonghua Yi Xue Za Zhi, 83*, 2114—2118.

Liddle, P. F., Kiehl, K. A., & Smith, A. M. (2001). Event-related fMRI study of response inhibition. *Human Brain Mapping, 12*, 100—109.

Linden, M., Habib, T., & Radojevic, V. (1996). A controlled study of the effects of EEG biofeedback on cognition and behavior of children with attention deficit disorder and learning disabilities. *Biofeedback and Self Regulation, 21*, 35—49.

Lou, H. C., Henriksen, L., Bruhn, P., Borner, H., & Nielsen, J. B. (1989). Striatal dysfunction in attention deficit and hyperkinetic disorder. *Archives of Neurology, 46*, 48—52.

Lubar, J. F. (1997). Neocortical dynamics: Implications for understanding the role of neurofeedback and related techniques for the enhancement of attention. *Applied Psychophysiology Biofeedback, 22*(2), 111—126.

Lubar, J. O., & Lubar, J. F. (1984). Electroencephalographic biofeedback of SMR and beta for treatment of attention deficit disorders in a clinical setting. *Biofeedback and Self Regulation, 9*, 1—23.

Lubar, J. F., & Shouse, M. N. (1976). EEG and behavioral changes in a hyperkinetic child concurrent with training of the sensorimotor rhythm (SMR): A preliminary report. *Biofeedback and Self Regulation, 1*, 293—306.

Lubar, J. F., Swartwood, M. O., Swartwood, J. N., & O'Donnell, P. H. (1995). Evaluation of the effectiveness of EEG neurofeedback training for ADHD in a clinical setting as measured by changes in T. O. V. A. scores, behavioral ratings, and WISC-R performance. *Biofeedback and Self Regulation, 20*, 83—99.

Makris, N., Biederman, J., Monuteaux, M. C., & Seidman, L. J. (2009). Towards conceptualizing a neural systems-based anatomy of attention-deficit/hyperactivity disorder. *Developmental Neuroscience, 31*, 36—49.

Makris, N., Biederman, J., Valera, E. M., Bush, G., Kaiser, J., Kennedy, D. N., et al. (2007). Cortical thinning of the attention and executive function networks in adults with attention-deficit/hyperactivity disorder. *Cerebral Cortex, 17*, 1364—1375.

Makris, N., Buka, S. L., Biederman, J., Papadimitriou, G. M., Hodge, S. M., Valera, E. M., et al. (2008). Attention and executive systems abnormalities in adults with childhood ADHD: A DT-MRI study of connections. *Cerebral Cortex, 18*, 1210—1220.

Mannuzza, S., Klein, R. G., Bessler, A., Malloy, P., & Hynes, M. E. (1997). Educational and occupational outcome of hyperactive boys grown up. *Journal of the American Academy of Child and Adolescent Psychiatry, 36*(9), 1222—1227.

Mataro, M., Garcia-Sanchez, C., Junque, C., Estevez-Gonzalez, A., & Pujol, J. (1997). Magnetic resonance imaging measurement of the caudate nucleus in adolescents with attention deficit hyperactivity disorder and its relationship with neuropsychological and behavioural measures. *Archives of Neurology, 54*, 963−968.

Mattes, J. A. (1980). The role of frontal lobe dysfunctionin childhood hyperkinesis. *Comprehensive Psychiatry, 21*, 358−369.

Menon, V., Adleman, N. E., White, C. D., Glover, G. H., & Reiss, A. L. (2001). Error-related brain activation during a Go/NoGo response inhibition task. *Human Brain Mapping, 12*, 131−143.

Mesulam, M. M. (1990). Large-scale neurocognitive networks and distributed processing for attention, language, and memory. *Annals of Neurology, 28*, 597−613.

Mick, E., & Faraone, S. V. (2008). Genetics of attention deficit hyperactivity disorder. *Child and Adolescent Psychiatry Clinics of North America, 17*, 261−284, vii−viii.

Monastra, V. J., Monastra, D. M., & George, S. (2002). The effects of stimulant therapy, EEG biofeedback, and parenting style on the primary symptoms of attention deficit/ hyperactivity disorder. *Applied Psychophysiology and Biofeedback, 27*, 231−249.

Monuteaux, M. C., Biederman, J., Doyle, A. E., Mick, E., & Faraone, S. V. (2009). Genetic risk for conduct disorder symptom subtypes in an ADHD sample: Specificity to aggressive symptoms. *Journal of the American Academy of Child and Adolescent Psychiatry, 48*, 757−764.

Morrison, J. R., & Stewart, M. A. (1974). Bilateral inheritance as evidence for polygenicity in the hyperactive child syndrome. *Journal of Nervous and Mental Disorders, 158*(3), 226−228.

Mostofsky, S. H., Cooper, K. L., Kates, W. R., Denckla, M. B., & Kaufmann, W. E. (2002). Smaller prefrontal and premotor volumes in boys with attention-deficit/ hyperactivity disorder. *Biological Psychiatry, 52*, 785−794.

Mostofsky, S. H., Reiss, A. L., Lockhart, P., & Denckla, M. B. (1998). Evaluation of cerebellar size in attention-deficit hyperactivity disorder. *Journal of Child Neurology, 13*, 434−439.

Neale, B. M., Lasky-Su, J., Anney, R., Franke, B., Zhou, K., Maller, J. B., et al. (2008). Genome-wide association scan of attention deficit hyperactivity disorder. *American Journal of Medical Genetics B Neuropsychiatric Genetics, 147B*, 1337−1344.

Nieoullon, A., & Coquerel, A. (2003). Dopamine: A key regulator to adapt action, emotion, motivation and cognition. *Current Opinion in Neurology, 16*(Suppl 2), S3−S9.

Oades, R. D., Lasky-Su, J., Christiansen, H., Faraone, S. V., Sonuga- Barke, E. J., Banaschewski, T., et al. (2008). The influence of serotonin and other genes on impulsive behavioral aggression and cognitive impulsivity in children with attention-deficit/ hyperactivity disorder (ADHD): Findings from a family-based association test (FBAT) analysis. *Behavior and Brain Functions, 4*, 48.

Ogdie, M. N., Bakker, S. C., Fisher, S. E., Francks, C., Yang, M. H, Cantor, R. M., et al. (2006). Pooled genome-wide linkage data on 424 ADHD ASPs suggests genetic heterogeneity and a common risk locus at 5p13. *Molecular Psychiatry, 11*, 5−8.

Overmeyer, S., Bullmore, E. T., Suckling, J., Simmons, A., Williams, S. C., Santosh, P., et al. (2001). Distributed grey and white matter deficits in hyperkinetic disorder MRI evidence for anatomical abnormality in an attentional network. *Psychological Medicine, 31*, 1425−1435.

Pavuluri, M. N., Yang, S., Kamineni, K., Passarotti, A. M., Srinivasan, G., Harral, E. M., et al. (2009). Diffusion tensor imaging study of white matter fiber tracts in pediatric bipolar disorder and attention-deficit/hyperactivity disorder. *Biological Psychiatry, 65*(7), 586−593.

Paus, T. (2001). Primate anterior cingulate cortex: Where motor control, drive and cognition interface. *Nature Reviews Neuroscience, 22*, 417−424.

Peter, I., Yelensky, R., Altshuler, D., & Daly, M. J. (2008). Estimation of the multiple testing burden for genome wide association studies of nearly all common variants. *Genetic Epidemiology*, *32*, 381–385.

Pliszka, S. R., Glahn, D. C., Semrud-Clikeman, M., Franklin, C., Perez, R., 3rd, Xiong, J., et al. (2006). Neuroimaging of inhibitory control areas in children with attention deficit hyperactivity disorder who were treatment naive or in long-term treatment. *American Journal of Psychiatry*, *163*, 1052–1060.

Posner, M. I., & Petersen, S. E. (1990). The attention system of the human brain. *Annual Review of Neuroscience*, *13*, 25–42.

Retz, W., Freitag, C. M., Retz-Junginger, P., Wenzler, D., Schneider, M., Kissling, C., et al. (2008). A functional serotonin transporter promoter gene polymorphism increases ADHD symptoms in delinquents: Interaction with adverse childhood environment. *Psychiatry Research*, *158*, 123–131.

Ribases, M., Ramos-Quiroga, J. A., Hervas, A., Bosch, R., Bielsa, A., Gastaminza, X., et al. (2009). Exploration of 19 serotoninergic candidate genes in adults and children with attention-deficit/hyperactivity disorder identifies association for 5HT2A. *DDC and MAOB. Molecular Psychiatry*, *14*, 71–85.

Roman, T., Schmitz, M., Polanczyk, G. V., Eizirik, M., Rohde, L. A., & Hutz, M. H. (2002). Further evidence for the association between attention-deficit/hyperactivity disorder and the dopamine-betahydroxylase gene. *American Journal of Medical Genetics*, *114*, 154–158.

Romanos, M., Freitag, C., Jacob, C., Craig, D. W., Dempfle, A., Nguyen, T. T., et al. (2008). Genome-wide linkage analysis of ADHD using high-density SNP arrays: Novel loci at 5q13.1 and 14q12. *Molecular Psychiatry*, *13*, 522–530.

Rommelse, N., Altink, M. E., Martin, N. C., Buschgens, C. J., Faraone, S. V., Buitelaar, J. K., et al. (2008). Relationship between endophenotype and phenotype in ADHD. *Behavior and Brain Functions*, *4*, 4.

Rossiter, T. (2004). The effectiveness of neurofeedback and stimulant drugs in treating AD/HD: Part II. Replication. *Applied Psychophysiology and Biofeedback*, *29*, 233–243.

Rossiter, T. R., & LaVaque, T. J. (1995). A comparison of EEG biofeedback and psychostimulants in treating attention deficit hyperactivity disorders. *Journal of Neurotherapy*, *1*, 48–59.

Rubia, K., Overmeyer, S., Taylor, E., Brammer, M., Williams, S. C., Simmons, A., et al. (1999). Hypofrontality in attention deficit hyperactivity disorder during higher-order motor control: A study with functional MRI. *American Journal of Psychiatry*, *156*(6), 891–896.

Rubia, K., Smith, A. B., Brammer, M. J., & Taylor, E. (2003). Right inferior prefrontal cortex mediates response inhibition while mesial prefrontal cortex is responsible for error detection. *Neuroimage*, *20*, 351–358.

Rubia, K., Smith, A. B., Brammer, M. J., Toone, B., & Taylor, E. (2005). Abnormal brain activation during inhibition and error detection in medication-naive adolescents with ADHD. *American Journal of Psychiatry*, *162*(6), 1067–1075.

Sandford, J. A., & Turner, A. (1995). *Manual for the intermediate visual and auditory continuous performance test*. Richmond, VA: Brain Train 727 Twin Ridge Lane.

Scheres, A., Milham, M. P., Knutson, B., & Castellanos, F. X. (2007). Ventral striatal hyporesponsiveness during reward anticipation in attention-deficit/hyperactivity disorder. *Biological Psychiatry*, *61*(5), 720–724.

Schmitz, M., Denardin, D., Silva, T. L., Pianca, T., Roman, T., Hutz, M. H., et al. (2006). Association between alpha-2a-adrenergic receptor gene and ADHD inattentive type. *Biological Psychiatry*, *60*, 1028–1033.

Schulz, K. P., Newcorn, J. H., Fan, J., Tang, C. Y., & Halperin, J. M. (2005). Brain activation gradients in ventrolateral prefrontal cortex related to persistence of ADHD in adolescent boys. *Journal of American Academy of Child and Adolescent Psychiatry, 44*(1), 47—54.

Seamans, J. K., & Yang, C. R. (2004). The principal features and mechanisms of dopamine modulation in the prefrontal cortex. *Progress in Neurobiology, 74,* 1—58.

Seidman, L. J., Valera, E. M., & Makris, N. (2005). Structural brain imaging of attention-deficit/hyperactivity disorder. *Biological Psychiatry, 57*(11), 1263—1272.

Seidman, L. J., Valera, E. M., Makris, N., Monuteaux., M. C., Boriel, D. L., Kelkar, K., et al. (2006). Dorsolateral prefrontal and anterior cingulate cortex volumetric abnormalities in adults with attention-deficit/hyperactivity disorder identified by magnetic resonance imaging. *Biological Psychiatry, 60,* 1071—1080.

Semrud-Clikeman, M. S., Filipek, P. A., Biederman, J., Steingard, R., Kennedy, D., Renshaw, P., et al. (1994). Attention-deficit hyperactivity disorder: Magnetic resonance imaging morphometric analysis of the corpus callosum. *Journal of the American Academy of Child and Adolescent Psychiatry, 33,* 875—881.

Semrud-Clikeman, M., Pliszka, S. R., Lancaster, J., & Liotti, M. (2006). Volumetric MRI differences in treatment-naive vs. chronically treated children with ADHD. *Neurology, 67,* 1023—1027.

Shafritz, K. M., Marchione, K. E., Gore, J. C., Shaywitz, S. E., & Shaywitz, B. A. (2004). The effects of methylphenidate on neural systems of attention in attention deficit hyperactivity disorder. *American Journal of Psychiatry, 161*(11), 1990—1997.

Shallice, T. (1988). *From neuropsychology to mental structure.* Cambridge: Cambridge University Press.

Shaw, P., Lerch, J., Greenstein, D., Sharp, W., Clasen, L., Evans, A., et al. (2006). Longitudinal mapping of cortical thickness and clinical outcome in children and adolescents with attention-deficit/hyperactivity disorder. *Archives of General Psychiatry, 63*(5), 540—549.

Sheehan, K., Lowe, N., Kirley, A., Mullins, C., Fitzgerald, M., Gill, M., et al. (2005). Tryptophan hydroxylase 2 (TPH2) gene variants associated with ADHD. *Molecular Psychiatry, 10,* 944—949.

Shouse, M. N., & Lubar, J. F. (1979). Operant conditioning of EEG rhythms and ritalin in the treatment of hyperkinesis. *Biofeedback and Self Regulation, 4,* 299—312.

Sieg, K. G., Gaffney, G. R., Preston, D. F., & Hellings, J. A. (1995). SPECT brain imaging abnormalities in attention deficit hyperactivity disorder. *Clinical Nuclear Medicine, 20,* 55—60.

Silk, T., Vance, A., Rinehart, N., Egan, G., O'Boyle, M., Bradshaw, J. L., et al. (2005). Fronto-parietal activation in attention-deficit hyperactivity disorder, combined type: Functional magnetic resonance imaging study. *British Journal of Psychiatry, 187,* 282—283.

Smith, E. E., & Jonides, J. (1999). Storage and executive processes in the frontal lobes. *Science, 283,* 1657—1661.

Sowell, E. R., Thompson, P. M., Welcome, S. E., Henkenius, A. L., Toga, A. W., & Peterson, B. S. (2003). Cortical abnormalities in children and adolescents with attention-deficit hyperactivity disorder. *Lancet, 362,* 1699—1707.

Spitzer, R. L., Williams, J. B., Gibbon, M., & First, M. B. (1992). The Structured Clinical Interview for DSM-III-R (SCID). I: History, rationale, and description. *Archives of General Psychiatry, 49,* 624—629.

Steinhausen, H-C. (2009). The heterogeneity of causes and courses of attention-deficit/hyperactivity disorder. *Acta Psychiatrica Scandinavica, 120,* 392—399.

Stevens, M. C., Pearlson, G. D., & Kiehl, K. A. (2007). An FMRI auditory oddball study of combined-subtype attention deficit hyperactivity disorder. *American Journal of Psychiatry, 164*(11), 1737—1749.

Still, G. (1902). The Goulstonian lectures on some abnormal physical conditions in children. Lecture 1. *Lancet*, i, 1008−1012 1077−1082, 1163−1168.

Strehl, U., Leins, U., Goth, G., Klinger, C., Hinterberger, T., & Birbaumer, N. (2006). Self-regulation of slow cortical potentials: A new treatment for children with attention-deficit/hyperactivity disorder. *Pediatrics, 118*(5), e1530−e1540.

Ströhle, A., Stoy, M., Wrase, J., Schwarzer, S., Schlagenhauf, F., & Huss, M. (2008). Reward anticipation and outcomes in adult males with attention-deficit/hyperactivity disorder. *Neuroimage, 39*(3), 966−972.

Suskauer, S. J., Simmonds, D. J., Fotedar, S., Blankner, J. G., Pekar, J. J., Denckla, M. B., et al. (2008). Functional magnetic resonance imaging evidence for abnormalities in response selection in attention deficit hyperactivity disorder: Differences in activation associated with response inhibition but not habitual motor response. *Journal of Cognitive Neuroscience, 20*(3), 478−493.

Swanson, J. M., Hinshaw, S. P., Arnold, L., Gibbons, R. D., Marcus, S., Hur, K., et al. (2007). Secondary evaluations of MTA 36-month outcomes: Propensity score and growth mixture model analyses. *Journal of the American Academy of Child and Adolescent Psychiatry, 46*(8), 1015−1027.

Tamm, L., Menon, V., & Reiss, A. L. (2006). Parietal attentional system aberrations during target detection in adolescents with attention deficit hyperactivity disorder: Event-related fMRI evidence. *American Journal of Psychiatry, 163*(6), 1033−1043.

Tamm, L., Menon, V., Ringel, J., & Reiss, A. L. (2004). Event-related FMRI evidence of frontotemporal involvement in aberrant response inhibition and task switching in attention-deficit/hyperactivity disorder. *Journal of the American Academy of Child and Adolescent Psychiatry, 43*, 1430−1440.

Tansey, M. A. (1984). EEG sensorimotor rhythm biofeedback training: Some effects on the neurologic precursors of learning disabilities. *International Journal of Psychophysiology, 1*, 163−177.

Tansey, M. A. (1985). Brainwave signatures − an index reflective of the brain's functional neuroanatomy: Further findings on the effect of EEG sensorimotor rhythm biofeedback training on the neurologic precursors of learning disabilities. *International Journal of Psychophysiology, 3*, 85−99.

Thompson, L., & Thompson, M. (1998). Neurofeedback combined with training in metacognitive strategies: Effectiveness in students with ADD. *Applied Psychophysiology and Biofeedback, 23*, 243−263.

Timmann, D., & Daum, I. (2007). Cerebellar contributions to cognitive functions: A progress report after two decades of research. *The Cerebellum, 6*, 159−162.

Vaidya, C. J., Austin, G., Kirkorian, G., Ridlehuber, H. W., Desmond, J. E., Glover, G. H., et al. (1998). Selective effects of methylphenidate in attention deficit hyperactivity disorder: A functional magnetic resonance study. *Proceedings of the National Academy of Sciences of the U S A, 95*, 14494−14499.

Valera, E. M., Faraone, S. V., Murray, K. E., & Seidman, L. J. (2007). Meta-analysis of structural imaging findings in attention-deficit/hyperactivity disorder. *Biological Psychiatry, 61*, 1361−1369.

van Steen, K., & Lange, C. (2005). PBAT: A comprehensive software package for genome-wide association analysis of complex family-based studies. *Human Genomics, 2*, 67−69.

Waldman, I. D., & Gizer, I. R. (2006). The genetics of attention deficit hyperactivity disorder. *Clinical Psychology Reviews, 26*, 396−432.

Walitza, S., Renner, T. J., Dempfle, A., Konrad, K., Wewetzer, C., Halbach, A., et al. (2005). Transmission disequilibrium of polymorphic variants in the tryptophan hydroxylase-2 gene in attention-deficit/hyperactivity disorder. *Molecular Psychiatry, 10*, 1126−1132.

Wang, B., Wang, Y., Zhou, R., Li, J., Qian, Q., Yang, L., et al. (2006). Possible association of the alpha-2A adrenergic receptor gene (ADRA2A) with symptoms of attention-deficit/hyperactivity disorder. *American Journal of Medical Genetics B Neuropsychiatric Genetics, 141B,* 130−134.

Wechsler, D. (1981). *Manual for Wechsler adult intelligence scale − revised.* San Antonio, TX: The Psychological Corporation.

Wigg, K. G., Takhar, A., Ickowicz, A, Tannock, R., Kennedy, J. L., Pathare, T., et al. (2006). Gene for the serotonin transporter and ADHD: No association with two functional polymorphisms. *American Journal of Medical Genetics B Neuropsychiatric Genetics, 141B,* 566−570.

Xu, X., Aysimi, E., Anney, R., Brookes, K., Franke, B., Zhou, K., et al. (2008). No association between two polymorphisms of the serotonin transporter gene and combined type attention deficit hyperactivity disorder. *American Journal of Medical Genetics B Neuropsychiatric Genetics, 147,* 1306−1309.

Zametkin, A. J., Nordahl, T. E., Gross, M., King, A. C., Semple, W. E., Rumsey, J., et al. (1990). Cerebral glucose metabolism in adults with hyperactivity of childhood onset. *New England Journal of Medicine, 323,* 1361−1366.

Zhou, K., Chen, W., Buitelaar, J., Banaschewski, T., Oades, R. D., Franke, B., et al. (2008). Genetic heterogeneity in ADHD: DAT1 gene only affects probands without CD. *American Journal of Medical Genetics B Neuropsychiatric Genetics, 147B,* 1481−1487.

Zhou, K., Dempfle, A., Arcos-Burgos, M., Bakker, S. C., Banaschewski, T., Biederman, J., et al. (2008). Meta-analysis of genome-wide linkage scans of attention deficit hyperactivity disorder. *American Journal of Medical Genetics B Neuropsychiatric Genetics, 147B,* 1392−1398.

CHAPTER 14

The Immediate Effects of EEG Neurofeedback on Cortical Excitability and Synchronization

Tomas Ros and John H. Gruzelier

Department of Psychology, Goldsmiths, University of London, London, UK

Contents

INTRODUCTION

In comparison with the much larger number of studies demonstrating long-lasting clinical and behavioral effects of neurofeedback (NFB), very few investigations have been carried out to date on the mechanisms and neurophysiological substrates of EEG-based NFB other than EEG measures. Most NFB involves multiple sessions repeated on at least a weekly basis, whose effects generally accumulate over time, reputedly as a result of neuroplastic changes in the brain (for peak performance at least eight sessions, for clinical application >20) (Doehnert, Brandeis, Straub, Steinhausen, & Drechsler, 2008; Hanslmayr, Sauseng, Doppelmayr, Schabus, & Klimesch, 2005; Lévesque, Beauregard, & Mensour, 2006). Over the years numerous studies have demonstrated behavioral as well as

Neurofeedback and Neuromodulation Techniques and Applications
DOI: 10.1016/B978-0-12-382235-2.00014-7

neurophysiological alterations after *long-term* NFB training, such as improvement in attention and cognitive performance and their accompanying EEG/ERP changes (Egner & Gruzelier, 2004; Gruzelier, Egner, & Vernon, 2006). However, to date and to the best of the authors' knowledge, no work exists or provides evidence for a causal and more direct temporal relationship between self-regulation of brain activity and concomitant short-term change in brain plasticity, or its mechanisms. This may possibly be due to a belief that the putative modulatory effect(s) that follow a discrete session of neurofeedback are too fine to be detected immediately thereafter, or alternatively, occur at some later stage, for example during sleep. However, as is common for all learning paradigms, NFB training occurs within a temporally distinct period or "session", and if it is ever to claim the grail of inducing lasting neuroplastic changes (and thus be taken seriously as a non-invasive tool for neuromodulation, such as rTMS and tDCS) (Wagner, Valero-Cabre, & Pascual-Leone, 2007), a stronger association is clearly warranted between a single training session and the reputed plasticity, if any, it engenders. Accordingly, there has been no demonstration to date of a chronologically direct neuroplastic effect following NFB. That is, of a robust and durable change in neurophysiological function immediately after discrete exposure to NFB. On the other hand, a substantial corpus of transcranial magnetic stimulation (TMS) literature purports significant and durable changes in brain plasticity following brain stimulation techniques such as rTMS and tDCS (Wagner, Valero-Cabre, & Pascual-Leone, 2007), hence similar investigations with NFB may ultimately enable more direct comparisons of effect size with other stimulation techniques.

Nowadays, the study of neuroplasticity in the intact human brain has been made possible with the advent of TMS. Here, evidence of neuroplastic change may be demonstrated non-invasively by an altered neurotransmission of the corticomotor projection to the hand, a method that has been physiologically validated by invasive recordings of human and animal corticospinal nerve impulses (Lazzaro, Ziemann, & Lemon, 2008). Although neuroplasticity appears to involve diverse cellular processes in the central nervous system (Nelson & Turrigiano, 2008), in TMS methodology it is operationally defined as a significant and lasting change in the motor evoked potential (MEP), evoked by a magnetic pulse, whose amplitude is representative of the strength of neurotransmission from motor cortex to muscle. A growing body of evidence (Lazzaro, Ziemann, & Lemon, 2008) indicates that MEPs from a single TMS pulse best reflect the overall responsiveness of the corticospinal pathway, or corticospinal excitability (CSE), whereas those originating from paired pulses (with interstimulus intervals of milliseconds) enable the discrimination of intracortical mechanisms, such as short intra-cortical inhibition (SICI) and facilitation (ICF), which are modulated by transynaptic neurotransmission (Ziemann, 2004).

Our initial hypothesis was that NFB-induced alpha (8−12 Hz) rhythm desynchronization, generally considered a marker of cortical activation (Neuper, Wörtz, & Pfurtscheller, 2006), would enhance both corticosp-inal excitability and intracortical facilitation, while effecting a reduction in intracortical inhibition. Conversely, low beta ("SMR", 12−15 Hz) syn-chronization, which has been associated with cortical deactivation (Oishi et al., 2007), sleep spindles (Sterman, 1996), and GABAergic function (Jensen et al., 2005), was expected to induce an opposite corticospinal and intracortical pattern. Although endogenous oscillations have thus far been implicated in many "on-going" functions such as binding and atten-tion (Schroeder & Lakatos, 2009), explicit evidence is still scarce on their role, if any, in neuroplasticity (Axmacher, Mormann, Fernández, Elger, & Fell, 2006). We therefore postulated that, in line with previous stimulation research, the more pronounced as well as persistent the oscillatory patterns would prove to be during NFB, the more substantial and long-lasting (plastic) would turn out to be their after effects.

METHODS

Participants

Twenty-four healthy participants (12 women, age 31 ± 5 years), all with normal or corrected-to-normal visual acuity, participated in the experi-ment. All were recruited via the participants' database of the Department of Psychology, University College London, and were *naive* to the neuro-feedback protocols used in this study. Experimental procedures were approved by the local ethics committee and in accordance with the Declaration of Helsinki.

Study Design

Subjects were randomly allocated to two protocol groups for a single 30 min-ute NFB session: alpha suppression (N = 12) or low beta enhancement (N = 12). For the purpose of testing hypotheses concerning protocol-specific effects on target EEG frequency components, subjects underwent resting EEG recordings for 3 minutes immediately before and after their

NFB training session. In order to test the hypotheses concerning the protocol-specific effects on corticospinal excitability (CSE), TMS motor evoked potential (MEP) responses were collected before (*pre*) and twice after (*post 1, post 2*) each NFB session, consecutively at right and left hand muscles.

Neurofeedback (NFB)

Apparatus and EEG Analysis

EEG signals were recorded using a NeXus-10 DC-coupled EEG amplifier using a 24-bit A—D converter (MindMedia, The Netherlands), and visual NFB training was carried out with the accompanying Biotrace + software interface on an Intel DualCore computer with a 15-inch screen. The EEG used for feedback was sampled at 256 Hz with Ag/Cl electrodes at the right first dorsal interosseous muscle (FDI) cortical representation/"hot spot" (approx. C3) referenced to the contralateral mastoid. The scalp area was carefully scrubbed with NuPrep abrasive gel, followed by application of Ten20 electrode paste. The ground electrode was placed on the right arm. The signal was IIR bandpass filtered to extract alpha (8—12 Hz) and low beta (12—15) amplitudes (μV peak-peak) respectively with an epoch size of 0.5 seconds. In the same way EEG was co-registered at the left FDI representation (approx. C4) referenced to its contralateral mastoid. IIR digital filtered (Butterworth 3rd order) EEG amplitude data of each band (delta (1—4 Hz), theta (4—7 Hz), alpha (8—12 Hz), low beta (12—15 Hz), beta (15—25 Hz), high beta (25—40 Hz), low gamma (40—60 Hz), and high gamma (60—120 Hz) were then exported at 32 samples/second and voltage-threshold artifacted for ocular, head movement, and EMG contamination. Outlying data points were rejected at >3 standard deviations using histogram analysis. Moreover, the Fast Fourier Transform (FFT) of raw (256 samples/sec) data was used in the calculation of *mean frequency* for each band. Averages of all measures were computed offline for 3 minute epochs, each defined as a training "period". Periods 1 and 12 consisted of feedback-free pre- and post-resting EEG measurements in the eyes-open condition. Periods 2—11 consisted of feedback training.

Neurofeedback Training Procedures

The ALPHA group aimed to suppress absolute alpha (8—12 Hz) amplitude, while the BETA group aimed to elevate absolute low beta amplitude (12—15 Hz). Accordingly, reward thresholds were set to be either 30% of the time above or below the initial alpha or low beta mean amplitude (baseline) respectively. The first baseline was recorded during a 3 minute eyes-open EEG recording at rest immediately before the start of feedback, and the second 3 minute recording was made immediately after the end of training. Subjects were given no explicit verbal instructions and were told to be guided by the feedback process instead. This was achieved via a collection of different visual displays/games whose control reflected the modulation of the trained EEG amplitude. Both protocols employed the same series of five Biotrace + software games, which were played in a random order for approximately 6 minutes each (Mandala, Space Invaders, Mazeman, Bugz, puzzles). In the case of the low beta down protocol a supplementary inhibit was coupled to excess mastoid and EMG activity to ensure low beta reward was not artifact-driven.

Neurofeedback Data Analyses

The degree of NFB-mediated EEG change for each subject was estimated by the *ratio* of EEG amplitudes between the neurofeedback EEG and the initial baseline EEG. This was calculated for each of the 10 training periods, and designated as change in the *training EEG*. Additionally, any pre-to-post change in the resting EEG following training was expressed by the ratio of the second divided by the first mean baseline amplitude, and designated as change in the *resting EEG*.

Transcranial Magnetic Stimulation (TMS): Apparatus and Procedure

The course of the experiment that was used to test the impact of NFB training on corticomotor measures of corticospinal excitability (CSE), short intracortical inhibition (SICI), and intracortical facilitation (ICF) is shown in Figure 14.1. TMS parameters (CSE, SICI, and ICF) were measured before (pre) and twice after NFB (post 1 and post 2). In random order, 78 TMS responses were measured, which required approximately 6 minutes per hemisphere. We evaluated the TMS parameters of both

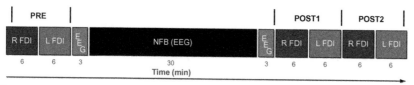

Figure 14.1 Scheme of the study. R FDI = trained left hemisphere, L FDI = untrained right hemisphere.

hemispheres, first left (trained) and then right (untrained) hemisphere, to investigate hemispheric effects of NFB. The post 1 measurement was performed circa 3—15 minutes after NFB training, and post 2 after 15—27 minutes. Well-established standard TMS paradigms were used to measure the corticospinal and intracortical parameters (Lazzaro, Ziemann, & Lemon, 2008). All measurements were carried out with two monophasic Magstim 200 magnetic stimulators (Magstim, Whitland, UK), which were connected with a "Y-cable" to a 70 mm figure-of-eight coil. We determined the cortical representation of the first dorsal interosseous muscles (FDI) for each hemisphere separately. The coil was placed flat on the skull with the handle pointing backward and rotated about 45° away from the midline. Resting motor threshold (RMT) intensity was defined as the lowest stimulator output intensity capable of inducing motor evoked potentials (MEPs) of at least 50 μV peak-to-peak amplitude in the FDI muscle in at least half of 10 trials. Active motor threshold (AMT) was defined as the intensity needed to evoke an MEP of about 200 mV during a 5—10% maximum voluntary contraction. Corticospinal excitability (CSE) was quantified by the amplitude of the motor evoked potential (MEP) elicited by a single test TMS pulse. The test pulse intensity was set to yield an average MEP amplitude of 1 mV at baseline (pre), and was kept constant throughout the experiment. Short latency intracortical inhibition and intracortical facilitation (SICI and ICF) were evaluated using the paired pulse protocol developed by Kujirai et al. (1993). In random trials the test pulse was preceded by a subthreshold conditioning pulse (80% AMT) with an interstimulus interval (ISI) of 2, 3, 10 or 12 ms. The test response was suppressed (SICI) at ISI = 3 ms; whereas facilitation occurred at ISI = 10 and 12 ms (ICF = mean of both time points). A run consisted of 78 stimuli given at approximately 0.25 Hz, where 48 paired-pulse (12 for each ISI) and 30 single-pulse MEPs were recorded. Single-pulse MEP amplitudes were normalized respectively as post 1 divided by pre, and post 2 divided by pre. For SICI and ICF the amplitude of the conditioned response was expressed as a percent of the amplitude of the test response alone. Ratios <1 indicate inhibition, whereas ratios >1 indicate facilitation.

Electromyographic Measures and Analysis

Surface electromyographic (EMG) recordings were made using a belly-tendon montage with Ag/AgCl-plated surface electrodes (9 mm diameter). Raw EMG signal was amplified and filtered using Digitimer D150 amplifiers (Digitimer Ltd, Welwyn Garden City, Herts, UK), with a time constant of 3 ms and a low–pass filter of 3 kHz. Signals were recorded via a CED 1401 laboratory interface (Cambridge Electronic Design Ltd, Cambridge, UK) and stored on a PC for later analysis using a sampling rate of 5 kHz.

Statistical Analyses

All statistical procedures were two–tailed with significance set at $\alpha = 0.05$. Protocol group EEG differences were examined with a GROUP × PERIODS (2 × 11) repeated measures ANOVA, from period 1 (baseline) to period 11. Within–group EEG was assessed by a one–way ANOVA with PERIODS as a repeated measures factor; post hoc Dunnett's test was used to detect significant changes from the baseline rest period. TMS measures of CSE, SICI, and ICF for each hemisphere were subjected to a GROUP × TIME (2 × 3) repeated measures ANOVA; Greenhouse–Geisser correction was used where necessary. Subsequent to reliable main effects, planned comparisons were conducted by Bonferroni corrected t-tests for long–term (>20 min) changes after NFB (post 2 − pre). A regression analysis was performed between normalized EEG (% baseline) vs. normalized TMS parameters (% baseline), as well as between training vs. resting EEG (% baseline). With regards to the weighted least squares (WLS) regression analysis, the reciprocal variance of the relevant training period amplitude (32 samples/sec) was used as each subject's weighting factor. Statistical analyses and structural equation modelling (SEM) were respectively carried out with SPSS 15.0 and Amos v7.0 (SPSS Inc., Chicago, IL, USA). For SEM we used maximum–likelihood estimation as well as bootstrapping (2000 samples, with a 95% bias–corrected confidence level). The final indirect model was also verified by an automatic specification search in the software. Chi–square (CMIN) and baseline fit measures (e.g. NFI) were used to estimate relative goodness–of–fit, along with parsimony measures (e.g. PNFI).

RESULTS

One–Way ANOVAs did not disclose any statistically significant differences (p <0.05) between protocol groups neither for age nor baseline measures of EEG band power (delta to high gamma), or TMS measures (RMT, single–pulse MEP, 3 ms SICI, and ICF) in either the trained or untrained hemispheres.

NFB Training Dynamic

Mean alpha and low beta amplitude during each 3 minute period of the neurofeedback training session is depicted in Figure 14.2, for the ALPHA and BETA groups respectively for each hemisphere. Period 1 denotes the eyes–open, feedback-free, baseline at rest. Mean ALPHA-group amplitude for the trained hemisphere exhibited a general decrease from baseline (9.08) to period 11 (8.50), with a minimum at 15–18 minutes, or period 7 (7.93, $t_{11} = 4.0$, $p = 0.002$), in line with training direction, and largely paralleled by the contralateral hemisphere. Paired t-test comparisons of baseline with period means revealed a significant reduction ($p < 0.05$) for all periods except periods 3, 9, and 11. For the BETA-group, whose aim on the other hand was to increase low beta, mean amplitude became statistically higher than baseline (5.95), uniquely between 24 and 27 minutes, or period 10 (6.62, $t_{11} = -2.4$, $p = 0.034$). No significant increases were observed in the contralateral hemisphere.

Across periods, within–subject EEG amplitude correlations between theta, alpha, low beta, and high beta EEG band pairs during training were consistently positive at the $p < 0.01$ level, within a range of $0.5 < r < 0.9$. In other words, amplitude increases/decreases in all EEG bands <25 Hz covaried in parallel with each other. Furthermore, for the ALPHA group, high gamma mean frequency (60–120 Hz) was *inversely* correlated with alpha amplitude during training ($r = -0.25$, $p < 0.01$). No significant online associations were detected between EEG bands and direct current

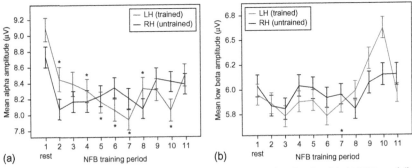

Figure 14.2 Time-course of the mean training EEG amplitudes for (a) ALPHA and (b) BETA groups, during a session of neurofeedback. Each session began with a 3-min baseline at rest (period 1), followed by 30 min of EEG feedback training (periods 2–11) on the left hemisphere (LH). * denote periods significantly different from baseline. Error bars represent SEM.

(DC) shifts, although the latter exhibited a negative correlation with period number ($r = -0.31$, p <0.01) in the ALPHA group.

TMS Main Effects

A GROUP × TIME (2 × 3) repeated measures ANOVA for the trained hemisphere CSE revealed a main TIME effect of significance for CSE ($F(2,44) = 6.8$, p < 0.01) and SICI ($F(2,44) = -4.3$, p = 0.03), while insignificant for ICF ($F(2,44) = 1.6$, p = 0.2). Interaction effects were not significant. No significant main effects were detected for the untrained hemisphere. Figure 14.3(a) depicts the mean effect of alpha suppression NFB training on corticospinal excitability (CSE) in the trained hemisphere. Single-pulse MEP amplitudes were significantly increased at post 2 compared to pre (130%, $t_{11} = -2.6$, p = 0.025), or circa 20 minutes after termination of NFB training. For the untrained hemisphere a similar albeit non-significant increase in MEP amplitudes was found post 2 (135%, $t_{11} = -1.691$, p = 0.12). Interestingly, no facilitatory effects were found just after (<10 min) NFB in the trained hemisphere (post 1), while an intermediate enhancement of 115% became manifest at around 10 minutes in the untrained hemisphere (Figure 14.3b, post 1, n.s.). A reliable trained hemisphere within-subject correlation between testing order (pre, post 1, post 2) and MEP amplitude was also detected ($r = 0.43$, p < 0.01). As detailed in Figure 14.4(a), we observed a significant and sustained decrease of intracortical inhibition (SICI 3 ms) at post

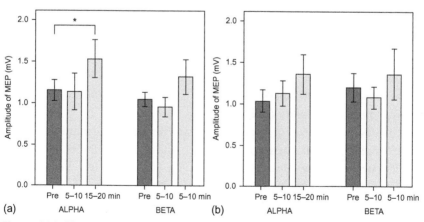

Figure 14.3 Mean corticospinal excitability (CSE) of (a) trained (left) hemisphere, and (b) untrained (right) hemisphere following the ALPHA and BETA protocols at times post 1 and 2. Error bars represent SEM.

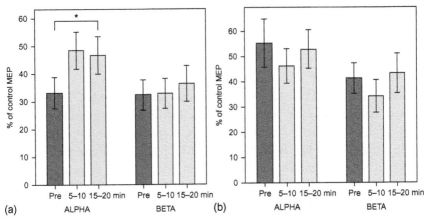

Figure 14.4 Mean short intracortical inhibition (SICI) of (a) trained (left) hemisphere, and (b) untrained (right) hemisphere following the ALPHA and BETA protocols at times post 1 and 2. Higher values signify lower SICI (disinhibition). Error bars represent SEM.

1 and post 2 uniquely in the trained hemisphere (post 1: 174%, $t_{11} = -3.5$, p <0.01; post 2: 165%, $t_{11} = -2.6$, p $= 0.023$). No other intracortical parameters were significantly altered following ALPHA protocol training.

As can be seen in Figure 14.3 depicting corticospinal excitability, no significant differences in CSE were found following low beta enhancement, although an initial decrease followed by increase was seen in both hemispheres at post 1 and post 2, respectively. No significant changes in SICI were observed in the trained (Figure 14.4a) or untrained hemisphere (Figure 14.4b).

TMS—EEG Relationships
Corticospinal Excitability (CSE)
Effective NFB training for each subject was defined by a training coefficient, or the Pearson correlation between the period number (1 to 11) and its corresponding mean EEG amplitude (alpha and low beta amplitude, for ALPHA and BETA groups respectively). This has previously (Gruzelier & Egner, 2005) proven to be a good estimator of the temporal consistency of either an increase or a decrease in the training EEG amplitude from baseline, which can be expressed in the range of −1 (steady decrease) and +1 (steady increase).

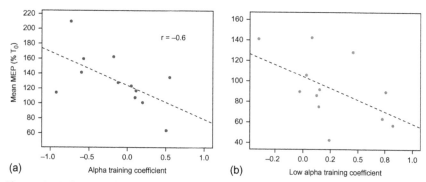

Figure 14.5 Scatter plots of each subject's (N = 12) training coefficient vs. mean single-pulse MEP change for (a) ALPHA group at post 2 and (b) BETA group at post 1.

As depicted in Figure 14.5a, a scatter plot of alpha training coefficient vs. post 2 MEP amplitude for the ALPHA group revealed a significant negative correlation ($r = -0.59$, $p = 0.044$), meaning that in general greater temporal consistency of alpha decrease from baseline is associated with greater increase in corticospinal excitability. Moreover, a parallel *positive* correlation was observed between high gamma mean frequency (60–120 Hz) training coefficient and MEP post 2 ($r = 0.62$, $p = 0.031$). No significant correlations were evident at post 1 ($r = -0.32$, n.s.). For the BETA protocol (Figure 14.5b), the correlation between reliable low beta synchronization and direction of MEP change was similarly negative at post 1, albeit less robust ($r = -0.53$, $p = 0.08$; weighted least-squares (WLS) regression $r = -0.62$, $p = 0.03$). This relationship was absent at post 2 ($r = -0.25$, n.s.).

Regarding the relation between TMS changes and absolute EEG parameters, first, no reliable relationships were evident between MEP change and absolute EEG amplitudes in any band, during any period of the neurofeedback session. However, when the EEG amplitudes were normalized as a percentage of their 3-min baseline value at rest (period 1), strong associations appeared, signalling that a change in the EEG was closely coupled to a change in MEP. Figure 14.6 illustrates the Pearson cross-correlation value between the post 2 MEP amplitude (outcome variable) and normalized alpha amplitude of each period (predictor variable) during neurofeedback in the ALPHA group. As anticipated, we observed mainly negative correlations between alpha power and MEP increase, with a gradual trend of increasing significance from the beginning of the session that reached a maximum at around the middle of the session,

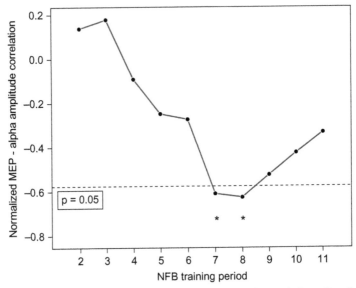

Figure 14.6 Post 2 MEP (%pre) vs. alpha amplitude (%pre) correlations, for all ALPHA periods.

during periods 7 ($r = -0.61$, $p = 0.35$) and 8 ($r = -0.63$, $p = 0.30$), or between 15 and 21 minutes of neurofeedback. Interestingly, period 7 also coincided with the minimum alpha amplitude during training (see Figure 14.2a).

The EEG amplitude ratio of the post-neurofeedback resting baseline and the pre-baseline (period 12/period 1) proved to be another successful predictor of post 2 MEP change in all bands investigated below *high* beta (delta: $r = -0.64$, $p = 0.03$; theta: $r = -0.7$, $p = 0.012$; alpha: $r = -0.71$, $p = 0.01$; low beta: $r = -0.62$, $p = 0.03$), suggesting that the more suppressed the slower EEG amplitudes were after NFB training the greater the enhancement of the MEP 20 minutes later. This also appeared to be positively the case for resting change in the high gamma mean frequency ($r = 0.53$, $p = 0.07$). Lastly, during periods 8, 9, and 10 correlations remained significantly positive ($r > 0.6$, $p < 0.05$) and predicted resting alpha amplitude change from *training* alpha amplitudes.

As seen in Figure 14.7, the overall implication is that a three-way significant association was thus established between core changes in the training EEG, the subsequent resting EEG, and corticospinal excitability.

Analogous analyses were performed on the BETA group for relationships between single-pulse MEP and low beta amplitudes, disclosing a

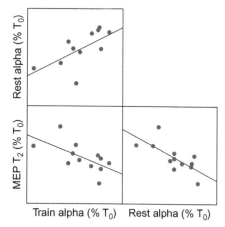

Figure 14.7 Matrix plot of training alpha (period 8 %pre), resting alpha (period 12 %pre), MEP (post 2 %pre) amplitudes. All correlations were significant at $r > |0.6|$, $p < 0.05$.

significant association similar to that found with ALPHA between resting low beta change and post 1 MEP (WLS $r = -0.58$, $p = 0.050$) as well as a borderline correlation between training period 7 and post 1 MEP (WLS $r = -0.52$, $p = 0.08$). Low beta amplitude during period 7 was in turn also tightly correlated with its subsequent change at rest (WLS $r = 0.67$, $p = 0.02$), mirroring closely but less reliably, the three-way relationship reported for the ALPHA group. No significant associations were observed between MEP and the remaining EEG bands in the BETA group (e.g. resting alpha vs. MEP post 1: WLS $r = -0.17$, $p = 0.60$).

In summary, pre-to-post increases in corticomotor excitability were positively (negatively) correlated with both the sustained time-course and relative degree of desynchronization (synchronization) of alpha and low beta rhythms.

SICI/ICF

For the ALPHA group, there was significant positive correlation ($r = 0.58$, $p = 0.050$) between alpha training coefficient and 3 ms SICI (% pre) change at post 1, suggesting that it was the weakest performers that had the greatest reductions in SICI. However, relatively robust correlations were discovered for the DC training coefficient and SICI post 1 ($r = -0.6$, $p = 0.04$), SICI post 2 ($r = -0.53$, $p = 0.07$), and ICF post 2 ($r = 0.79$, $p < 0.01$). Moreover ICF post 2 (but not post 1) change was inversely proportional with SICI at post 1 ($r = 0.63$, $p = 0.03$) and post 2 ($r = 0.72$, p <0.01), suggesting that SICI decreases may have preceded ICF increases. No significant links were apparent for the BETA group; however, negative associations of marginal statistical significance were observed between ICF at post 1 and the low beta training coefficient ($r = -0.51$, $p = 0.09$) and resting (period 12) low beta amplitude ($r = -0.52$, $p = 0.08$). Resting alpha amplitude (in the BETA group) was uncorrelated ($r = 0.14$, $p = 0.67$).

Path Analysis

To investigate the possible causal relationships between training EEG, resting EEG, and MEP amplitudes, we conducted a path analysis of the three-way correlates linking these variables from our experimental data. Figure 14.8 shows the Path Analysis results for ALPHA training during period 7 and MEP at post 2, mirroring Figure 14.7. For ALPHA group training periods 6, 7, 8, and 9, regression coefficients were consistently higher ($r > 0.5$) in the Path Analysis for the two indirect pathways (dark gray) of training EEG to resting EEG, and resting EEG to MEP, compared to the direct pathway (light gray) of training EEG to MEP ($r < 0.5$) as shown in Figure 14.8. Accordingly, a bootstrap test (see Methods for

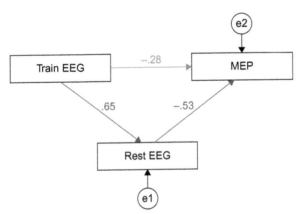

Figure 14.8 Path Analysis of the hypothesized causal relationship between observed training EEG, subsequent resting EEG and corticospinal excitability (MEP) measures. Here, the indirect pathway (dark gray arrows) emerges as a better predictor of the training EEG effect on MEP than the direct pathway (light gray arrow). ALPHA group standardized regression coefficients are illustrated for normalized training alpha (period 7), resting alpha (second baseline), and single-pulse MEP amplitudes at post 2 in the trained hemisphere. Unobserved residual (error) variables are denoted by e1 and e2.

details) revealed a statistically significant ($p < 0.05$) *indirect* effect of training EEG on MEP, *mediated* via the resting EEG change. Moreover, deletion of the training EEG to MEP direct pathway resulted in a better-fit (chi-square $= 1.1$, df $= 1$, $p = 0.3$) and greater parsimony (change in PNFI $= 0.31$). We then applied this final model to the BETA group relationships described above (low beta amplitude period 6 vs. MEP post 1), which turned out analogous to the ALPHA group, confirming a good-fit mediation model (chi square $= 0.4$, df $= 1$, $p = 0.5$), with the indirect effect having a marginal bootstrap significance of $p = 0.08$.

Overall, these modeling results suggest that the general NFB effect may be better explained by its action on the resting/spontaneous EEG, which is in turn a more direct reflection of cortical excitability.

DISCUSSION

In summary, sustained neurofeedback-mediated EEG changes in the ALPHA group (Figure 14.2a) resulted in a statistically reliable (>20 min) overall increase in corticospinal excitability (130%) (Figure 14.3a) and decrease in short intracortical inhibition (174%) (Figure 14.4a), when compared to the negligible longer-lasting changes in the BETA group which showed less evidence of learning. Most importantly, correlation analyses revealed robust relationships between the historical activity of certain brain rhythms during neurofeedback and the resultant change in corticospinal excitability. Specifically during neurofeedback, alpha ($8-12$ Hz) desynchronization (Figure 14.5a) coupled with increased mean frequencies of high gamma rhythms ($60-120$ Hz), was tightly correlated with long-term potentiation-like (>20 min) enhancement of single-pulse motor evoked potentials. In contrast, neurofeedback involving low beta ($12-15$ Hz) synchronization was inversely correlated with short-term depression-like (>5 min) reductions of corticospinal excitability (Figure 14.5b). Thirdly, in both groups, changes in resting EEG amplitudes were *predicted by* the neurofeedback training EEG, and were also a *predictor of* the later motor evoked potential amplitudes (Figure 14.7).

In this experiment, the longer-term neuroplastic effects following alpha desynchronization are highly unlikely to be consequences of basic changes in psychological arousal after neurofeedback, as the within-subject motor evoked potential data denotes a significant positive correlation between amplitude and elapsed time following training, while the reverse would be otherwise expected (moreover, the BETA group did not demonstrate equivalent changes, discounting the likelihood of a placebo effect). Bearing in mind that neuroplastic induction may have already begun mid-session (see Figure 14.6, where correlations are highest around 20 min), such a progressive dynamic could also be suggestive of a time course involving cellular cascades known to occur during early long-term potentiation (Cooke & Bliss, 2006). In contrast, short-term potentiation amplitudes are markedly extinguished by 15−20 min (Schulz & Fitzgibbons, 1997). A reduction in alpha band power has commonly been found to be associated with increased cortical excitability (Sauseng, Klimesch, Gerloff, & Hummel, 2009), cortical metabolism (Oishi et al., 2007), attention (Fries, Womelsdorf, Oostenveld, & Desimone, 2008), and behavioral activation (Rougeul-Buser & Buser, 1997). Critically, in the current study a negative correlation between low-end frequencies (especially alpha) and high gamma mean frequencies during neurofeedback was also detected, as well as a positive correlation between the latter and single-pulse MEP increase. This is supported by recent reports linking high-frequency oscillations (HFO) or higher gamma activity with learning (Ponomarenko, Li, Korotkova, Huston, & Haas, 2008) and attention (Fries, Womelsdorf, Oostenveld, & Desimone, 2008), as well as with increased BOLD activity (Niessing et al., 2005), neuronal depolarization and firing rate (Grenier, Timofeev, & Steriade, 2001; Niessing et al., 2005). Interestingly, the ALPHA group reduction in short intracortical inhibition at post 1 and 2 may be attributed to a decrease in cortical GABAergic transmission (Hallett, 2007). This could possibly be the system's intrinsic reaction in order to further facilitate plasticity, as previous reports have found an antagonistic relationship between inhibitory and excitatory transmission on motor plasticity and long-term potentiation (Bütefisch et al., 2000; Komaki et al., 2007). At present, however, we can neither confirm nor rule out the release of endogenous neuromodulators as an interacting mechanism for the observed effects. One potential candidate may be noradrenaline, which is released during attentive behavior (Berridge & Waterhouse, 2003; Rougeul-Buser & Buser, 1997) and has previously been reported to enhance long-term potentiation (Harley, 1987), desynchronize alpha rhythms (Rougeul-Buser & Buser, 1997), and increase corticospinal excitability and decrease short intracortical inhibition concomitantly (Ziemann, 2004).

As low beta learning was less effective it is possible that it was associated with an inappropriate training approach in some subjects which was perhaps more desynchronizing than synchronizing, and therefore con-founded the group result; hence the slightly increased corticospinal excit-ability observed later on. This is supported by the negative correlations found between low beta training and MEP, which remain in line with findings that low beta synchronization is associated with motor-cortical deactivation (Oishi et al., 2007) and inhibition (Zhang, Chen, Bressler, & Ding, 2008). The finding that electrical stimulation of sensori-motor cortex at 10 Hz leads to long-term depression (Werk, Klein, Nesbitt, & Chapman, 2006) may be related to the short-term depression-like effect observed in this study at a slightly higher, albeit correlated, fre-quency of 12–15 Hz. Moreover, it has recently been observed that longer durations of 10 Hz repetitive TMS lead to long-term depression-like effects (Jung, Shin, Jeong, & Shin, 2008).

It is tempting to compare the average effect sizes in this study with those of existing non-invasive brain stimulation protocols used to induce neuroplasticity. Repetitive magnetic (Ziemann et al., 2008) and direct current (Nitsche & Paulus, 2001) stimulation investigations report average corticospinal excitability increases of around 150%, which is comparable to the range we observed following alpha desynchronization. Remarkably, this may indicate that regardless of whether endogenous or exogenous techniques are used, they appear to impact on a common neural substrate, which is intrinsic to the brain. However, numerous exogenous protocols induce after effects that last for periods up to an hour or more. Therefore a question of scientific and therapeutic importance is, how long can endogenously driven effects last?

Another intriguing question is whether the observed plasticity effects are a direct consequence of longer-term changes to the dynamics of "rest-ing" or spontaneous rhythms (Sauseng et al., 2009), and associated thalamocortical networks (Steriade & Timofeev, 2003; Thut & Miniussi, 2009). This seems a tempting account in light of the significant three-way correlations between amplitude changes in training EEG, subsequent rest-ing EEG, and the motor evoked potential (Figure 14.7). Moreover, path analysis and structural equation model results (Figure 14.8) point to an indirect effect of neurofeedback (via the resting EEG) on the single-pulse motor evoked potential. If ultimately confirmed, this would suggest that the brain indeed "shapes itself" (Rudrauf, Lutz, Cosmelli, Lachaux, & Le Van Quyen, 2003), whereby past activities perpetually influence or bias future (baseline) states of processing (Silvanto, Muggleton, & Walsh, 2008). In this case, the notion of a "background" or baseline brain state would cease to be informative, as it would be continually in flux and shaped by past/present activity. We hope that future studies will elucidate these complex activity-dependent relationships further.

The novel finding that short intracortical inhibition was positively correlated with slow shifts in DC potential are compatible with the established view that slow cortical negativities are a marker of increased excitability and/or cortical disinhibition (Niedermayer & Lopes Da Silva, 1999). As this was for the ALPHA group only, this relationship awaits replication, and supports the online/offline use of TMS full-band EEG coregistration. The lack of relation of paired-pulse or DC measures with oscillatory EEG in this study is especially noteworthy. The latter effect has been documented previously and may suggest physiologically separate mechanisms of action (Kotchoubey, Busch, Strehl, & Birbaumer, 1999). We have to acknowledge that our recording conditions were suboptimal, as we did not additionally short-circuit the skin (Vanhatalo, Voipio, & Kaila, 2005); although random fluctuations of skin/sweat voltages would be unlikely to account for this phenomenon. Overall our results remain consistent with traditional evidence from both cellular and non-invasive studies reporting that very high frequency stimulation usually induces synaptic potentiation whereas lower frequencies may engender synaptic depression (Cooke & Bliss, 2006). It is well-established that EEG activity is generated by the summed electrical fluctuations of postsynaptic potentials (Niedermayer & Lopes Da Silva, 1999), and so may potentially be a close correlate of changes in synaptic transmission frequency or dendritic activity (Williams, Wozny, & Mitchell, 2007). Higher frequencies could reflect denser temporal incidence of EPSPs and hence greater influx of calcium (a trigger of long-term potentiation) through voltage-gated ion channels (Na^+, Ca^{2+}). Intracellularly, second messengers such as Cam Kinase II have also been found to be sensitive to the frequency of calcium oscillations (De Koninck, 1998). On the other hand, a recent study observed that zero net-current extracellular high-frequency stimulation in cultured neurons gave rise to an overall depolarization of the cell membrane (Schoen & Fromherz, 2008), which could hypothetically lower activation thresholds for voltage-gated ion channels. However, our data did not reveal significant changes in the resting motor threshold (considered to reflect changes in membrane excitability), making a case for a transsynaptic effect more likely. On the whole, the activity-dependent relationships observed in this study, together with the cited works above, vouch for the possible involvement of endogenous oscillations in the mediation of synaptic plasticity (Steriade & Timofeev, 2003). Latest findings that appear to support this role report neuroplasticity induction based on slow-wave sleep, sleep spindle (Rosanova & Ulrich, 2005), and theta (Huang, Edwards, Rounis, Bhatia, & Rothwell, 2005) endogenous rhythms.

In light of the initial neurophysiological evidence presented in this study, a repetitive alpha suppression protocol could theoretically be of significant therapeutic value in clinical cases where the pathophysiology consists of poor corticospinal activation and/or increased inhibition; in a motor disorder such as stroke, for example. Moreover, as other methods of neuromodulation are reported to facilitate motor learning by inducing increases in cortical excitability (Ziemann et al., 2008), this particular protocol may be potentially useful in enhancing practice-dependent motor performance in healthy subjects (Ros et al., 2009). Lastly, whilst additionally supporting previous clinical applications of neurofeedback (Heinrich, Gevensleben, & Strehl, 2007), a similar NFB approach aimed at cortical activation may eventually prove to be appropriate for brain disorders exhibiting low cortical excitability or elevated slow-wave EEG power, such as attention-deficit hyperactivity disorder (ADHD) (Lubar, 1991), traumatic brain injury (Thatcher, 2000), and depression (Korb, Cook, Hunter, & Leuchter, 2008).

In conclusion, our results provide a first basis for the "missing link" between the historical long-term training effects of neurofeedback and direct validation of neuroplastic change after an individual session of training.

REFERENCES

Axmacher, N., Mormann, F., Fernández, G., Elger, C. E., & Fell, J. (2006). Memory formation by neuronal synchronization. *Brain Research Reviews, 52*(1), 170–182.

Berridge, C., & Waterhouse, B. (2003). The locus coeruleus-noradrenergic system: Modulation of behavioral state and state-dependent cognitive processes. *Brain Research Reviews, 42,* 33–84.

Bütefisch, C. M., Davis, B. C., Wise, S. P., Sawaki, L., Kopylev, L., Classen, J., et al. (2000). Mechanisms of use-dependent plasticity in the human motor cortex. *Proceedings of the National Academy of Sciences of the United States of America, 97*(7), 3661–3665.

Cooke, S. F., & Bliss, T. V. (2006). Plasticity in the human central nervous system. *Brain, 129*(Pt 7), 1659–1673.

De Koninck, P. (1998). Sensitivity of CaM Kinase II to the Frequency of Ca^{2+} Oscillations. *Science, 279*(5348), 227–230.

Doehnert, M., Brandeis, D., Straub, M., Steinhausen, H., & Drechsler, R. (2008). Slow cortical potential neurofeedback in attention deficit hyperactivity disorder: is there neurophysiological evidence for specific effects? *Journal of Neurophysiology, 115*(10), 1445−1456.

Egner, T., & Gruzelier, J. H. (2004). EEG biofeedback of low beta band components: frequency-specific effects on variables of attention and event-related brain potentials. *Clinical Neurophysiology, 115*(1), 131−139.

Fries, P., Womelsdorf, T., Oostenveld, R., & Desimone, R. (2008). The effects of visual stimulation and selective visual attention on rhythmic neuronal synchronization in macaque area V4. *Journal of Neuroscience, 28*(18), 4823−4835.

Grenier, F., Timofeev, I., & Steriade, M. (2001). Focal synchronization of ripples (80-200 Hz) in neocortex and their neuronal correlates. *Journal of Neurophysiology, 86*(4), 1884−1898.

Gruzelier, J., & Egner, T. (2005). Critical validation studies of neurofeedback. *Child and Adolescent Psychiatric Clinics of North America, 14*(1), 83−104, vi.

Gruzelier, J., Egner, T., & Vernon, D. (2006). Validating the efficacy of neurofeedback for optimising performance. *Progress in Brain Research, 159*, 421−431.

Hallett, M. (2007). Transcranial magnetic stimulation: a primer. *Neuron, 55*(2), 187−199.

Hanslmayr, S., Sauseng, P., Doppelmayr, M., Schabus, M., & Klimesch, W. (2005). Increasing individual upper alpha power by neurofeedback improves cognitive performance in human subjects. *Applied Psychophysiology and Biofeedback, 30*(1), 1−10.

Harley, C. W. (1987). A role for norepinephrine in arousal, emotion and learning? Limbic modulation by norepinephrine and the Kety hypothesis. *Progress in Neuro-psychopharmacology and Biological Psychiatry, 11*(4), 419−458.

Heinrich, H., Gevensleben, H., & Strehl, U. (2007). Annotation: neurofeedback - train your brain to train behaviour. *Journal of Child Psychology and Psychiatry, 48*(1), 3−16.

Huang, Y., Edwards, M. J., Rounis, E., Bhatia, K. P., & Rothwell, J. C. (2005). Theta burst stimulation of the human motor cortex. *Neuron, 45*(2), 201−206.

Jensen, O., Goel, P., Kopell, N., Pohja, M., Hari, R., Ermentrout, B., et al. (2005). On the human sensorimotor-cortex beta rhythm: sources and modeling. *NeuroImage, 26* (2), 347−355.

Jung, S. H., Shin, J. E., Jeong, Y., & Shin, H. (2008). Changes in motor cortical excitability induced by high-frequency repetitive transcranial magnetic stimulation of different stimulation durations. *Clinical Neurophysiology, 119*(1), 71−79.

Komaki, A., Shahidi, S., Lashgari, R., Haghparast, A., Malakouti, S. M., Noorbakhsh, S. M., et al. (2007). Effects of GABAergic inhibition on neocortical long-term potentiation in the chronically prepared rat. *Neuroscience Letters, 422*(3), 181−186.

Korb, A. S., Cook, I. A., Hunter, A. M., & Leuchter, A. F. (2008). Brain electrical source differences between depressed subjects and healthy controls. *Brain Topography, 21*(2), 138−146.

Kotchoubey, B., Busch, S., Strehl, U., & Birbaumer, N. (1999). Changes in EEG power spectra during biofeedback of slow cortical potentials in epilepsy. *Applied Psychophysiology and Biofeedback, 24*(4), 213−233.

Kujirai, T., Caramia, M. D., Rothwell, J. C., Day, B. L., Thompson, P. D., Ferbert, A., et al. (1993). Corticocortical inhibition in human motor cortex. *Journal of Physiology, 471*, 501−519.

Lazzaro, V. D., Ziemann, U., & Lemon, R. N (2008). State of the art: Physiology of transcranial motor cortex stimulation. *Brain Stimulation, 1*(4), 345−362.

Lévesque, J., Beauregard, M., & Mensour, B. (2006). Effect of neurofeedback training on the neural substrates of selective attention in children with attention-deficit/hyperactivity disorder: A functional magnetic resonance imaging study. *Neuroscience Letters, 394*, 216−221.

Lubar, J. F. (1991). Discourse on the development of EEG diagnostics and biofeedback for attention-deficit/hyperactivity disorders. *Biofeedback and Self-Regulation, 16*(3), 201−225.

Nelson, S. B., & Turrigiano, G. G. (2008). Strength through diversity. *Neuron, 60*(3), 477−482.

Neuper, C., Wörtz, M., & Pfurtscheller, G. (2006). ERD/ERS patterns reflecting sensorimotor activation and deactivation. *Progress in Brain Research, 159,* 211−222.

Niedermayer, E., & Lopes Da Silva, F. (1999). *Electroencephalography: Basic principles, clinical applications and related fields* (4th ed.) Baltimore, MD: Williams & Wilkins.

Niessing, J., Ebisch, B., Schmidt, K. E., Niessing, M., Singer, W., Galuske, R. A., et al. (2005). Hemodynamic signals correlate tightly with synchronized gamma oscillations. *Science, 309*(5736), 948−951.

Nitsche, M. A., & Paulus, W. (2001). Sustained excitability elevations induced by transcranial DC motor cortex stimulation in humans. *Neurology, 57*(10), 1899−1901.

Oishi, N., Mima, T., Ishii, K., Bushara, K. O., Hiraoka, T., Ueki, Y., et al. (2007). Neural correlates of regional EEG power change. *NeuroImage, 36*(4), 1301−1312 doi: 10.1016/j.neuroimage.2007.04.030

Ponomarenko, A. A., Li, J., Korotkova, T. M., Huston, J. P., & Haas, H. L. (2008). Frequency of network synchronization in the hippocampus marks learning. *The European Journal of Neuroscience, 27*(11), 3035−3042 doi: 10.1111/j.1460-9568.2008.06232.x

Ros, T., Moseley, M. J., Bloom, P. A., Benjamin, L., Parkinson, L. A., Gruzelier, J. H., et al. (2009). Optimizing microsurgical skills with EEG neurofeedback. *BMC Neuroscience, 10*(1), 87 doi: 10.1186/1471-2202-10-87

Rosanova, M., & Ulrich, D. (2005). Pattern-specific associative long-term potentiation induced by a sleep spindle-related spike train. *Journal of Neuroscience, 25*(41), 9398−9405 doi: 10.1523/JNEUROSCI.2149-05.2005

Rougeul-Buser, A., & Buser, P. (1997). Rhythms in the alpha band in cats and their behavioural correlates. *International Journal of Psychophysiology, 26*(1−3), 191−203.

Rudrauf, D., Lutz, A., Cosmelli, D., Lachaux, J., & Le Van Quyen, M. (2003). From autopoiesis to neurophenomenology: Francisco Varela's exploration of the biophysics of being. *Biological Research, 36*(1), 27−65.

Sauseng, P., Klimesch, W., Gerloff, C., & Hummel, F. C. (2009). Spontaneous locally restricted EEG alpha activity determines cortical excitability in the motor cortex. *Neuropsychologia, 47*(1), 284−288.

Schoen, I., & Fromherz, P. (2008). Extracellular stimulation of mammalian neurons through repetitive activation of Na^+ channels by weak capacitive currents on a silicon chip. *Journal of Neurophysiology, 100*(1), 346−357.

Schroeder, C. E., & Lakatos, P. (2009). Low-frequency neuronal oscillations as instruments of sensory selection. *Trends in Neurosciences, 32*(1), 9−18.

Schulz, P. E., & Fitzgibbons, J. C. (1997). Differing mechanisms of expression for short- and long-term potentiation. *Journal of Neurophysiology, 78*(1), 321−334.

Silvanto, J., Muggleton, N., & Walsh, V. (2008). State-dependency in brain stimulation studies of perception and cognition. *Trends in Cognitive Sciences, 12*(12), 447−454.

Steriade, M., & Timofeev, I. (2003). Neuronal plasticity in thalamocortical networks during sleep and waking oscillations. *Neuron, 37*(4), 563−576.

Sterman, M. B. (1996). Physiological origins and functional correlates of EEG rhythmic activities: implications for self-regulation. *Biofeedback and Self-Regulation, 21*(1), 3−33.

Thatcher, R. W. (2000). EEG operant conditioning (biofeedback) and traumatic brain injury. *Clinical EEG (electroencephalography), 31*(1), 38−44.

Thut, G., & Miniussi, C. (2009). New insights into rhythmic brain activity from TMS-EEG studies. *Trends in Cognitive Sciences, 13*(4), 182−189.

Vanhatalo, S., Voipio, J., & Kaila, K. (2005). Full-band EEG (FbEEG): an emerging standard in electroencephalography. *Clinical Neurophysiology*, *116*(1), 1−8.

Wagner, T., Valero-Cabre, A., & Pascual-Leone, A. (2007). Noninvasive human brain stimulation. *Annual Review of Biomedical Engineering*, *9*, 527−565.

Werk, C. M., Klein, H. S., Nesbitt, C. E., & Chapman, C. (2006). Long-term depression in the sensorimotor cortex induced by repeated delivery of 10 Hz trains in vivo. *Neuroscience*, *140*(1), 13−20.

Williams, S. R., Wozny, C., & Mitchell, S. J. (2007). The back and forth of dendritic plasticity. *Neuron*, *56*(6), 947−953.

Zhang, Y., Chen, Y., Bressler, S., & Ding, M. (2008). Response preparation and inhibition: The role of the cortical sensorimotor beta rhythm. *Neuroscience*, *156*(1), 238−246.

Ziemann, U. (2004). TMS and drugs. *Clinical Neurophysiology*, *115*(8), 1717−1729.

Ziemann, U., Paulus, W., Nitsche, M. A., Pascual-Leone, A., Byblow, W. D., Berardelli, A., et al. (2008). Consensus: Motor cortex plasticity protocols. *Brain Stimulation*, *1*(3), 164−182.

CHAPTER 15

Enduring Effects of Neurofeedback in Children

Robert Coben[1], Martijn Arns[2], and Mirjam E.J. Kouijzer[3]
[1]Neurorehabilitation and Neuropsychological Services, Massapequa Park, New York, USA
[2]Research Institute Brainclinics, Nijmegen, and Utrecht University, Department of Experimental Psychology, Utrecht, The Netherlands
[3]Behavioral Science Institute, Radboud University Nijmegen, Nijmegen, The Netherlands

Contents

INTRODUCTION

The benefits of neurofeedback as a treatment for children with developmental disorders have been demonstrated. Neurofeedback has shown efficacy for a wide variety of developmental disorders such as autism, ADHD, epilepsy, and dyslexia (Coben & Padolsky, 2007; Egner & Sterman, 2006; Evans & Park, 1996; Hammond, 2007; Leins et al., 2007; Lubar, et al., 2005). Further, to our knowledge there is no study that has reported any detrimental side effects as a result of neurofeedback treatment.

Preliminary research suggests that neurofeedback is an effective therapy for reducing core symptoms in children with both autism and ADHD (Arns et al., 2009; Coben & Padolsky, 2007; Heinrich, Gevensleben, Freisleder, Moll & Rothenberger, 2004; Jarusiewicz, 2002). Neurofeedback is a therapy that teaches clients to regulate their brain activity to work in a new, more efficient way through the use of underlying operant conditioning paradigms. This treatment involves providing a subject with visual and/or auditory "feedback" for particular neural behaviors

Neurofeedback and Neuromodulation Techniques and Applications
DOI: 10.1016/B978-0-12-382235-2.00015-9

(Monastra, Monastra, & George, 2002). Through conditioning the subject is taught to inhibit EEG frequencies that are excessively generated and augment frequencies that are deficient. With continuous training and coaching, individuals are taught to maintain brainwave patterns concurrent with healthy neural functioning. Recently, Walker, Kozlowski, and Lawson (2007) presented evidence demonstrating the ability of neurofeedback training to successfully train neural functioning to more normal states as well as simultaneously demonstrating reductions in pathological symptoms. For more in-depth information regarding neurofeedback the interested reader is referred to Hammond (2007).

Neurofeedback was originally assessed as a useful therapy by Barry Sterman in 1970 at the Neuropsychiatric Institute of UCLA (Sterman et al., 1970). Later, Lubar and Shouse (1976) reported distinct positive EEG and behavioral changes in a hyperkinetic child with ADHD after training the sensorimotor EEG rhythm (SMR: 12–14 Hz). Since then there has been an increasing quantity of published research indicating positive effects of neurofeedback with a variety of disorders, including ADHD. Recently, Monastra et al. (2002) assessed more than 100 children with ADHD, and found that neurofeedback was capable of significantly reducing core symptoms of ADHD. Arns et al. (2009) performed a meta-analysis encompassing over 15 studies and a total sample size of more than 1100 children, and concluded that neurofeedback is an effective form of treatment for subjects with ADHD. Moreover, recent investigations have found the results of neurofeedback training to be comparable to the clinical gains achieved through medication in children (Fox, Tharp, & Fox, 2005). However, unlike medications, there has been no report of any unwanted or negative side effects as a result of treating ADHD with neurofeedback training.

The efficacy of neurofeedback for autistic children was initially assessed in a study by Jarusiewicz (2002) in which she reported a 26% decrease in autistic symptoms in an experimental group and a 3% reduction in a wait-list control group. More recently, Coben & Padolsky (2007) found similar, yet more impressive results, reporting a 40% decrease in core autistic symptoms as a result of neurofeedback therapy. Similar to the findings in regards to ADHD, to our knowledge there is no evidence of neurofeedback training producing any detrimental or unwanted side effects in children with autism spectrum disorders (ASD).

In this chapter we discuss evidence for long-term effects of neurofeedback. Over the course of three series of studies we examined the efficacy of neurofeedback training for children with autism as well as children with ADHD. We hypothesized that neurofeedback creates effective as well as enduring positive clinical changes in children with autism and ADHD.

NEUROFEEDBACK AS A TREATMENT FOR CHILDREN WITH ADHD

Recently the 8-year follow-up results from a very large NIMH sponsored trial on different treatments for ADHD have been published [the NIMH Collaborative Multisite Multimodal Treatment Study of Children with Attention-Deficit/Hyperactivity Disorder (ADHD), abbreviated as MTA (Molina et al., 2009)]. This study compared four different treatments in 579 children. These were initially randomly assigned to: (1) systemic medication management; (2) multi-component behavior therapy; (3) a combination of (1) and (2); and (4) usual community care. The first results after 14 months initially showed that the medication and combined groups showed the greatest improvements in ADHD and ODD symptoms. However, half of these effects had dissipated 10 months after the treatment was completed. More importantly, after 8 years follow-up, there were no differences to be found between these four groups, indicating that the initial treatments to which the children were randomly assigned, did not predict functioning 6−8 years later. This multi-centre large-scale study hence clearly demonstrates a lack of long-term effects for either stimulant medication, multi-component behavior therapy or multimodal treatment (Molina et al., 2009). Furthermore, in general, response rates to stimulant medication in ADHD are estimated to be between 70 and 90% (see Hermens, Rowe, Gordon, & Williams (2006) for an overview).

These results clearly show that at present there is no commonly accepted treatment modality that has sufficient long-term efficacy for children with ADHD, and there is a need for new treatments with better long-term outcomes. In the next paragraphs we provide evidence that neurofeedback may be as effective and have more enduring effects than any of the presently commonly used treatment approaches for ADHD.

As noted above, in 1976 Lubar and Shouse were the first to report on EEG and behavioral changes in a hyperkinetic child after training the sensorimotor EEG rhythm (SMR: 12−14 Hz). In 2004, Heinrich et al. were the first to report positive results after Slow Cortical Potential (SCP) neurofeedback in the treatment of ADHD. SCP neurofeedback is different from the above-mentioned neurofeedback approach in that changes in the polarity of the EEG are rewarded (i.e. positivity vs. negativity in the EEG), and a discrete reward scheme is used. Incidentally, both SCP neurofeedback and SMR neurofeedback approaches have been successfully used in treating epilepsy as well [for an overview also see Egner & Sterman, (2006)], and it has been suggested that both regulate cortical excitability (Arns et al., 2009; Kleinnijenhuis, Arns, Spronk, Breteler & Duysens, 2008). Several studies have compared theta-beta training and SCP training using both within-subject (Gevensleben et al., 2009b) and between-subject (Leins et al., 2007) designs, and both neurofeedback approaches showed comparable effects on different aspects of ADHD such as inattention, hyperactivity, and impulsivity. A recent meta-analysis investigating the effects of neurofeedback used data from 15 published studies with a total sample size of 1194 children with ADHD. Based on this study (Arns et al., 2009) it was concluded that neurofeedback for the treatment of ADHD met the evidence-based criteria for Level V: Efficacious and Specific. This study also addressed some of the criticisms made in the past. In this meta-analysis, long-term effects were not addressed at length.

Some studies have considered long-term effects of neurofeedback and found that the skill to modulate EEG activity in the required direction is still preserved over time [6 months: (Leins et al., 2007); and 2 years: (Gani, Birbaumer & Strehl, 2008)]. Given the treatment potential already mentioned, these long-term findings make neurofeedback a very interesting and promising treatment for ADHD. In the following paragraphs we will in a more quantitative way report on the long-term effects of neurofeedback.

LONG-TERM EFFECTS OF NEUROFEEDBACK

Some of the earliest studies of neurofeedback with ADHD considered long-term effects. Lubar (1991) reported follow-up results on the initial case mentioned above (Lubar & Shouse, 1976) demonstrating that the effects were sustained over time, and the child was still performing well without medication. In the Monastra, Monastra, and George (2002) study, all 100 ADHD children were medicated and 51 children also received neurofeedback. Interestingly, when the medication was removed at the end of treatment, only the subjects who had completed neurofeedback were able to sustain their improvements. The qEEG measurements also showed a significant decrease in cortical slowing of the individuals who had completed neurofeedback, but not in the subjects who had only received medication.

Several controlled studies that investigated the effects of neurofeedback in ADHD reported follow-up results as well. Heinrich et al. (2004) performed a 3-month follow-up for a SCP training group and found all criterion measures improving further (Heinrich, personal communication: unpublished results; Arns et al., 2009). Strehl and colleagues showed that at 6-month follow-up scores in impulsivity, inattention, and hyperactivity were improved even further as compared to the end of treatment (Leins et al., 2007; Strehl et al., 2006). Furthermore, a 2-year follow-up for this study (Gani et al., 2008) showed that all improvements in behavior and attention turned out to be stable. Test results for attention and some of the parents' ratings once more improved significantly. In addition, EEG self-regulation skills turned out to be preserved, indicating that these children were still able to successfully regulate their brain activity.

In order to visualize these effects further we have plotted the effects for inattention and hyperactivity in Figure 15.1. The weighted average is an average of the scores of all three studies, and then weighted for the number of subjects per study. This figure clearly shows that the effects of neurofeedback improve further over time. Both measures are based on a DSM-based questionnaire. For impulsivity there were too few data to make a sensible comparison.

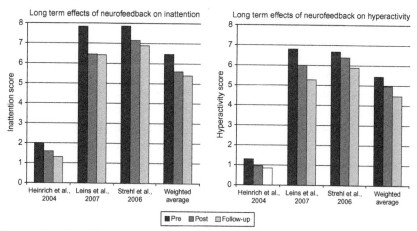

Figure 15.1 The effects of neurofeedback over time for three controlled studies for inattention (left) and hyperactivity (right). The study by Heinrich et al. performed 3 months follow-up and the other two studies performed 6 months follow-up. Note that the effects of neurofeedback tend to improve further over time (as opposed to the effects of medication, which are not sustained when the medication is stopped).

In 2009 one of the largest multi-site randomized controlled trials on neurofeedback in ADHD was published by Gevensleben (Gevensleben et al., 2009b). This study incorporated data from more than 100 subjects. Post-qEEG data from this sample showed that the neurofeedback-trained group — but not the control group — showed reduced EEG theta power (Gevensleben et al., 2009a), thereby demonstrating the specificity of this intervention. The 6-month follow-up data from this study (Gevensleben et al., 2010) showed that the beneficial effects that resulted from neurofeedback were maintained at follow-up.

Based on the totality of the limited data available, it may be concluded that the clinical effects of neurofeedback remain stable over time, and may improve further with time. This is in contrast to current treatments such as medication management and multicomponent behavior therapy [(as explained in the introduction based on the NIMH-MTA trial (Molina et al., 2009)]. However, more large-scale, controlled studies with longer follow-up will be required to solidify these conclusions.

Investigations have also been conducted in recent years on the long-term enduring effects of neurofeedback for conditions other than ADHD. For example, neurofeedback has been shown to be ameliorative in nature for subjects with autism and the lasting effects of this treatment have been increasingly examined.

NEUROFEEDBACK AS A TREATMENT FOR CHILDREN WITH ASD

The first study of Kouijzer and colleagues (Kouijzer, de Moor, Gerrits, Congedo, & van Schie, 2009) investigated the effects of neurofeedback in children with autism. It included 14 children aged from 8 to 12 years with a diagnosis of Pervasive Developmental Disorder — Not Otherwise Specified (PDD-NOS). Excluded were children with an IQ score below 70, children using medication, and children with a history of severe brain injury or co-morbidity such as ADHD or epilepsy. Participants were divided into treatment and wait-list control group according to the order of applying. The first seven participants who applied were assigned to the treatment group; the control group included seven participants who were recruited out of a larger group of children who applied later, and matched participants in the treatment group on diagnosis, sex, and intelligence test scores. During baseline (Time1), all participants were evaluated using qEEG and a range of executive function tasks, and parents completed behavior questionnaires (CCC and Auti-R). After neurofeedback training (Time2), or a comparable time interval for the wait-list control group, qEEGs and data on executive functions and social behavior were re-collected. One year after ending treatment (Time3), follow-up data including qEEGs, executive function tasks, and behavior questionnaires were collected in the treatment group. Participants in the wait-list control group did not participate in the follow-up, because they had started neurofeedback training. Participants in the treatment group had neuro-feedback training twice a week, until 40 sessions were completed. In each session participants were rewarded when inhibiting theta power (4−8 Hz) and increasing low beta power (12−15 Hz) at scalp location C4 according to a protocol including seven 3-min intervals of neurofeedback training separated by 1-min rest intervals.

After 40 sessions of neurofeedback, 70% of the participants in the treatment group had effectively decreased theta power, $ps < 0.05$ and $rs = -0.496$ to -0.771, and increased low beta power, $ps < 0.05$ and $rs = 0.218$ to 0.529. Repeated measures MANOVA on the executive functions data collected at Time1 and Time2 revealed a significant inter-action between treatment and control group, indicating improvement of participants in the treatment group on tasks measuring attention skills, $F(1,11) = 8.437$, $p < 0.05$, $\eta_\rho^2 = 0.434$, cognitive flexibility, $F(1,11) = 5.602$, $p < 0.05$, $\eta_\rho^2 = 0.3373$; set-shifting, $F(1,11) = 5.081$, $p < 0.05$, $\eta_\rho^2 = 0.316$; concept generation/inhibition $F(1,11) = 4.890$, $p < 0.05$, $\eta_\rho^2 = 0.308$ (verbal inhibition) and $F(1,11) = 5.064$, $p < 0.05$, $\eta_\rho^2 = 0.315$ (motor inhibition), and planning, $F(1,11) = 7.198$, $p < 0.05$, $\eta_\rho^2 = 0.396$. Using repeated measures MANOVA to compare questionnaire data collected at Time1 and Time2 revealed a significant interaction effect between treatment and control group, indicating improvement in non-verbal com-munication, $F(1,12) = 5.505$, $p < 0.05$, $\eta_\rho^2 = 0.314$, and general commu-nication, $F(1,12) = 5.379$, $p < 0.05$, $\eta_\rho^2 = 0.310$. Time2 Auti-R questionnaire data evaluating changes in behavior over the last six months showed significant improvement in social interactions, $F(1,12) = 17.775$, $p < 0.05$, $\eta_\rho^2 = 0.618$, communication skills, $F(1,12) = 29.054$, $p < 0.05$, $\eta_\rho^2 = 0.725$, and stereotyped and repetitive behavior, $F(1,12) = 7.782$, $p < 0.05$, $\eta_\rho^2 = 0.414$ for the treatment group, but not for the control group, $ps > 0.05$.

One-year follow-up data demonstrated enduring effects of neurofeed-back treatment (Kouijzer, de Moor, Gerrits, Buitelaar, & van Schie, 2009). Repeated measures MANOVA on the executive function task scores at Time2 and Time3 indicated maintenance of cognitive flexibility, planning skills, and verbal inhibition, $ps < 0.05$, improvement of attention, $F(1,6) = 16.248$, $p < 0.05$, $\eta_\rho^2 = 0.765$, and marginally significant improvement of motor inhibition, $F(1,6) = 4.560$, $p = 0.086$, $\eta_\rho^2 = 0.477$. No significant decreases in executive function skills were found after one year. Repeated measures MANOVA comparing Time1 and Time 3 data confirmed maintenance of these effects. Analysis revealed significant increases of all executive functions that improved after neurofeedback treatment, i.e. attention skills, $F(1,6) = 39.201$, $p < 0.05$, $\eta_\rho^2 = 0.887$, cognitive flexibility, $F(1,6) = 27.802$, $p < 0.05$, $\eta_\rho^2 = 0.848$ (set-shifting), and $F(1,6) = 18.540$, $p < 0.05$, $\eta_\rho^2 = 0.788$ (concept generation), inhibition, $F(1,6) = 15.458$, $p < 0.05$, $\eta_\rho^2 = 0.756$ (verbal inhibition) and $F(1,6) = 10.696$, $p < 0.05$, $\eta_\rho^2 = 0.681$ (motor inhibition), and planning, $F(1,6) = 21.420$, $p < 0.05$, $\eta_\rho^2 = 0.811$. Figure 15.2 shows Time1, Time2, and Time3 scores of the treatment group on tests for attention, cognitive flexibility, inhibition, and planning.

Analysis of behavior questionnaires filled out by parents at Time2 and Time3 showed no loss of non-verbal communication and general communication (CCC), $ps > 0.05$, social interactions, communication skills, and stereotyped and repetitive behavior (Auti-R), $ps > 0.05$. Comparing Time1 and Time3 behavior questionnaires (CCC) confirmed the positive effect for non-verbal communication, $F(1,6) = 7.125$, $p < 0.05$, $\eta_\rho^2 = 0.543$, but not for general communication, $F(1,6) = 2.745$,

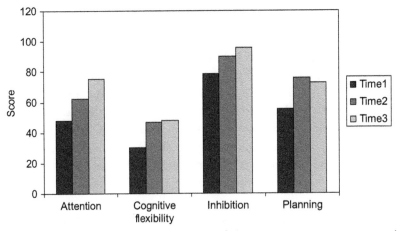

Figure 15.2 Time1, Time2, and Time3 data of the treatment group on executive function tasks.

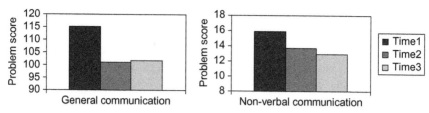

Figure 15.3 Time1, Time2, and Time3 data of the treatment group on social behavior.

$p = 0.149$, $\eta_\rho^2 = 0.314$. Figure 15.2 shows Time1, Time2, and Time3 questionnaire data (CCC) for general communication and non-verbal communication of the treatment group. Detailed information about the results of this study can be found in the original paper (Kouijzer, de Moor, Gerrits, Buitelaar et al., 2009).

In a second study of Kouijzer and colleagues (Kouijzer, van Schie, de Moor, Gerrits, & Buitelaar, 2010) several methodological improvements were implemented to better identify the effects of neurofeedback. A randomized wait-list control group design was used, and the study was conducted at the schools of the participants (N = 20). Participants were 8−12 years old and had diagnoses of autism, Asperger's disorder or PDD-NOS. Participants in the treatment group had 40 individual neurofeedback sessions using an individualized treatment protocol based on an initial qEEG. However, all treatment protocols included theta inhibition at fronto-central scalp locations. Treatment response was evaluated by qEEG measures taken during rest and task conditions, a range of executive function tasks, and social behavior questionnaires filled out by parents and teachers. All data were collected before (Time1) and after treatment (Time2) and at 6 months follow-up (Time3).

Results of the study showed that 60% of participants decreased theta power within 40 sessions of neurofeedback, $ps < 0.05$ and $rs = -0.387$ to -0.832. Additionally, repeated measures MANOVA on qEEG data revealed a significant interaction between treatment and control group, indicating a decrease in theta power in the treatment group in two out of four qEEG conditions, i.e. eyes closed, $F(1,14) = 4.883$, $p < 0.05$, $\eta_\rho^2 = 0.259$, and hand movement, $F(1,14) = 7.856$, $p < 0.05$, $\eta_\rho^2 = 0.359$. Repeated measures MANOVA on Time1 and Time2 executive function data showed a significant interaction between treatment and control group for cognitive flexibility, indicating improvement in cognitive flexibility in the treatment group compared to the control group,

$F(1,18) = 4.652$, $p < 0.05$, $\eta_\rho^2 = 0.205$. Repeated measures MANOVA showed a significant interaction effect for social interactions and communication skills, indicating that parents of participants in the treatment group reported significant improvement in social interactions and communication skills, $F(1,18) = 9.874$, $p < 0.05$, $\eta_\rho^2 = 0.367$, whereas less or no improvement was reported by parents of children in the control group. However, teachers of participants in the treatment group did not report any greater improvement in social behavior after neurofeedback treatment compared to reports of teachers of participants in the control group, $F(1,18) = 0.341$, $p = 0.566$, $\eta_\rho^2 = 0.019$.

Analysis of the 6-month follow-up data revealed enduring effects of neurofeedback treatment. Repeated measures MANOVA was used to compare the scores on executive function tasks at Time2 and Time3 and showed no significant changes, $F(1,18) = 0.186$, $p = 0.671$, $\eta_\rho^2 = 0.010$, suggesting that participants maintained the same levels of executive functioning for at least 6 months. Repeated measures MANOVA comparing Time1 and Time3 data confirmed the previously described effects by revealing a significant increase of cognitive flexibility for the treatment group but not for the control group, $F(1,18) = 5.499$, $p < 0.05$, $\eta_\rho^2 = 0.234$. Figure 15.4 shows Time1, Time2, and Time3 scores of the treatment and control group on cognitive flexibility.

Repeated measures MANOVA comparing the scores on behavioral questionnaires at Time2 and Time3 showed no effects of group or time,

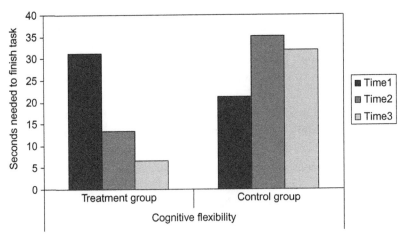

Figure 15.4 Time1, Time2, and Time3 data of treatment and control group on cognitive flexibility.

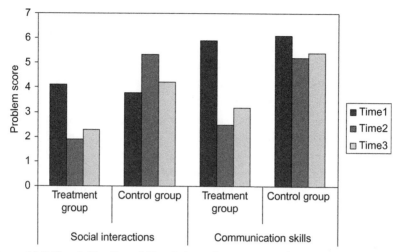

Figure 15.5 Time1, Time2, and Time3 data of treatment and control group on social behavior.

$F(1,18) = 1.099$, $p = 0.380$, $\eta_\rho^2 = 0.180$, indicating maintenance of the effects in social behavior that were reached 6 months earlier. Repeated measures MANOVA comparing Time1 and Time3 questionnaire data confirmed this effect by showing a significant interaction, suggesting decreases in problem scores on behavior questionnaires for the treatment group, but not for the control group, $F(1,18) = 4.871$, $p < 0.05$, $\eta_\rho^2 = 0.223$. Figure 15.5 shows Time1, Time2, and Time3 questionnaire data of social interactions and communication skills of treatment and control group. More detailed information about the results of this study can be found in the original paper (Kouijzer, de Moor, Gerrits, Buitelaar et al., 2009).

Both studies discussed above indicate maintenance of the effects in executive functions and social behavior from 6 months to 1 year after ending neurofeedback treatment.

ENDURING BEHAVIORAL AND NEUROPSYCHOLOGICAL BENEFITS OF NEUROFEEDBACK IN ASD

A similar study with findings that can be considered complementary to those of Kouijzer and colleagues was recently conducted by Coben at his New York clinic. This study assessed 20 patients with ASD in order to investigate long-term clinical effects of neurofeedback in terms of behavioral and neuropsychological measures. The subject pool for this study was predominately male (male 16; female 4) and all Caucasian. The mean age was 9.53, with a range of 5–10. Most subjects (80%) were medication-free, with only one subject taking more than two medications. Handedness was mostly right-handed (N = 16) with one left-handed and three ambidextrous subjects.

Subjects were administered parent rating scales, including the Autism Treatment Evaluation Checklist (ATEC; Rimland & Eldelson, 2000), the Personality Inventory for Children (PIC-2; Lachar & Gruber, 2001), the Behavior Rating Inventory of Executive Function (BREIF; Gioia, Isquith, Guy & Kenworthy, 2000), and the Gilliam Asperger's Disorder Scale (GADS; Gilliam, 2001). Subjects were also administered neuropsychological assessments covering domains of attention/executive functioning, language, and visuo-spatial processing. After baseline assessments were collected all subjects underwent at least 40 sessions of neurofeedback training, with an average of 64.5 completed sessions among all subjects. Upon completion of therapy, subjects were re-evaluated and pre- and post-treatment scores were compared for significance. After re-evaluation, neurofeedback was withheld for 5–22 months (M = 10.1 months) while no other treatments were administered. Following this break in treatment, subjects were evaluated once again in the same fashion as previously described. Their latter scores were then compared to scores obtained at the end of active neurofeedback training (Time 2).

All statistical computations were performed in the statistical package SPSS. Scores prior to treatment on parent rating scales were compared for significance to scores obtained after treatment had ended. Analysis of pre- and post-scores obtained from the ATEC revealed significant changes following neurofeedback training (two-sample t test, $t = 11.302$, d.f. 19, $p < 0.000$). Likewise, changes in scores on the GADS prior to and following treatment were found to be significant (two-sample t test, $t = 8.332$, d.f. 19, $p < 0.000$). Significant changes were also found to be present following treatment among scores from the BRIEF (two-sample t test, $t = 5.370$, d.f. 19, $p < 0.000$) as well as the PIC-2 (two-sample t test, $t = 6.320$, d.f. 19, $p < 0.000$). Interestingly, when subjects were re-assessed following a period of no neurofeedback training (range 5–22 months), no significant changes were found on any parent rating scale administered (see Figure 15.6). This suggests that changes in parent ratings that were improved by neurofeedback training remained stable during this follow-up period.

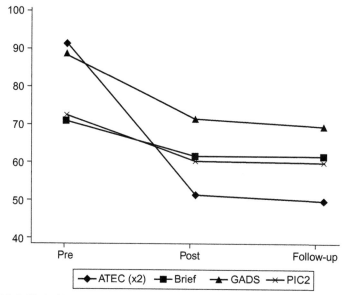

Figure 15.6 Clinical improvements among subjects as assessed by the parents rating scales of ATEC, BRIEF, GADS, and PIC-2 for pre-, post-treatment, and follow-up periods.

Neuropsychological evaluations encompassing the domains of attention, executive functioning, language, and visuo-spatial processing were also analyzed for significant differences. Significant changes from pre- to post-treatment scores were found among all three domains assessed: attention/executive functioning (two-sample t test, $t = -5.297$, d.f. 19, $p < 0.000$), language (two-sample t test, $t = -2.235$, d.f. 10, $p < 0.049$) and visuo-spatial processing (two-sample t test, $t = -5.308$, d.f. 18, $p < 0.000$). Interestingly, significant therapeutic changes were also found after subjects were re-evaluated after a lengthy (5–22 months) absence from neurofeedback training. These occurred in the areas of attention (two-sample t test, $t = -3.021$, d.f. 19, $p < 0.007$), language (two-sample t test, $t = -2.347$, d.f. 10, $p < 0.041$) and visuo-spatial processing (two-sample t test, $t = -3.568$, d.f. 18, $p < 0.002$) (see Figure 15.7). This would suggest that neurofeedback training not only led to objective gains in neuropsychological functioning, but that these enhancements in functioning continued to improve over the follow-up period when no treatment was being received.

The results of this present study were quite interesting. First, our findings add to the wealth of studies that have shown that from pre- to

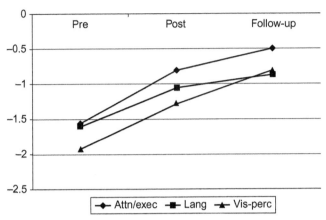

Figure 15.7 Graph showing the clinical improvements among the domains of attention/executive functioning, language, and visuo-spatial processing as assessed by neuropsychological evaluations at pre-, post-treatment and follow-up periods.

post-treatment conditions, neurofeedback is an effective therapy for treating individuals with autistic spectrum disorders. Additionally, these results show that this treatment was effective in limiting autistic behavioral deficits as well as deficits of a more neuropsychological nature. Furthermore, as our analysis shows, there were no significant increases in autistic pathology when subjects were re-evaluated after neurofeedback was withheld. This finding supports previously found evidence that neurofeedback is capable of creating stable changes within autistic subjects that are not likely to rapidly degrade when treatment ends (Coben & Padolsky, 2007; Jarusiewicz, 2002).

Of potentially even greater interest, this study found that during the period in which subjects were receiving no treatment, positive clinical neuropsychological gains were still being manifested within the domains of attention, executive functioning, language, and visuo-spatial processing. Thus, even without continued treatment subjects apparently were continuing to improve in these realms. An important implication of this finding is that neurofeedback may indeed change the autistic brain to work in novel and more efficient ways, and these changes may continue to progress even after the treatment has ended. This finding helps further the claim that neurofeedback creates specific neurophysiological changes within the autistic brain (Coben, Sherlin, Hudspeth & McKeon, 2009 [study under review]). This is in stark contrast to other commonly administered treatments for autism. For example, Lovaas et al. (1973) performed a study in which Applied Behavioral Analysis (ABA) was administered to a group of children with autism. Upon completion of ABA training the experimenters reported positive gains in terms of clinical improvements in behavioral deficits. Subjects were then re-evaluated 1–4 years later, and subjects who did not continuously receive ABA training had significantly regressed. As our current findings demonstrate, there is no evidence of regression among any of our subjects receiving neurofeedback training. In terms of drug therapies there is no evidence to our knowledge that would indicate that medications result in enduring clinical gains for subjects with autism when medication is withheld. In fact, numerous studies indicate that prolonged medication use has detrimental effects on autistic individuals (Anderson et al., 2009; Malone et al., 2002).

In terms of the limitations of the current study, the participants consisted of a selected pool of subjects. Subjects were placed in groups by choice of the experimenter rather than by random assignment. When subjects are chosen in that manner there may be a degree of selection bias associated. We would also recommend that this experiment be replicated with more neuropsychological assessments and parent rating scales included in order to more widely assess the effects of neurofeedback training. This type of investigation could broaden the present findings, and help determine if there are other correlations or significant predictors we might not have considered. Also, we would recommend a study with a greater gap between the end of treatment and re-evaluation of subjects. Doing this, we believe, would help to assess nature and extent of any positive clinical gains found in subjects when they are no longer receiving treatment, as well as test more fully the limits of enduring effects of neurofeedback treatment.

DISCUSSION

The current chapter provided evidence that neurofeedback is a therapy capable of creating enduring changes in children with both autism and ADHD. This was found across all experiments reviewed. This coupling of multiple studies converging upon a singular finding, namely the enduring clinical effects of neurofeedback, serves to provide strong evidence that neurofeedback is effective for children with developmental disorders. Moreover, these findings provide evidence that neurofeedback is not only effective in children with developmental disorders, but also is capable of leading to long-lasting positive changes in these subjects.

A therapy that can lead to long-lasting effects for children with developmental disorders (and perhaps continuing improvement even after the treatment is stopped) is an enormous asset for children with developmental disorders. Most contemporary treatments require prolonged and lengthy treatment sessions. For example, ABA training can require up to 40 hours a week over several months to be effective (Howard et al., 2005). Furthermore, drug therapies usually require years of medication in order to maintain efficacy. In addition, some children require incremental increases in dosages over a period of years for medication use to be clinically viable. Our current results and those of others discussed in this chapter indicate that neurofeedback therapy can reach clinical efficacy relatively quickly, and positive gains can be retained for months after treatment has stopped. Outside of the clinical implications, there are ancillary benefits supporting the use of neurofeedback. For example, the financial aspects of this treatment should be considered. Presently, the United States alone spends upwards of $3.2 million for the care and treatment for a single individual with autism, a figure that equates to $35 billion annually (Ganz, 2006). Similarly, the overall cost for treatment of ADHD in the United States is $30 billion annually (Birnbaum et al., 2000). A treatment such as neurofeedback with positive effects that can endure over time has great potential to relieve some of the fiscal burdens associated with these disorders.

Results of the studies reviewed in this chapter also provide evidence for the safety of neurofeedback. All studies reported no instances of subjects worsening or showing any side effects while undergoing this treatment over an extended period of time. Moreover, there was no evidence of negative side effects when neurofeedback was ceased. In fact, the opposite was found across all studies. This, again, is contradictory to other interventions, most notable drug therapies, which have documented adverse reactions within this population and often have failed to demonstrate positive effects on primary symptoms (Kidd, 2002). For example, complaints of excessive weight gain, drowsiness, and fatigue have been reported by children with ASD and ADHD while taking Risperdal (risperidone) (McCraken et al., 2002); and it has been reported that children taking risperidone at relatively high doses may become susceptible to developing facial dystonia (Zuddas et al., 2000). Likewise, research into the administration of fluoxetine has been found to produce side effects such as restlessness, hyperactivity, agitation, decreased appetite, and insomnia (Cook et al., 1992). Investigations into other contemporary treatments (i.e. diet and chelation therapies) have failed to yield adequate evidence in regard to their safety or efficacy (Doja & Roberts, 2005; Harrison-Elder et al., 2006; McDougle et al., 2000). Recently, Dr Susan Hyman and colleagues (2010) of the University of Rochester performed the single largest randomized study on the effects of casein- and whey-free diets as a treatment for autism. The results of this study found no therapeutic benefits in withholding whey or casein proteins from an autistic child's diet.

We speculate that the enduring effects of neurofeedback in children with developmental disorders are the result of this treatment's ability to change the brain in a therapeutic manner. Recently, Coben and colleagues reported specific neurophysiological changes in terms of coherence within and between specific neural regions following neurofeedback treatment for children with ASD (Coben, Sherlin, Hudspeth, & McKeon, 2009 [study under review]). We would argue that neurofeedback training causes specific neurophysiological changes within the brain, which in turn contribute to the long-lasting effects of this treatment, and this fosters the continued growth and development of cognitive functions. Moreover, we suggest that more research be conducted into the precise neural areas clinically affected by neurofeedback in an effort to more fully understand the efficacy of neurofeedback for children with developmental disorders.

In summary, results of the studies examined add to the growing wealth of investigations into the efficacy of neurofeedback as a treatment for children with developmental disorders. Moreover, these results have found this treatment to be effective over an extended period of time. Consistent with these results we recommend future studies be conducted that assess the enduring effects of neurofeedback over even longer treatment spans.

ACKNOWLEDGMENT

We acknowledge Hartmut Heinrich for providing us with the unpublished follow-up data from his study. We also acknowledge the support from Ute Strehl in providing us with the data from her studies.

REFERENCES

Anderson, G., Scahil, L., McCracken, J., McDougle, C., Aman, M., Tierney, E., et al. (2009). Effects of short- and long-term Risperidone treatment on prolactin levels in children with autism. *Journal of Biological Psychiatry, 61*(4), 545−550.

Arns, M., de Ridder, S., Strehl, U., Breteler, M., & Coenen, A. (2009). Efficacy of neurofeedback treatment in ADHD: The effects on inattention, impulsivity and hyperactivity: A meta-analysis. *Clinical EEG and Neuroscience: Official Journal of the EEG and Clinical Neuroscience Society (ENCS)*, 40(3), 180—189.

Birnbaum, H. G., Kessler, R. C., Lowe, S. W., Secnik, K., Greenberg, P. E., Leond, S. A., et al. (2000). Cost of attention deficit-hyperactivity disorder (ADHD) in the US: Excess cost of persons with ADHD and their family members in 2000. *Current Medical Research and Opinion*, 21(2), 195—205.

Coben, R., & Padolsky, I. (2007). Assessment-guided neurofeedback for autistic spectrum disorder. *Journal of Neurotherapy*, 11, 5—23.

Coben, R., Sherlin, L., Hudspeth, W. J., & McKeon, K. (2009). Connectivity guided EEG biofeedback for autism spectrum disorder: Evidence of neurophysiological changes. *Journal of Autism and Developmental Disorders* [under review]

Cook, E. H., Rowlett, R., Jaselskis, C., & Leventhal, B. L. (1992). Fluoxetine treatment of children and adults with autistic disorder and mental retardation. *Journal of American Academy of Child & Adolescent Psychiatry*, 31, 739—745.

Doja, A., & Roberts, W. (2005). Immunizations and autism: A review of the literature. *Canadian Journal of Neurological Sciences*, 33, 341—346.

Egner, T., & Sterman, M. B. (2006). Neurofeedback treatment of epilepsy: From basic rationale to practical application. *Expert Review of Neurotherapeutics*, 6(2), 247—257.

Evans, J. R., & Park, N. S. (1996). Quantitative EEG abnormalities in a sample of dyslexic persons. *Journal of Neurotherapy*, 2(1), 1—5.

Fox, D. J., Tharp, D. F., & Fox, L. C. (2005). Neurofeedback: An alternative and efficacious treatment for attention deficit hyperactivity disorder. *Journal of Applied Psychophysiology and Biofeedback*, 30(40), 364—373.

Gani, C., Birbaumer, N., & Strehl, U. (2008). Long term effects after feedback of slow cortical potentials and of theta-beta-amplitudes in children with attention deficit/hyperactivity disorder (ADHD). *International Journal of Bioelectromagnetism*, 10(4), 209—232.

Ganz, M. (2006). The costs of autism. In S. Moldin & J. L. Rubenstein (Eds.), *Understanding autism: From basic neuroscience to treatment* (pp. 476—498). New York, NY: CRC Press.

Gevensleben, H., Holl, B., Albrecht, B., Schlamp, D., Kratz, O., Studer, P., et al. (2009a). Distinct EEG effects related to neurofeedback training in children with ADHD: A randomized controlled trial. *International Journal of Psychophysiology: Official Journal of the International Organization of Psychophysiology*, 74(2), 149—157.

Gevensleben, H., Holl, B., Albrecht, B., Schlamp, D., Kratz, O., et al. (2010). Neurofeedback training in children with ADHD: 6-month follow-up of a randomised controlled trial. *European Child and Adolescent Psychiatry*, doi 10.1007/s00787-010-0109-5

Gevensleben, H., Holl, B., Albrecht, B., Vogel, C., Schlamp, D., Kratz, O., et al. (2009b). Is neurofeedback an efficacious treatment for ADHD? A randomised controlled clinical trial. *Journal of Child Psychology and Psychiatry, and Allied Disciplines*, 50(7), 780—789.

Gilliam, J. E. (2001). *Gilliam Asperger's Disorder Scale: Examiner's manual* Austin, TX: Pro-Ed.

Gioia, G. A., Isquith, P. K., Guy, S. C., & Kenworthy, L. (2000). *Behavior Rating Inventory of Executive Function*. Lutz, FL: Psychological Assessment Resources, Inc.

Hammond, D. C. (2007). What is neurofeedback? *Journal of Neurotherapy*, 10(4), 25—36.

Harrison-Elder, J., Shankar, M., Shuster, J., Theriaque, D., Burns, S., & Sherrill, L. (2006). The gluten-free, casein-free diet in autism: Results of a preliminary double blind clinical trial. *Journal of Autism and Developmental Disorders*, 36, 413—420.

Hayman, S. et al. (2010) The gluten-free and casein-free (GFCF) diet. A double-blind, placebo controlled challenge study. Paper presented at the International Society for Autism Research 2010 conference, Philadelphia, PA.

Heinrich, H., Gevensleben, H., Freisleder, F. J., Moll, G. H., & Rothenberger, A. (2004). Training of slow cortical potentials in attention-deficit/hyperactivity disorder: Evidence for positive behavioral and neurophysiological effects. *Biological Psychiatry, 55* (7), 772−775.

Hermens, D. F., Rowe, D. L., Gordon, E., & Williams, L. M. (2006). Integrative neuroscience approach to predict ADHD stimulant response. *Expert Review of Neurotherapeutics, 6*(5), 753−763.

Howard, J. S., Sparkman, C. R., Cohen, H. G., Green, G., & Stanislaw, H. (2005). A comparison of intensive behavior analytic and eclectic treatments for young children with autism. *Research in Developmental Disabilities, 26*, 359−383.

Jarusiewicz, B. (2002). Efficacy of neurofeedback for children in the autistic spectrum. A pilot study. *Journal of Neurotherapy, 6*(4), 39−49.

Kidd, P. M. (2002). Autism, an extreme challenge to integrative medicine. Part II: Medical Management. *Alternative Medical Review, 7*(6), 472−499.

Kleinnijenhuis, M., Arns, M. W., Spronk, D. B., Breteler, M. H. M., & Duysens, J. E. J. (2008). Comparison of discrete-trial based SMR and SCP training and the interrelationship between SCP and SMR networks: Implications for brain-computer interfaces and neurofeedback. *Journal of Neurotherapy, 11*(4), 19−35.

Kouijzer, M. E. J., de Moor, J. M. H., Gerrits, B. J. L., Buitelaar, J. K., & van Schie, H. T. (2009). Long-term effects of neurofeedback treatment in autism. *Research in Autism Spectrum Disorders, 3*, 496−501.

Kouijzer, M. E. J., de Moor, J. M. H., Gerrits, B. J. L., Congedo, M., & van Schie, H. T. (2009). Neurofeedback improves executive functioning in children with autism spectrum disorders. *Research in Autism Spectrum Disorders, 3*, 145−162.

Kouijzer, M. E. J., van Schie, H. T., de Moor, J. M. H., Gerrits, B. J. L., & Buitelaar, J. K. (2010). Neurofeedback treatment in autism. Preliminary findings in behavioral, cognitive, and neurophysiological functioning. *Research in Autism Spectrum Disorders, 4*(3), 386−399.

Lachar, D., & Gruber, C. P. (2001). *The Personality Inventory for Children* (2nd ed.) Los Angeles, CA: Western Psychological Services.

Leins, U., Goth, G., Hinterberger, T., Klinger, C., Rumpf, N., & Strehl, U. (2007). Neurofeedback for children with ADHD: A comparison of SCP and theta/beta protocols. *Applied Psychophysiology and Biofeedback, 32*(2), 73−88.

Lovaas, I., Koegel, R., Simmons, J. Q., & Long, J. S. (1973). Some generalization and follow-up measures on autistic children in behavior therapy. *Journal of Applied Behavior Analysis, 6*(1), 131−166.

Lubar, J. F. (1991). Discourse on the development of EEG diagnostics and biofeedback for attention-deficit/hyperactivity disorders. *Applied Psychophysiology and Biofeedback, 16*(3), 201−225.

Lubar, J. F., & Shouse, M. N. (1976). EEG and behavioral changes in a hyperkinetic child concurrent with training of the sensorimotor rhythm (SMR): A preliminary report. *Biofeedback and Self-Regulation, 1*(3), 293−306.

Lubar, J. F., Swartwood, M. O., Swatwood, J. N., & O'Donnell, P. H. (2005). Evaluation of the effectiveness of EEG neurofeedback training for ADHD in a clinical setting as measured by changes in TOVA scores, behavioral ratings, and WISC-R performance. *Applied Psychophysiology and Biofeedback, 20*, 83−99.

Malone, R. P., Maislin, G., Choudhury, M. S., Gifford, C., & Delaney, M. A. (2002). Risperidone treatment in children and adolescents with autism: Short- and long-term safety and effectiveness. *Journal of the American Academy of Child and Adolescent Psychiatry, 41*(2), 140−147.

McCraken, J. T., McGough, J., Shah, B., Cronin, P., Hong, D., Aman, M. G., et al. (2002). Risperidone in children with autism and serious behavioral problems. *New England Journal of Medicine, 9*, 3−14.

McDougle, C. J., Scahill, L., McCracken, J. T., Aman, M. G., Tierney, E., & Arnold, L. E. (2000). Research units on pediatric psychopharmacology (RUPP) autism network. Background and rationale for an initial controlled study of risperidone. *Child and Adolescent Psychiatric Clinics of North America, 9*(1), 201–224.

Molina, B. S., Hinshaw, S. P., Swanson, J. M., Arnold, L. E., Vitiello, B., Jensen, P. S., et al. (2009). The MTA at 8 years: Prospective follow-up of children treated for combined-type ADHD in a multisite study. *Journal of the American Academy of Child and Adolescent Psychiatry, 48*(5), 484–500.

Monastra, V. J., Monastra, D. M., & George, S. (2002). The effects of stimulant therapy, EEG biofeedback, and parenting style on the primary symptoms of attention-deficit/hyperactivity disorder. *Applied Psychophysiology and Biofeedback, 27*(4), 231–249.

Rimland, B., & Eldelson, S.M. (2000). Autism treatment evolution checklist (ATEC). Retrieved May 12, 2010 from www.autismeval.com/ari-atec/report1.html.

Strehl, U., Leins, U., Goth, G., Klinger, C., Hinterberger, T., & Birbaumer, N. (2006). Self-regulation of slow cortical potentials: A new treatment for children with attention-deficit/hyperactivity disorder. *Pediatrics, 118*(5), e1530–1540.

Sterman, M. B., Howe, R. D., & Macdonald, L. R. (1970). Facilitation of spindle-burst sleep by conditioning of electroencephalographic activity while awake. *Science, 167,* 1146–1148.

Walker, J. E., Kozlowski, G. P., & Lawson, R. (2007). A modular activation/coherence approach to evaluating clinical/qEEG correlations and for guiding neurofeedback training: modular insufficiencies, modular excesses, disconnections, and hyperconnections. *Journal of Neurotherapy, 11,* 25–44.

Zuddas, A., Dimartino, A., Muglia, P., & Cianchetti, C. (2000). Long-term risperidone for pervasive developmental disorder: Efficacy, tolerability, and discontinuation. *Journal of Child Adolescent Psychopharmacology, 10*(2), 79–90.

INDEX

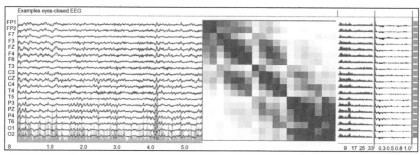

Figure 2.5 From left to right: about 5.5 s of eyes-closed EEG recorded at the standard 19 leads described by the 10–20 electrode placement system, the 19 × 19 correlation matrix of EEG time-series, the power spectra (red plot: 1 Hz–32 Hz), autocorrelation function (blue plot: lag = 0–1 s) and Hurst exponent (green bars) of the 19 EEG signals. The entries of the correlation matrix are color coded, with white coding correlation equal to zero and red (blue) coding correlation equal to 1 (−1). The entries in diagonal are the autocorrelations, hence they all equal 1. Note that electrode T3 is much less correlated to other electrodes as compared to the others. This is because it contains a considerable amount of muscle artifacts (as seen also from the high-frequency content of the power spectrum and the flat autocorrelation function), which does not distribute through the head to other electrodes. (Please refer to Chapter 2, page 34).

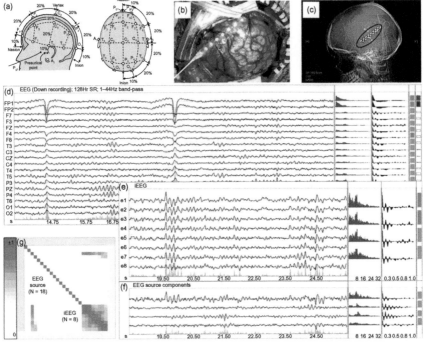

Figure 2.6 A tinnitus patient was implanted with two rows of eight extradural intracranial recording electrodes. Nineteen scalp electrodes (EEG) and the intracranial electrodes (iEEG) were recorded simultaneously with a common reference positioned on the vertex. (a) Position of the 19 electrodes on the scalp (10—20 system). (b) Demonstration of the surgical procedure to insert the extradural electrodes. (c) Computerized tomography of the patient's head showing the location of the electrodes (over the left secondary auditory cortex). (d) Example 9 seconds of the scalp EEG data. (e) Example 7 seconds of the intracranial data. (g) Four of the 18 sources estimated from scalp EEG data only with time-course corresponding exactly to the extradural recording in (e). (g) Correlation matrix between the 18 sources estimated from the scalp EEG and the eight extradural recordings (iEEG). The first source in (f) is strongly correlated with the iEEG, which can be seen also from the time-course. The source localization of the first source by sLORETA confirmed that the source is generated by the secondary auditory cortex (data not shown here; see Van der Loo et al., 2007). (Please refer to Chapter 2, page 38).

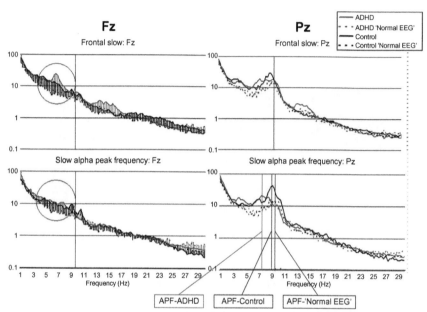

Figure 4.2 This figure clearly shows that the sub-group with a slowed alpha peak frequency (bottom), present parietally, also show elevated "theta EEG power" at frontal sites. However, this is not true "frontal slow", but simply the effect of the slowed alpha peak frequency. This demonstrates that a raised theta/beta ratio at least also includes the slow APF sub-group, which neurophysiologically is a different group, as demonstrated later with respect to treatment outcome to stimulant medication. *(From Arns, Gunkelman, Breteler, & Spronk (2008); reproduced with permission.)* (Please refer to Chapter 4, page 86).

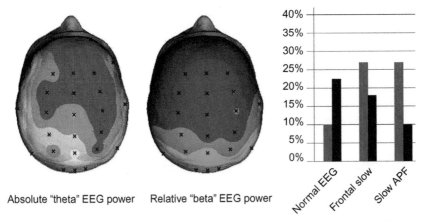

Absolute "theta" EEG power   Relative "beta" EEG power

Figure 4.3 The averaged brain activity of 275 ADHD patients compared to a matched control group. The figure left shows the increased theta ($p < 0.0001$) and right the decreased relative beta power ($p < 0.0001$). Note the frontocentral localization. The graph on the right shows that when inspecting the individual data sets only 25% of children with ADHD (red) indeed exhibit "real frontal slow" or frontal theta. Finally, about the same percentage exhibit a slow APF pattern, which after filtering will show up as "theta" but in fact is alpha, as explained below. (Please refer to Chapter 4, page 89).

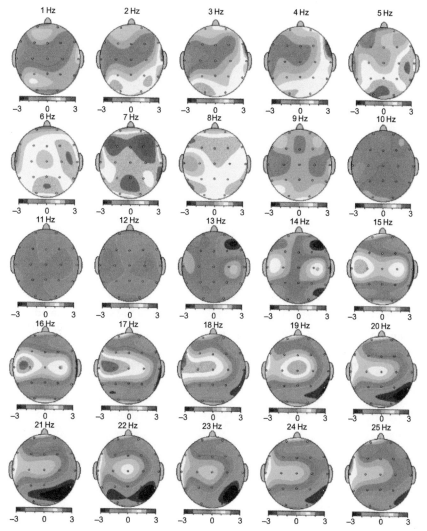

Figure 7.2 qEEG — Example 7.6. (Please refer to Chapter 7, page 199).

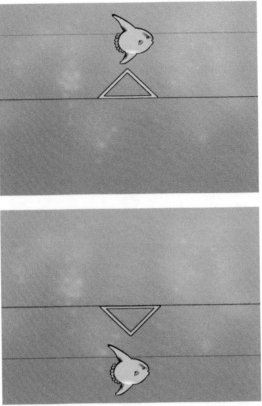

Figure 8.1 Example of SCP feedback training screens for negativity ("Activation", upper panel) and positivity ("Deactivation", lower panel). *(By kind permission of neuroConn GmbH, Germany.)* (Please refer to Chapter 8, page 212).

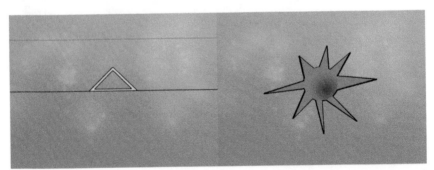

Figure 8.2 Example of SCP transfer training screen for negativity—activation task (left panel). Example of SCP visual feedback reward for successful activation or deactivation (right panel). *(By kind permission of neuroConn GmbH, Germany.)* (Please refer to Chapter 8, page 213).

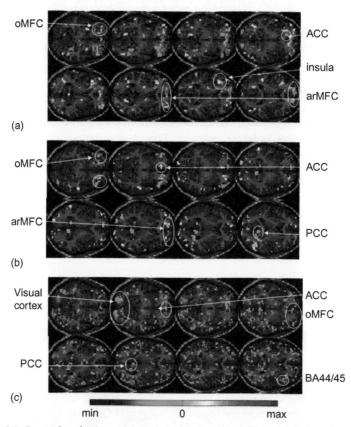

Figure 9.2 Exemplary brain activation maps generated from a single subject whole brain SVM classification showing discriminating voxels for: (a) happy vs. disgust classification, (b) happy vs. sad classification, and (c) disgust vs. sad classification. Brain regions: oMFC, orbital medial frontal cortex; arMFC, anterior rostral MFC (based on Amodio & Frith, 2006); OFC, orbitofrontal cortex; ACC, anterior cingulate cortex; PCC, posterior cingulate cortex. (Please refer to Chapter 9, page 242).

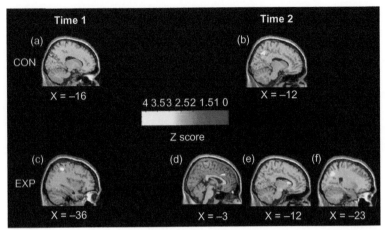

Figure 13.1 Statistical activation maps at Time 1 and Time 2 produced by the Interference minus Neutral contrast. Images are sagittal sections for the data averaged across subjects. At Time 1, significant loci of activation were detected in the left superior parietal lobule for both the CON (a) and EXP (c) groups. At Time 2, activations were also noted in this cortical region for the CON (b) and EXP (f) groups. In addition, for the EXP group only, significant loci of activation were measured in the right ACcd (d), as well as the left caudate nucleus and left substantia nigra (e). *(Reproduced from Beauregard & Lévesque (2006) by permission of Springer Science + Business Media.)* (Please refer to Chapter 13, page 365).

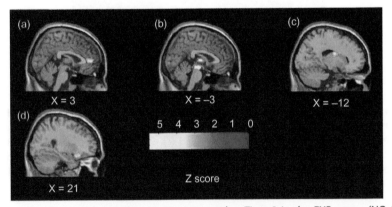

Figure 13.2 Statistical activation maps measured at Time 2 in the EXP group (NO-GO minus GO contrast). Significant loci of activation were measured in the right ACcd (a), left thalamus and left substantia nigra (b), left caudate nucleus (c), and right ventrolateral prefrontal cortex (d). *(Reproduced from Beauregard & Lévesque (2006) by permission of Springer Science + Business Media.)* (Please refer to Chapter 13, page 366).